ACCIDENTS IN HISTORY:
INJURIES, FATALITIES AND SOCIAL RELATIONS

THE WELLCOME INSTITUTE SERIES IN THE HISTORY OF MEDICINE

Forthcoming Titles

Operative Chymist: A Biography of Thomas N. R. Morson
Anthony F. P. Morson

Fantasy Surgery
Ann Dally

Medicine and Morals in the Enlightenment:
John Gregory, Thomas Percival and Benjamin Rush
Lisbeth Haakenssen

Academic enquiries regarding the series should be addressed
to the editors W. F. Bynum and Roy Porter at
the Wellcome Institute for the History of Medicine,
183 Euston Road, London NW1 2BE, UK

ACCIDENTS IN HISTORY: INJURIES, FATALITIES AND SOCIAL RELATIONS

Edited by Roger Cooter and Bill Luckin

Rodopi

Amsterdam – Atlanta, GA 1997

First published in 1997
by Editions Rodopi B. V., Amsterdam – Atlanta, GA 1997.

Design and Typesetting by Christine Buckley, the Wellcome Trust.
Printed and bound in The Netherlands by Editions Rodopi B. V.,
Amsterdam – Atlanta, GA 1997.

British Library Cataloguing in Publication Data
A catalogue record for this book is available from the British Library
ISBN 90-420-0104-6 (Bound)

Cooter, Roger and Luckin, Bill
Accidents in History: Injuries, Fatalities and Social Relations/Roger
Cooter and Bill Luckin, – Amsterdam – Atlanta, GA: Rodopi. – ill.
(Clio Medica 41/ ISSN 0045-7183;
The Wellcome Institute Series in the History of Medicine)

Front cover: The engraving by J. Pass shows a patient being carried
through the gates of Guy's Hospital on a stretcher, 1816.
Wellcome Institute Library, London.

Printed in The Netherlands

for Karl Figlio, friend and mentor

Contents

Acknowledgements

Some of these chapters were first presented to a one-day conference on 'Accidents in History' held at the Institute for Historical Research in October 1991, sponsored by the Society for the Social History of Medicine. Summaries of the conference papers are published in *Social History of Medicine,* volume 4 (1991), pp. 196–202. We are grateful to all the participants for their stimulating contributions. We are also grateful to the Society for the History of Technology for permission to reprint, in a slightly modified form, Arthur McEvoy's paper, 'Working Environments' which first appeared in the Supplement to *Technology and Culture,* volume 36 (1995), pp. S145–S172. Our thanks also to Kate Baker for skilful word processing; and, not least, to the Wellcome Trust for encouragement and support.

Notes on Contributors

Robert Campbell is Principal Lecturer in Philosophy and Deputy Head of Humanities at the Bolton Institute. He is the co-author, with D. Collinson, of *Ending Lives* (1988) and, with A. Kitson, of *The Ethical Organisation* (1996). His main area of interest is applied philosophy.

Roger Cooter is University Reader at the Wellcome Unit for the History of Medicine, in the Centre for the History of Science, Technology and Medicine, at the University of Manchester. He has published widely in the social history of science and medicine. The author of *The Cultural Meaning of Popular Science* (1984); *Phrenology in the British Isles* (1989); and *Surgery and Society in Peace and War* (1993), he has also edited *Studies in the History of Alternative Medicine* (1988) and *In the Name of the Child: Health and Welfare, 1880–1940* (1991).

Judith Green is a Senior Lecturer at South Bank University, London. She has researched and published on primary care, the organization of health services and the sociology of accidents.

John F. Hutchinson is Professor of History at Simon Fraser University in British Columbia and is the author of *Politics and Public Health in Revolutionary Russia, 1890–1918* (1990) and *Champions of Charity: War and the Rise of the Red Cross* (1996). His current research interests include the development of urban ambulance services, and the politics of international health between 1919 and 1949.

Bill Luckin is Professor in Urban and Cultural Studies at the Bolton Institute, and an Associate of the Centre for the History of Science, Technology and Medicine, University of Manchester. The author of *Pollution and Control: A Social History of the Thames in the Nineteenth Century* (1986), and *Questions of Power: Electricity and Environment in Inter-war Britain* (1990), he has also published on quantitative aspects of epidemics, and on various aspects of environmental, social, cultural and urban history.

Arthur F. McEvoy is Professor of Law and History at the University of Wisconsin – Madison. He is the author of *The Fisherman's Problem: Ecology and Law in the California Fisheries* (1986).

Dietrich Milles (PhD, Privatdozent) is head of the Sozialpolitisches Archiv at the Zentrum für Sozialpolitik (University of Bremen). His latest work, *Gesundheitsrisiken, Industriegesellschaft und soziale Sicherungen in der Geschichte,* was published in 1993. He is currently working on *The Risk-Biography and the Historical Changes of the Insurance-System* with the Sub-Projekt D1 at the Special Research Centre 186 in Bremen.

Roy Porter is Professor in the social history of medicine at the Wellcome Institute for the History of Medicine. He is currently working on a general history of medicine, on the history of Bethlem Hospital and on the Enlightenment in Britain. Recent books include *Doctor of Society: Thomas Beddoes and the Sick Trade in Late Enlightenment England* (London: Routledge, 1991) and *London: A Social History* (Hamish Hamilton, 1994).

Joel Tarr is the Richard S. Caliguiri Professor of Urban and Environmental History and Policy at Carnegie Mellon University. He has published widely in the areas of urban and environmental history. A book of his collected environmental essays, *The Search for the Ultimate Sink: Urban Pollution in Historical Perspective* has been recently published.

Mark Tebeau is a PhD candidate in Social History at the Carnegie Mellon University. He is currently completing a social and cultural history of firefighting and fire protection in American cities for his dissertation, entitled '"Eating Smoke": Masculinity, Technology, and the Politics of Urbanization, 1850–1950'.

1

Accidents in History: An Introduction

Roger Cooter and Bill Luckin

Whether considered domestically or globally, from the perspective of child or parent, worker or sportsperson, driver, pilot or passenger, accidents can seem nearly as pervasive as the air we breathe. They have been legislated against and made the object of psychological, statistical, and epidemiological study. They have provided a base for medical organization and professionalization, and generated a massive insurance industry. And they have cut deeply into the GNP of the modern nation state. But although they have also been fictionalized and filmed, they have not been seriously or substantially historicized. With the exception of air itself, there is hardly a comparable subject in which historical investment has been so meagre. For all the interest in representations, accidents remain historically unrepresented. Within histories of philosophy, sociology, demography, political economy, culture, technology, medicine, religion, psychology, literature, mentalité, labour, urban design, transport, and everyday material life, 'accidents' – if we take the trouble to look for them – are conspicuous only by their absence. The plea of a writer in 1813 for 'something [to] be said, in *earnest*, about ... ACCIDENTS – those frequent sources of *deep* and *lasting* Misery', still rings true.[1]

Whiggish and internalist preoccupations in economic history and the history of technology are partly to blame. Still predominantly concerned with quantification and the tacit step-by-step evolution of one technique or mode of production into its 'logical' 'successor', neither discipline has left much room for the discussion of accidents, except rhetorically in methodological debates over change, where the 'accidental', or the unintentionally consequential, sometimes vies with the structurally permissible.[2] Nor has the history of medicine yet placed the accident in a convincing historiographical context. Despite the move to contextualism, it is still rare to see phenomena presented in their full economic, social, legal and medical complexity. The too frequent equation of a social history of the accident with the history of occupational health – which highlights institutional and administrative structures rather than the social experience of sudden death or injury – has been equally debilitating. There are analogies here with other tendencies in medical history: the concentration, for example, on infectious disease, and on professional and therapeutic change, rather than the social location and socio-medical condition of patients.[3] Parallels can also be made with those genres of labour history which have substituted the growth and development of trade unionism for the social experience of work. Here, too, the institutional has been allowed to force out the experiential and the contingent.

Yet more than the sins of historians lie behind the failure of accidents to attain even the status of a 'minority interest'. As conventionally understood, a technological, corporeal, or 'natural' accident is ahistorical, almost by definition. It is the 'irruption of the unpredictable',[4] an isolated event unconnected to wider systems or structures, a matter of chance, fate or providence. Such an image has even been a frame for history, as in Michael Harrington's *The Accidental Century* (1966), which argues that our times – including our ideologies and beliefs – have been shaped haphazardly by unplanned technology. The historian is hardly helped, moreover, by turning to the dictionary itself; however pursued etymologically, the 'accident' seems ever destined to slide into ambiguity, defying any fixity of meaning. Although it does not follow that the accident is therefore unhistoricizable – etymologies, after all, *are* histories – the weight of the dictionary, as it were, leans against the project.

So too does the lack of definitional precision between an 'accident' and a 'misfortune', 'misadventure', 'mishap', 'injury', 'casualty', 'crisis', 'emergency' and 'disaster'. According to the anthropologist of disasters, Michael Barkun, accidents and disasters *can* be sharply distinguished from one another. Accidents may 'severely affect ... but ... not lead to fundamental social change', whereas disasters do; and accidents may temporarily change environments, whereas disasters transform them.[5] Barkun thus writes accidents out of history as insignificant happenings. But who is to say which is accident and which disaster – and when? As Charles Perrow reminds us in *Normal Accidents*, 'minor accidents can cascade into major unanticipated catastrophes'.[6] In making his distinction, Barkun was thinking mainly of modern man-made, non-localized (or even localizable) 'horrific' events – the economic depression of the 1930s, the two world wars, the Holocaust. But here, surely, as the cultural historian of technology Rosalind Williams has observed, there arises the question of the play of modern imagination in the definition and interpretation of a disaster, and, by extension, an accident.[7] Moreover, as the political critic of science and technology, Les Levidow reminds us, in a review of yet another edition of Dexter Masters' novel, *The Accident* (1955), 'imagination' in this area can scarcely be non-political. Construing Chernobyl as 'an accident' but the bombings of Hiroshima and Nagasaki as 'experiments' belies political complexions and understandings, as well as raising further definitional ambiguities.[8]

Even if the grounds for Barkun's distinctions held good for the present, there is no reason to suppose that they are appropriate for the past. Unlike Barkun, historical actors *did* see accidents as significant. Crucially, they sought to distinguish, not between 'the accidental' and 'the disastrous', but between the man-made and the 'natural', and between those tragedies for which an individual or community might be held responsible and those to which no blame could be attached. Implicated among these distinctions is the paradox that compounds the difficulty of historicizing the accident – the fact that accidents may seem to be random and arbitrary, yet at the same time be expected or preordained. 'Though they are often said to be *casual* [as opposed to uniform] in their occurrence,' remarked Newton Bosworth, in his *The Accidents of Human Life* (1813),

> [accidents] are all produced by their proper causes, as much so as the most regular and uniform appearances in nature. They are only called accidents, because previous circumstances did not appear to indicate them, or, in simpler terms, because they come upon us unawares. (iii–iv)

Although Bosworth and his peers could not possibly 'exclude the idea of an overruling Providence, extending to the minutest events, as well as to the greatest', they were inclined to attribute accidents to 'inattention, ignorance, or presumption',[9] that is, to *human* rather than *divine* causation. Whichever, accidents were fraught with moral meaning.

The rise of statistics in the mid-nineteenth century secularized accidents as expected events, though it in no way extricated them from morality and ideology. Man-made industrial accidents in particular were increasingly seen as a part of the expected and 'normal' flow and structure of everyday social life – endogenous rather than exogenous to human motivations, actions and processes. But they continued to be attributed in part to carelessness and recklessness (later 'fatigue' and 'proneness')[10] and regarded to varying degrees as preventable.

It might be supposed that these tensions between providence and precaution, chance and predictability, blamelessness and accountability, fate and intervention, the random and the structural, and the natural and the fabricated render the subject well suited to a postmodern gaze. Accidents, like wars, appear to challenge the logic of linear positivist explanations of progress and to mock the metanarratives of philosophy and sociology.[11] Here, surely, are the fragments, contingencies and irreductions so beloved of post-structuralist discourse analysts. Not only is there no archive labelled 'accidents', but neither is there a stable subject.

For even more obvious reasons, however, no such postmodern turning has occurred. The accident, far from being irreducible (or appearing so symbolically), is in reality the stable object of an exquisite actuarial reduction. 'Within the next 33 minutes someone in the United Kingdom will be killed as a result of an accident', insurance vendors typically remind us[12] – cashing in, like fellow agents for the last century and a half, on the statistical 'normalization' of the accident, or the transformation of the once unknowable workings of chance into calculations that reinforce the predictability of everyday economic and technological life. In recent years this calculus has gained greater intellectual and commercial strength through innumerable deliberations on 'risk'. Tellingly, Ulrich Beck's *Risk Society* (1992) is subtitled 'towards a new *modernity*', not 'postmodernity', and has even been criticized as just 'another *apologia* for science'.[13]

This is not the place to enter into a critique of 'risk', whether prefixed by 'acceptable', suffixed by 'perception', or deployed as a synonym for 'hazard', 'danger' or 'peril'.[14] Suffice it to make three historically-oriented points. First, the risk industry has tended further to marginalize the history of the accident, stimulating, instead, historical thought on the origins of probability theory and the philosophy of statistics.[15] Secondly, the now voluminous literature on risk reflects a fearfulness among society at large of environmental hazards which, in the past, were mainly experienced (industrially and domestically) by the working class. Last, but not least, what is mystified through the discussion of 'risk' is precisely that which was occluded as a result of the nineteenth-century statistical normalization of the accident: an understanding of these happenings and the discussions around them as socially and politically laden, rather than as 'natural' and 'neutral'.[16]

It is important to recall that accidents became normalized and legitimated in the nineteenth century in synchronization with the extension of automatically driven machinery. This was a process which went hand in hand with claims that the sites where mishaps were most likely to occur were inherently predictable and manipulable. However, the full social cost of accidents was never admitted by business and government. To have done so might have starkly revealed disillusionment with the industrial system *as* a system. Certainly, any acknowledgement of the volume of death and injury in factories, mines, building sites and shipyards, would have drawn attention to the astonishingly low status given to the issue of safety within society as a whole. Implicitly and explicitly, therefore, both business and the state accentuated the normalization of the accident. Although the volume of accidents became well-known and the accident-causing potential of certain technologies and labour processes recognized, the extent of such injuries and fatalities could be reckoned a part of the 'natural order' of industrial society. Through the very act of labelling these injuries and fatalities 'accidents', blame was shifted away from the labour process and even, eventually (through workmen's compensation legislation), from the fault of individual workers.

One of the few articles to pursue the history of this 'neutralization' process is Karl Figlio's 'What is an Accident?'.[17] Pitched at a deep conceptual level, Figlio's article is also uniquely expansive in chronological terms. Although the workmen's compensation legislation of the late nineteenth century provides a focus, it serves as an end-point, rather than the beginning usually depicted in 'social policy' histories of the topic.

In pre-modern society, Figlio argues, very few chance events were ever perceived as 'accidental'. Rather, they were 'symbolically important indicators of social integrity and disruption'.

> When something occurs in such a setting, either fortune or misfortune, it is expected. Something like that was about to happen and not necessarily to anyone in particular, though 'just deserts' might frequently be commented upon. An injury, an illness, or some other misfortune, brings relief from the rising community temperature. Nothing could happen by accident, when every event is scrutinized for its place in the dense fabric of expectation. (184)

But between the sixteenth and nineteenth centuries, he continues, these meanings and certitudes began to be eroded under the twin pressures of capitalism and the legal forms and procedures that legitimated the new economic ideology. Surveying coroners' records, Figlio concludes that three terms – *deodand*, *malfeasance* and *nonfeasance* – were crucial both to the shaping of the modern law of contract and to the emergence of the kinds of 'normalized' and 'neutralized' accidents that would later become conventional in industrial society. *Deodand* – a curious mixture of act and 'accident' whereby the animate or inanimate objects or instruments with the closest 'causal' connection to a violent death were compelled to be forfeited to the authorities – was intermediate between 'traditional society' and the emergent capitalist order. It implied intent, yet the event occasioning the death was held to be unforeseen and not malicious. *Malfeasance* and *nonfeasance* seem to be less revealing than *deodand* as indices of explicitly cosmological transition, and Figlio's main concern with them is as part shapers of the changes in master-and-servant relationships that would lead, in due course, to the seeming 'neutrality' and 'naturalness' of formal contracts between employer and employee, and of such 'accidents' as might occur within them. Thus, 'even in relations between equals, when a contracted set of actions, agreed by consenting parties, had an unexpected outcome or ancillary consequence, the claim to recompense lay in showing misconduct (*malfeasance*)'. During the sixteenth century, however, the 'legal formalism for establishing the terms of contract and its breach – *assumpit* – began to apply to cases of not doing (*nonfeasance*) as well as to *malfeasance*'.[18] From this point on, Figlio's task becomes less daunting. Focusing on the late nineteenth- and early twentieth-century Workmen's Compensation Acts, he claims that

> at a specifiable moment, an event led to injury or disease; it was an accident – an unforeseen and unintended breach in natural, social and personal history. If it happened at work, it probably lay within the field of the labour contract, and the question arose as to whether or not risk was an implied term of contract. The contract-form of social relations put *nonfeasance* on a par with *malfeasance* so that doing or intending nothing became a kind of causality. (201–2)

And finally, and daringly, 'such an event was an accident – a breach of contract', and hence was compensational without implying liability.

For our purposes here, two general points may be made about Figlio's theoretically sophisticated and elegantly argued essay. First, at the level of evidence, the discourses that are reported and commented upon are almost exclusively legalistic: the corollary is that the experiences and worldviews of those actually involved in 'accidents' – however defined or historicized – are marginalized. Second, in juxtaposing 'traditional society' against an emergent, contract-based capitalist order in Britain between the sixteenth and nineteenth centuries, Figlio seems to exclude the possibility of 'uneven cosmological development' outside the legalistic framework. What requires emphasis is that those who came into contact with the formal apparatus of the Workmen's Compensation Acts were still very much a minority. Elsewhere, accidents were, to borrow Figlio's own mode of analysis, rendered institutionally impossible by 'dense networks of expectation and meaning' that continued to sustain and uphold the highly conservative rural hierarchy. Thus, in remote areas of Britain until well into the nineteenth century, the providential, the pre-Christian and the neo-animistic continued to exercise a powerful hold over the collective imagination.[19] The thrust of Figlio's argument tends to be generated by its own end-point: the neo-collectivist Workmen's Compensation Acts. This is certainly too subtle a piece of work to be designated 'Whiggish', but the *coup de grâce* – 'Such an event was an accident, a breach of contract' – implicitly excludes all those who continued to work wholly or partly outside the 'protection' of 'progressive' contractual frameworks.

Negatively, then, Figlio's pioneering contribution reminds us that one of the primary concerns of the social historian of accidents must be with the uncompensated individual victim, in terms of his or her experience of injury. The need for such a perspective is all the greater in that, even today, there is a tendency to prioritize the circumstances surrounding the accident over the experience itself, thus allowing it to be socially pacified and politically neutralized (much as pain-killers tranquillize the injured person and transform him or her into a 'patient'). Thus domestic and street accidents, in particular, are 'naturalized' or rendered politically benign by focusing on the emergency services. The result, as with the statistical normalization of industrial and environmental accidents, is loss of both political and historical insight.

For one thing, the 'naturalization' of the domestic accident disguises socio-economic inequality. Whether in seventeenth-century Norwich or twentieth-century Calcutta, it is highly likely that some sectors of the community rather than others will suffer a greater incidence of accidental injury or death purely as a result of differences in income and class/caste. For another thing, the very use of the term 'domestic' for such events further mystifies them. It reinforces a consensus that such mishaps are less preventable than industrial injuries (hence more 'natural'), at the same time that it sustains the idea that these are happenings that are indeed exclusively 'domestic'. But the home has more often than not been a place of productive labour; 'domestic accidents' were thus more likely to occur in the homes of the poor than in those of the relatively affluent when – from at least the late seventeenth century onwards – the homes of the latter were increasingly devoted to 'withdrawal from labour'.[20] Moreover, tiredness, leading to inattentiveness and delayed reaction-time, has been a permanent and threatening presence in the dwellings of the poor, with undersupervised babies and toddlers comprising the most tragically affected groups of victims. Finally, since the mid nineteenth century, homes have become increasingly 'industrialized',[21] with networked utilities such as gas and electricity precipitating novel genres of accidents within the domestic sphere.[22]

The 'naturalization' of the domestic accident also deprives us of insights into the history of class and gender. Barbara Hanawalt shows that in medieval London one half of all accidental deaths among women, but only a fifth among men, occurred in the home or adjoining buildings. The other 50 per cent of women's fatal accidents took place in the street, in water, and in churches, while the remaining four-fifths of men's fatal accidents happened in shops (16 per cent) and public spaces (60 per cent).[23] Medieval Londoners were more at risk in their leisure than at work and, here again, Hanawalt shows, there were significant differences between the sexes: '33 percent of men's accidental deaths and 8 percent of women's accidental deaths occurred in the evening or at night'.[24] There were, in addition, differences in the accident rate between village- and town-based toddlers and children. The younger age group in the capital had *fewer* accidents than those in rural areas, partly, it seems, because they were better supervised by parents and community.[25]

There is no reason to suppose that coroners' records and similar material for other times and places would be any less revealing[26] – and not only on the material conditions of social life. There may have been men and women during the early modern period who utterly rejected a fatalistic or providential interpretation of 'accidents'. Even in 1813, at the time of the famous Felling Colliery disaster near Newcastle, some may have anticipated the view of the techno-chronicler Humphrey Jennings over a century later, that attributing such a calamity to fate or to God constituted 'a conception à la Calvin to depress the people'.[27] As we know little in detail about the secularization of the accident in law and medicine,[28] so we know even less about when workers, or impoverished householders, began to conceive of accidents as 'inevitable' only in relation to (alterable) socio-economic conditions. The study of working-class biographies, newspapers, gossip, old wives-tales and folklore might all prove useful here. So, too, might be the analysis of popular literature and drama, the sermons preached over fatal accidents, and the wealth of public inquiries in more recent times.

But secularization must not be assumed; nor should it necessarily be cast in positivistic terms. Implicit in the kind of quantitative urgency that obsessed the medical statistician, William Farr, was the belief that 'the accident' would disappear from popular cosmology once the 'truth' about probability was accepted.[29] Such a belief was premised on the assumption that the 'normalized' and de-individualized, or de-Providentialized accident had already established itself in popular culture, and had significantly altered consciousness. As we have indicated, however, this was not necessarily the case, not even in 'industrialized' Britain. Although in the late twentieth century 'accidents' no longer function as measures of social integration or disruption in the west, they continue to be perceived in terms of deserved 'come-uppance' or, by Buddhists and non-Buddhists alike, as the cosmic consequence of bad *karma*. Medical sociologists report that in contemporary western culture an individual sense of personal responsibility or self-blame for illness is greater than that for minor injuries attributable to accidents (the cause of which can be 'othered').[30] But seriously debilitating accidents are still likely to give rise to the question 'why me?', and invoke notions of punishment for earthly sins.[31]

No one has yet sought to apply 'thick' description or controlled historical sociology to the effects of accidents on communities,[32] and neither have accidents been systematically studied demographically as a branch of the history of 'public death'.[33] Still lacking is knowledge of the kinds of sources that might throw light on the incidence of fatal and non-fatal accidents, and on their shifting prevalence over time and place. Variations according to age and gender, between industries, and in relation to the impact of new and changing technologies have yet to be investigated.[34] In the case of England and Wales, statistics contained in the annual *Reports* of the Registrar-General are far from definitive. Moreover, as Judith Green points out in her contribution to this volume, the history of the shifting classifications of 'violent death' in those documents and, later, in the publications of the World Health Organization demand careful epistemological analysis.[35] Why 'accidents' were initially compounded with statistics on suicide and executions clearly needs unpacking.

There are links between the demographic history of the accident, the 'rise of statistics', and the history of the accident insurance industry – links commercial and ideological which, as Roger Cooter notes in his chapter, are important for understanding the rise of consciousness in relation to accidents, but which, as yet, have not received the historical research they deserve. The insurance industry, in turn, connects to the unwritten history of accidents in medical and surgical practice, which again connects with the insurance industry via suits for malpractice.[36] Professional performance in medicine and insurance is closely related to psychological expertise and norms. The latter interact with accidents not only through the study of an (unhistoricized) 'proneness', but also through the medico-legal construction of 'railway spine' (or 'traumatic neurasthenia', 'traumatic' or 'accident neurosis' and on down to 'Post-Traumatic Stress Disorder'),[37] as well as through fundamental and, indeed, 'everyday' concepts such as the 'Freudian slip'.[38]

The history of the accident, like the plight of the 'ordinary patient' or that of the 'unskilled worker' will doubtless never become fully visible. Nor does it seem probable that we shall ever know completely either the biographies of the individuals involved in such events, or the aggregate of 'normalized' or 'predictable' mishaps during any given historical period. What is clear, however, is that the historicization of the accident is possible, and that the project is open to a wide variety of analytical frameworks and approaches. Such is the point underlined in the chapters that follow.

The first three probe the myriad epistemological, social and political roots of the 'accidental'. Each of these chapters is important for distinguishing and carving out routes between determinism, neo-determinism, providentialism and 'pure' contingency. Beginning with the word itself, the social philosopher Robert Campbell provides a set of base positions for thinking about what an 'accident' is, and, more specifically, what an accident may not be. The medical sociologist Judith Green problematizes the term still further in her historical account of the classification of accidents. Emphasizing the extent to which accidents are administratively defined and shaped by both the state and the legal system, she also shows how this construction has been fitted into sociological discourse. Like Campbell, she engages with Figlio's arguments. Arthur McEvoy's chapter introduces different problems, and sets old ones on their head, by construing the workplace site of accidents as an ecological system with the worker's body at its core. Within an extensive scrutiny of the history of technology, he 'denaturalizes' the industrial accident by bringing it into sharp social, political and legal relief.

The subsequent six chapters intersect these and other conceptual and historiographical questions surrounding accidents in history. Their perspectives are more rooted in time and place, however. Roy Porter, concentrating on eighteenth-century Britain, explores not only the secularization of accidents, but also the extent of medicalization. Roger Cooter extends this discussion, proposing that much of the explanation for the wave of interest in accident provision he detects in Britain during the last third of the nineteenth century hinges less on medicalization than on militarization. John Hutchinson, endorsing this view whilst challenging Cooter's 'ideological' casting of events, extends the framework for discussion further still by looking comparatively to developments in accident provision on the Continent.

The crucial 'cultural moment' in the history of accidents that Cooter and Hutchinson explore is approached in Dietrich Milles' chapter from the perspective of the German state's intervention into industrial medicine. Informed by the work of Ulrich Beck, Milles explicates the development of German accident insurance in order to connect present-day concerns with risk to the ideological and technological origins of industrial society. In the concept of 'industrial pathogenicity' he locates a critical point of differentiation.

The chapter by Joel Tarr and Mark Tebeau is no less preoccupied with the structuring of risk than that by Milles, and during some of the same decades. Its reference is not to the German industrial worker, however, but to the arguably 'separate sphere' of the American housewife. Here the object is to establish conceptual and empirical linkages between the supposed 'liberation' set in train by the technological 'revolution' of the home, and the emergence of the housewife as the 'superintendent' of that new terrain saddled with responsibility for 'domestic safety'.

From concerns with gender and accident prevention we turn, finally, to the relations between accidents and war. Bill Luckin's chapter connects two seemingly disparate sets of events: the preparation for resistance to the Nazi bombing of urban areas in Britain at the beginning of World War II, and the 'slaughter' on the roads set in train by air-raid precautions. Motor vehicle accidents in this context provide a forum for relating technologies of 'peace' and 'war', as well as for casting discussion of accidents in terms of a class structure in crisis.

From a variety of perspectives, then, these essays challenge the common tendency to regard accidents as beyond the pale of serious study. Through a number of different contexts, they open to socio-historical inquiry that which has hitherto been considered irrelevant or, at best, politically, ideologically and discursively inscrutable. In the course of moving the subject to centre-stage they expose, paradoxically, that there are no 'accidents' in history, just as there are no coincidences. The 'accident', they reveal, far from being 'accidental' or wholly arbitrary in occurrence and meaning is, in fact, historically contingent, as well as germane to our understanding of some of the most fundamental features of social, political, cultural and material life.

Acknowledgements

Our thanks to Steve Sturdy for many useful and incisive comments.

Notes

1. Newton Bosworth, *The Accidents Of Human Life; With Hints For Their Prevention, Or The Removal Of Their Consequences* (London: Allen and Co., 1813), iii.
2. See, for example, David Landes, 'What Room for Accident in History? Explaining Big Changes by Small Events', *Economic History Review*, xlvii (1994), 637–56.
3. Agendas on *how* to write medical history 'from below' threaten to torpedo the project itself. But see Mary Fissell, *Patients, Power and the Poor in Eighteenth Century Bristol* (Cambridge: Cambridge University Press, 1991), chapter 8; Roy Porter (ed.), *Patients and Practitioners: Lay Perceptions of Medicine in Pre-Industrial Society* (Cambridge: Cambridge University Press, 1985); and Roy Porter and Dorothy Porter, *In Sickness and in Health: The British Experience 1650–1850* (London: Fourth Estate, 1988).
4. Robert Castel, 'From Dangerousness to Risk', in Graham Burchell, Colin Jones and P. Miller (eds), *The Foucault Effect: Studies In Governmentality* (London: Harvester/Wheatsheaf, 1991), 285.
5. Michael Barkun, *Disaster and the Millennium* (New Haven: Yale University Press, 1974), 50ff.
6. Charles Perrow, *Normal Accidents: Living with High-Risk Technologies* (New York: Basic Books, 1984), 10.
7. Rosalind Williams, *Notes on the Underground: An Essay on Technology, Society and the Imagination* (Cambridge, MA: MIT Press, 1990), 200. On the changing concept and definition of 'disaster', see Peter Curson, 'Introduction' to John I. Clarke *et al.* (eds), *Population and Disaster* (Oxford: Blackwell, 1989), 1–23.
8. Les Levidow, 'Nuclear Accidents By Design', *Science as Culture*, ix (1990), 99–109.
9. Bosworth, *op.cit.* (ref. 1), iv.

10. See Anson Rabinbach, *The Human Motor: Energy, Fatigue and the Origins of Modernity* (Berkeley: University of California Press, 1990); and Peter Froggatt and J.A. Smiley, 'The Concept of Accident Proneness: A Review', *British Journal of Industrial Medicine*, 24 (1964), 1–12. For exemplification of the psychologization of accidents in these terms, see Arnold Wilson and Hermann Levy, *Workmen's Compensation* (London: Oxford University Press, 1939), vol. 2, chapter 2.
11. See Daniel Pick, *War Machine: The Rationalisation of Slaughter in the Modern Age* (New Haven: Yale University Press, 1993).
12. Undated letter (c.1992) from the Royal Bank of Scotland to all investors, quoting the Office of Population Censuses and Surveys (1991 *Monitor*). Our thanks to Steve Sturdy for this reference.
13. By the post-modern sociologist Zygmunt Bauman, 'The Solution as Problem', *Times Higher Education Supplement*, 13 Nov. 1992, 35, cited in Les Levidow, 'De-reifying Risk', *Science as Culture*, xx (1994), 440–56.
14. On the manifold expressions of 'risk' which now threaten to empty the concept of all meaning, see 'definitions of risk', in George Cvetkovich and Timothy C. Earle, 'Environmental Hazards and the Public', *Journal of Social Issues*, xlviii (1992), 5. See also Castel, *op.cit.* (ref. 4), especially 282, and Francois Ewald, 'Insurance and Risk', in Burchell *et al.*, *op.cit.* (ref. 4), 197–210, at 199.
15. Most notably in the work of Ian Hacking. See his *The Emergence of Probability: A Philosophical Study of Early Ideas About Probability, Induction and Statistical Inference* (Cambridge: Cambridge University Press, 1975); and *idem*, *The Taming of Chance* (Cambridge: Cambridge University Press, 1990).
16. On the political negotiation and social construction of the perception of 'risk', see Karl Dake, 'Myths of Nature: Culture and the Social Construction of Risk', *Journal of Social Issues*, xlviii (1992), 21–37. See also Sheldon Krimsky and Dominic Golding (eds), *Social Theories of Risk* (London/New York: Praeger, 1992). It remains to be seen if the same will come to be said of the parallel (and related) growth of interest in trauma. 'Trauma studies' are now nearly as voluminous as those on 'risk' and are beginning to be converged upon by historians of different types; to date, however, psychology and medicine seem the driving force.
17. In Paul Weindling (ed.), *The Social History of Occupational Health* (London: Croom Helm, 1985), 180–206.
18. Figlio, 'What is an Accident?', 183.
19. See James Obelkevich, *Religion and Rural Society: South Lindsey, 1825–1875* (Oxford: Clarendon Press, 1975), 259–313.
20. For regional and local detail, see Richard G. Wilson, *Gentlemen Merchants: The Merchant Community in Leeds, 1700–1830* (Manchester: Manchester University Press, 1971); John Foster, *Class Struggle and the Industrial Revolution: Early Industrial Capitalism in Three English Towns* (London:

Weidenfeld & Nicolson, 1974); and Peter Earle, *The Making of the English Middle Class: Business, Society and Family Life in London, 1660–1730* (London: Methuen, 1989).

21. See Ruth Schwartz Cowan, *More Work for Mother: The Ironies of Household Technology from the Open Hearth to the Microwave* (new edition, London: Free Association, 1989). See also Dolores Hayden, *The Grand Domestic Revolution: A History of Feminist Designs for American Homes, Neighborhoods and Cities* (Cambridge, MA: MIT Press, 1981).
22. On accidents from the latter source, see Bill Luckin, *Questions of Power: Electricity and Environment in Inter-war Britain* (Manchester: Manchester University Press, 1990).
23. Barbara Hanawalt, *Growing Up In Medieval London: The Experience of Childhood in History* (New York: Oxford University Press, 1993), 75.
24. *Ibid.*, 77.
25. *Ibid.*, 63–7.
26. Such material cannot be used uncritically however. As Richard Wall has pointed out with regard to Hanawalt's use of coroners' records, implicit to it is the assumption that actions which resulted in an accidental death were representative of *all* actions, and that they thereby allow the patterns of daily life to be reconstructed. 'Burnt Girls and Drowned Boys: Some Inequalities in Death in England and Wales, Germany and the United States', paper presented to the conference on 'Accidents in History', 13 Oct. 1990: summary in *Social History of Medicine*, iv (1991), 200–1.
27. Humphrey Jennings, *Pandaemonium 1660–1886: The Coming of the Machine as Seen by Contemporary Observers*, edited by Mary-Lou Jennings and Charles Madge (London: Andre Deutsch, 1934), 134. For one of the contemporary sermons on the Felling disaster, see Roger Cooter's chapter in this volume, note 1.
28. Much greater is our knowledge of the secularization of suicide. See Michael MacDonald and T.R. Murphy, *Sleepless Souls: Suicide in Early Modern England* (Oxford: Clarendon Press, 1990) which references the major sociological and historical sources.
29. J.M. Eyler, 'William Farr and the Cholera: The Sanitarian's Disease Theory and the Statistician's Method', *Journal of the History of Medicine*, xxviii (1973), 79–100; *idem*, *Victorian Social Medicine: The Ideas and Methods of William Farr* (Baltimore: Johns Hopkins University Press, 1979). See also Michael J. Cullen, *The Statistical Movement in Early Victorian Britain: The Foundations of Empirical Social Science* (Hassocks, Sussex: Harvester, 1975); Theodore M. Porter, *The Rise of Statistical Thinking 1820–1900* (Princeton, N.J.: Princeton University Press, 1980); and *idem*, *Trust in Numbers: The Pursuit of Objectivity in Science and Public Life* (Princeton, N.J.: Princeton University Press, 1995).
30. See, for example, Jocelyn Cornwell, *Hard-Earned Lives: Accounts of Health and Illness from East London* (London: Tavistock, 1984), 130 *et passim.* On eighteenth-century distinctions between 'natural' and

'deserved' illness, see Alfons Labisch, *Homo Hygienicus: Gesundheit und Medizin in der Neuzeit* (Frankfurt: Campus Verlag, 1992). See also, *idem*, 'Doctors, Workers and the Scientific Cosmology of the Industrial World: The Social Construction of "Health" and the "Home Hygienicus"', *J. Contemporary History*, xx (1985), 599–615.

31. Cf. Cotton Mather, *Days of Humiliation. Times of Affliction and Disaster. Nine Sermons for Restoring Favor with an Angry God, 1696–1727*. Facsimile reprint and introduction by George Harrison Orians (Gainesville: Scholar's Facsimiles and Reprints, 1970).
32. Clifford Geertz, 'Thick Description: Toward an Interpretive Theory of Culture', in Geertz, *Interpretation of Cultures* (New York: Basic Books, 1973). For contemporary sociological studies of communities which have suffered disasters, see Samuel Henry Prince, *Catastrophe and Social Change, Based Upon a Sociological Study of the Halifax Disaster* (PhD thesis, University of New York, 1920); Allen H. Barton, *Communities in Disaster: A Sociological Analysis of Collective Stress Situations* (New York: Doubleday, 1969); and *idem*, *Social Organization Under Stress: A Sociological Review of Disaster Studies* (Washington, DC: National Academy of Sciences, National Research Council, 1963).
33. See Gil Elliot, *Twentieth Century Book of the Dead* (London: Allen Lane, 1972), 175ff. Elliot, perhaps only facetiously, calculates that 'with a budget of say £100,000 ... half a dozen people of assorted disciplines and with access to other specialists' he could 'over a period of three to five years put the whole area of macro-violence on a sound statistical basis, give it historical roots and link it to the wider field of public death in the underdeveloped and ecological senses, expand the matrix of concepts and factual detail in conjunction with a continuous research activity into current and future events, and supply the social sciences in general with a wealth of enlightening and research-stimulating information.' (209)
34. An exception is Margaret J. Mettert, *Industrial Injuries to Women in 1930 and 1931 compared with Injuries to Men* (Washington, D.C.: GPO, 1935).
35. See, also, for the debate on the nature and level of violence in early modern English society, Susan Dwyer Amussen, 'Punishment, Discipline, and Power: The Social Meaning of Violence in Early Modern England', *Journal of British Studies*, xxxiv (1995), 1–34.
36. The few histories we possess of medicine and the law have little to say on the matter of accidents; nor do we find accidents indexed in contemporary texts, such as Marilynn Rosenthal, *The Incompetent Doctor: Behind Closed Doors* (Milton Keynes: Open University Press, 1995), or Patricia M. Danzon, *Medical Malpractice: Theory, Evidence, and Public Policy* (Cambridge, MA: Harvard University Press, 1985), which largely concern themselves with the issue of professional protection.

37. See Esther Fischer-Homberger, *Die Traumatische Neurose. Vom Somatischen Zum Sozialen Leiden* (Berne: Hans Huber, 1975); Wolfgang Schivelbusch, *The Railway Journey: The Industrialization of Time and Space in the 19th Century* (Leamington Spa: Berg, 1986), especially chapter 9: 'Railway Accident "Railway Spine" and Traumatic Neurosis'; and Michael Clark, '"Traumatic Neurasthenia"' and Eric M. Caplan, 'Trains, Brains and Sprains: Railway Spine and the Origins of Psychoneuroses', *Bulletin of the History of Medicine,* lxix (1995), 387–419; Thomas Keller, 'Railway Spine Revisited: Traumatic Neurosis or Neurotrauma?', *Journal of the History of Medicine and Allied Sciences,* 1 (1995), 507–24; and the 'British Workmen's Compensation Acts, c.1900–c.1935', paper presented to the Conference on 'Accidents in History', 13 Oct. 1990, summary in *Social History of Medicine,* iv (1991), 197–8. For some of the contemporary sources on the psychological effects of railway accidents, see Roger Cooter's chapter in this volume, note 42.
38. On Freud and the psychology of the accident, see Judy Green, 'Some Problems in the Development of a Sociology of Accidents', in Sue Scott *et al.* (eds), *Private Risks and Public Dangers,* Explorations in Sociology no. 43 (Aldershot: Avebury, 1992), 20, 26, and 30–31.

2

Philosophy and the Accident

Robert Campbell

'accident (æks_dent), *sb.* [a.Fr. *accident:* -L. *accidens, -ent*, sb. properly pr. pple. of *accid-_re* to fall, to happen.'
(*Oxford English Dictionary*)

Introduction

An accident may be defined as something which 'happens'. But since all happenings 'happen', this is scarcely helpful. Things happen 'deliberately', 'intentionally', 'predictably', 'by mistake', 'by chance', 'unexpectedly', 'through the inexorable workings of fate'; they are 'providential', 'unfortunate', 'disastrous', 'tragic' or 'catastrophic'. They may also be 'haphazard' or happen 'at random' or they may be 'acts of God'. Where are we to fit 'accidentally' into an adverbial taxonomy of happenings?

These qualifications belong to different categories. Some relate to agency and the ways in which our plans and projects compare with actual outcomes – 'intentionally' and 'by mistake'. Others are epistemological – 'predictably', 'unforeseeably'. We may be passing judgement on the value or disvalue of the event, as when, for example, we call it 'providential' or 'unfortunate'. I want to argue that the concept of the accidental combines elements from all of these categories making claims, simultaneously, about agency, epistemology and value.

Let me describe an accident to you.[1] On 6 March, 1987 at around 7.00 p.m. the *Herald of Free Enterprise* left the Belgian port of Zeebrugge bound for Dover. Shortly afterwards she capsized and sank, leaving a third of the hull still above water. It seems that the bow doors of the roll-on roll-off ferry had been left open allowing water to pour on to the car deck. The assistant bosun, part of whose duties it was to close the bow doors, was later found to have been asleep in his cabin. The ferry company was also criticized for the lack of effective procedures and guidelines to ensure that this could not happen. One hundred and fifty passengers and thirty-eight crew lost their lives.[2]

What made this an 'accident'? Clearly none of the ship's crew or the operating company had intended or expected that this should happen. Nor had the ship been designed with the view that it would (though it was subsequently claimed that it, and ships like it, had not been carefully enough designed so that it would not). The incident was, however, far from being inexplicable. Indeed, given information about the design of the ship and the state of its bow doors as it left the port, it could have been predicted that there was a high risk that the ferry would sink. It was not predicted because it was neither intended nor expected that the bow doors would be left open. The bosun, who had slept through the call to 'harbour stations' which should have prompted him to close the bow doors, was not actually responsible for ensuring that they were. The doors could have been, and often were, closed by many other members of the crew. The chief officer, who *was* responsible for ensuring that they were closed, was, however, also required to be on the bridge during 'harbour stations', from which position neither he nor the ship's master could tell whether the doors had actually been closed or not. Probably none of the crew had any idea of the possible drastic consequences of leaving the doors open, and, indeed, the *Herald* had sailed successfully on a number of occasions in this condition. However, the instability of such ferries in these circumstances was well known. The lack of internal watertight bulkheads on the car deck meant that any water taken on board could easily and rapidly destabilize the entire vessel. The *Herald* needed thirty minutes for a successful evacuation, but capsized in ninety *seconds* and sank in another one hundred and fifty. All the information necessary to predict the incident was available though it did not coexist in any one person's head and was, therefore, effectively 'hidden'.

Why are we concerned about such accidents? We were concerned about Zeebrugge principally because of the loss of life. But total deaths in the UK from all causes in the preceding year came to 581,203 and in that year over 4,000 people committed suicide.[3] Suicide did not make the headlines that year in Britain, however, even though Zeebrugge was, and was expected to be, a one-off event and the problem of suicide remains with us on a continuing basis (3,893 deaths in 1991).[4] So loss of life cannot be the only factor.

From this point of view it is interesting to compare the statistics on suicide with the homicide rate. Murder always hits the headlines and the detection, conviction and punishment of murderers is a perennial subject of public debate. Yet only 255 people were murdered in Britain in 1991,[5] compared to the 3,893 who committed suicide. This suggests very strongly that the degree of public interest and concern is not related only to the numbers involved. For the significant difference between suicide and homicide in this regard is the fact that suicides, for the most part, intend their deaths (at the time, and however misguidedly). Suicide is not seen as interfering in the control we normally think we exercise over the course and shape of our lives[6] – despite the undoubted fact that at least some apparent attempts were not intended to end in death. Murder, on the other hand, is the paradigm case of such interference and it is easy to see how survivors of attempts and victims of other crimes of violence will often find that the most lingering psychological damage they suffer arises from the loss of autonomy they feel as a result.

Accidents are also interventions in the control we (perhaps wrongly) believe we have over the large part of our lives. They frustrate and, sometimes, vitiate our plans and projects for ourselves. This is precisely because they are neither intended nor expected. The clearest evidence that this is what concerns us about them lies in the extensive apparatus we set up in the attempt to control accidents or to ameliorate their worst effects. Legal recovery is possible in tort or negligence and there are also statutory procedures for compensation. The criminal law in part aims to prevent and/or to deter criminal injuries and damage, and there are numerous institutions set up to foster accident prevention – health and safety at work, in the home and on the roads.

Of course, not all interruptions to the control we have over our lives are, or would naturally be described as, 'accidents'. We do not worry about strokes of good fortune, though there are, of course, 'happy accidents'; the implied oxymoron is significant. It is not just lack of control that matters, but the intervention of pain, misery, distress and loss. Our reaction to this is often a need to blame, to ascribe responsibility. Sometimes this is bad faith – the attempt to evade our own responsibility – but it can also be a rational search for a responsible agent which can be prevented from allowing such a thing to happen again. Sometimes a sense of justice or fairness is involved. Misfortunes are an affront to our worth and dignity. Those who allow accidents to happen fail to treat those potentially harmed with respect, showing, apparently, an absence of that care to which we are entitled because we are, or ought to be, as important as anyone else. When human agents are involved, accidents are, *prima facie*, failures of respect or care or both, until it can be shown that there was no negligence.

Accidental Death: The Scale of the Problem

In 1991 total deaths registered in the UK were 570,044, a crude rate of 11.2 per thousand population. As might be expected, more than half of these were aged 75 and over, and in this group the commonest cause of death was heart disease. In people younger than this (15–64) cancer was the most frequent cause of death, accounting for 36,907 of the 97,194 deaths in this age range. But of the 1,165 5–14 year-olds who died in Britain in 1991, 587 died in accidents, and accidents were also the most frequent cause of death in those aged between 15 and 34 (2,870 out of 9,490, compared to the next most common cause of death – cancer – which accounted for 1,459). For those between 35 and 44, accidents were the third commonest cause of death but still nearly as significant in numerical terms as cancer and heart disease. Only in those aged 45 and over do accidents steadily decline in importance compared to the others, becoming the eighth most frequent cause of death in those aged 85 and over and the seventh overall.[7]

It is easy to be misled by such figures. The mortality rate for human beings is a hundred per cent. The risk of dying as one gets older is increased not just by external, contingent factors, but by the very fact of getting older. The significance of accidents as a cause of death lies not in their relative number but in the fact that they are not linked to increasing age, though they are, as we have seen, age-related. They are the most significant cause of death in age groups whose risk of death from other causes is otherwise very low. From the age of 1 to 34 you are more likely to die in an accident than from any other cause.[8]

One may speculate about the reasons for this, though the evidence is suggestive. Of the 4,408 people who died in British motor vehicle traffic accidents in 1991, the single largest group comprised young men aged 15–24 (959). Accidents kill more children under four than any other cause and motor vehicle accidents account for nearly half of those accidents.[9] Separate figures for accidents at work and sporting and leisure accidents are not available, but these must take their biggest toll of those who are most involved in them – those of working age who are relatively fit and active. Industrial accidents almost certainly affect younger workers more than others because younger workers are also more inexperienced and, by definition, less mature.

Accidents and Social Class

Accidents as a cause of mortality are also related to social class, which is rather more surprising. The Black Report found that, when infant mortality in Britain was measured against parents' occupational class, the most marked gradients were for deaths from accidents and respiratory disease. Infants (children up to 12 months of age) in social class V were five times as likely to die from accidental causes than those in social class I. Similar disparities were noted in children aged 1–14 years and in adults (though in the latter group it is far more marked in men than in women).[10] The reason for this, the authors conclude, is that:

> Households in occupational classes IV and V simply lack the means to provide their children with as high a level of protection as that which is to be found in the average middle-class home. This can mean both material and non-material resources.[11]

Furthermore:

> Men engaged in manual occupations routinely confront a much higher degree of risk to health and physical well-being in their work than their non-manual counterparts. These risks are manifold. They may result in direct loss of life either suddenly in the form of accidents or in an attenuated manner through long-term exposure to dust or poisonous substances in the workplace.[12]

The *Report* makes this striking observation:

> These substantial differences demonstrate the non-random nature of these events. While the death of an individual child may appear as a random misfortune, the overall distribution clearly indicates the social nature of the phenomena.[13]

We think of accidents as random events, as things which just happen without a pattern. It is, therefore, surprising to realize that they are not distributed among the population randomly, but according to factors which we recognize as social ones, factors thrown up by the nature of the society which we have created. That means that we are, as a society, collectively responsible for that distribution because it shows that it is in our power to change it. This responsibility is clearly collective rather than individual, not only because no single individual can have caused it, but also because it lies beyond the power of any single individual *to* change it. The old legal principle of tort law, that where there is no fault, a loss should lie where it falls, seems wholly inapplicable here, if this is correct. For such losses seem not to fall at random, but on specific groups of people to whom the state owes a duty of care to protect, so far as it is able to.

Another way of putting this might be to point out that, although accidents have always been seen as raising technical problems of prevention and avoidance, they also have an inescapably ethical and political dimension which has to do with our collective responsibility for the groups they most affect. That, in turn, raises questions about how we deal with the consequences of the pattern of accidents for which we are responsible. I have looked, so far, only at accidents and mortality. Clearly that is only the tip of an iceberg of which illness, disability, distress, discomfort and physical and financial loss will form by far the greater part. Are we to continue to let such losses lie where they fall, or, if not, how is compensation to be arranged? On whom should the cost of taking such preventative measures as might be effective fall? In Britain in 1991, 4,408 people died in road traffic accidents.[14] They were all avoidable. Banning motor cars, lorries and motorcycles would have saved all of those lives, though at a considerable cost. Are those lives worth that cost? Clearly we do not think so, or we would have urged the state to pay it. Or, perhaps, the idea that they are avoidable has never occurred to us.

Causation and Accidents

There is a view that everything which happens has a cause, that a cause is something which determines or necessitates its effect – that an effect follows *necessarily* from its cause. Therefore everything which happens, happens necessarily; it could not have happened otherwise. This is determinism. It is not the same as fatalism. Fatalism is the view that what will happen *will* happen whatever anyone tries to do; what is fated is unavoidable. Determinism, on the contrary, says what is done *will* affect what will happen. If action A is performed, it will cause C, D and E to happen. If on the other hand B is performed, then F, G and H will happen, but C, D and E will not. However, it is true, according to determinism, that the outcome of the choice between A and B is determined in advance of the choice by its preceding conditions. A fatalist will say: 'I'm fated either to pass this exam or fail it, so it does not matter whether I revise or not: whatever is fated will happen.' For a determinist this is quite wrong. Determinism says that if I do not revise then my failure will have been caused by my lack of revision. If I do revise and I pass, then my passing will have been caused by revising. So it *does* matter whether I revise or not. But it is also true, according to determinism, that whether I revise or I do not revise is caused by some prior fact, such as my laziness which in turn is caused by my genetic make-up or my upbringing and so on.

Both the fatalist and the determinist might be thought to agree that nothing is ever an accident. For the fatalist this is because there is a grand design, a pattern of events which will occur whatever anyone does to prevent it. This may be correct, but it is important to realize that it is not the same view as determinism and would not follow even if determinism were true. Fatalism is a matter of faith for there is no evidence that would support it. It may even be wholly vacuous since it would seem to be compatible with any future possibilities whatsoever.

For the determinist there is no grand design but, nonetheless, it might seem that nothing happens by accident. If everything is determined then there is an internal necessity in events that could, in principle, make them predictable, if we knew enough about them and the laws which govern their behaviour. Thus, on this view, everything which happens, happens necessarily; nothing happens which could not have been foreseen and, therefore, there are no accidents. This is a mistake. An accident is not something which *cannot* be foreseen, but something which *was not* foreseen. Just because something *can* be foreseen does not mean that it will be. Accidents are not uncaused events; an uncaused event is a miracle, not an accident. On the contrary, we expect an accident to have causes. We frequently try very hard to determine the causes of accidents, in the hope of preventing them in the future.

There is also something odd in the implication that what is determined can always be foreseen. For what does 'determined' mean here? It does not, in most causal contexts, mean 'logically necessary'. What is determined is not foreseeable in the sense that it can be logically deduced. As Hume pointed out,[15] causal statements are not logically necessary, whatever other kind of necessity might be attributed to them. Genuinely logically necessary statements are tautologous – they are truisms – and seldom have the cognitive content of genuine causal statements. 'It is either raining or it is not', or 'All black birds are black' are two typical examples of logically necessary statements which tell us virtually nothing about the weather or ornithology. Such statements are entirely foreseeable and it is easy to see why they are. Those causal statements which come closest to the firmness of the logically necessary tend to be both very general and rather abstract: 'Raising pure water to a temperature of 100°C under normal (sea-level) atmospheric pressure will cause it to boil'. This is based on the regularities of ordinary experience purified by qualification and idealization in order to preserve it from falsity. Thus we come close to making it definitionally – and hence logically – true of water that this is how it behaves. The necessity is ideal rather than actual, though, for we know that many different factors can intervene in practice to falsify such a claim – the water will not be pure, neither the temperature nor the pressure can be guaranteed, and so on. Ordinarily, the causal claims we make are even more subject to qualification and exception: 'Wearing silver jewellery will turn your skin black'. Often this is so; it depends on the purity of the silver, the sweatiness of the skin, the length of time the article is worn, the closeness of its contact with the skin, and so on. It therefore, quite often, is also not so. Such a claim is more useful as a retrospective explanation – a diagnosis – than a prediction of what will happen. 'The black mark on your finger is caused by the silver ring you were wearing; it is not life-threatening. It will wash off.' It might still be claimed that the defeasibility – or even impossibility – of prediction in such cases is due to ignorance and that, in principle, whether your silver ring will leave a black mark on your finger is foresee*able* even if not actually foreseen. But foreseeable *by whom*? Many things we fail to foresee we know, nonetheless, to be foreseeable because, on other occasions, we have foreseen just that, or a relevantly similar thing. But, equally, we know that we, ordinary human beings, are not able to foresee many things; they are not foreseeable *by us*. They are too remote in the future or depend on the correlation of too many variables for us to be able to predict them. But that does not, of course, mean that we think they are not determined; they do have causes and their causes are sufficient to explain their occurrence.

Chaos Theory raises other problems[16] with foreseeability and causation. Except in very simple cases events occur not in causal chains but in trees which proliferate exponentially. We should not look on causes like this: A causes B which causes C which causes D ... but like this:

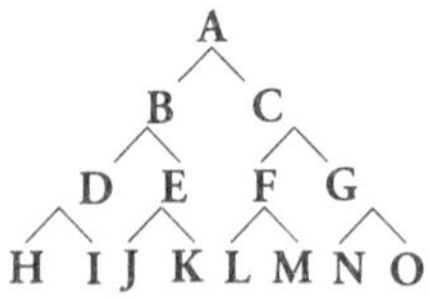

A causes B and C; B causes D and E whereas C causes F and G; D, in turn, causes H and I, E causes J and K, F causes L and M and G causes N and O; and so on. Within three steps the single cause A has produced eight independent effects each of which will produce two more, making sixteen in all and so on. This is a simplified model which assumes that each cause will have only two effects. This seems unrealistically small and the causal tree is likely in reality to be even more complex than this. The claim is that any action will, in a very short space of time, have had so many consequences which themselves will have had consequences that even the most unimaginably large and powerful computer could not track or model them. Reality is not foreseeable, not because events are not caused, but because it is so complex as to be beyond the computations our predictions would require.

If accidents were to be defined as caused but unforeseen events, therefore, then it would seem that if Chaos Theory is correct, everything is an accident. This is clearly absurd. In the first place, even within Chaos Theory, predictability *does* exist, albeit within a relatively restricted time-frame; how restricted depends, presumably, on the complexity of the phenomena in question. In the second place some totally unforeseeable events, such as the timing and extent of the hurricane force winds which occur on average every two or three hundred years in this country, tend to be classed as 'acts of God' rather than accidents. The reason for this is that human agency is not involved. It seems to be true that accidents, as they are normally thought of, involve some kind of error in human action; where we reclassify 'acts of God' as accidents, it is because we wish to emphasize the involvement of human error in making them worse than they would otherwise have been if not in actually bringing them about.

> The cause of a great famine in India may be identified by the Indian peasant as the drought, but the World Food Authority may identify the Indian government's failure to build up reserves as the cause and the drought as a mere condition.[17]

It seems to be true, therefore, that events have causes and, if that is all determinism means, then determinism is probably true. If determinism implies, in addition, that all events are, in principle, foreseeable, then it is probably either false or vacuous. But that does not mean that we will always be wrong in our expectations about what will happen, only that those expectations are probabilistic – not certain – and that we have to deal with likelihood not necessity here. Accidents are not uncaused events, nor is it true that, if every event has a cause, there can be no true accidents. Accidents are caused but unexpected events (or the repercussions of events) involving human agency – events whose likelihood we did not see or, if we did, did not rate very highly.

Responsibility and Accidents

But clearly, not all unexpected events are accidents even when a human agent is involved. Someone who attacks and seriously injures another may not expect them to die; but if they do, and they do so as a result of the attack, it would hardly do to call their death an accident. For though the death may not have been foreseen, it ought to have been and only a refusal to consider consequences could have failed to encompass it. This is the difference between carelessness or negligence and recklessness, between failing in a duty of care we owe to others and disregarding it altogether. The line is often difficult to draw and in many cases it is drawn out of policy or pragmatism rather than principle, but it distinguishes the accidental from the malicious and deliberate and, in doing so, distinguishes compensation from punishment.

Nonetheless, it is clearly too simple to suggest that we divide events involving human agency into those for which someone is responsible, and the rest which are accidents. Certainly it is true that the paradigm case of something which is *not* an accident is the deliberate action which brings about what it was intended to achieve or, at the least, what was not unlooked for. So the 'accidental' is closely tied to the idea of *control*, as was noted earlier. What we control successfully is non-accidental; the accidental appears where there is imperfect control or no control at all. But this does not mean that we have no responsibility for what we do not control, for it is also obviously true that accidents *can* be someone's responsibility, blame can be attributed for bringing them about.

We need to make a distinction which ordinary language does not make entirely clear but which is nevertheless uncontroversial – between responsibility and liability. We may be responsible for things for which we are not liable, for which we may, for example, have a good excuse or a defence. (It is also possible, though this is rarer, to be liable for things for which we are not, in a strict sense, responsible: as, for example, when we assume liability for the actions of another as parent, guardian or, sometimes, employer – what the law calls 'vicarious liability'.) In this sense we are *responsible* for those things which only happened because we acted, or failed to act, as we did. The rest – what would have happened anyway whatever we did – we are not responsible for (though we may, rarely, be liable for some of them). The class of things for which we are, therefore, responsible is a very large one since it includes the non-occurrence of everything we failed to do as well as the results of what we did do. Thankfully, though responsible, we are not *liable* for everything in that class; it includes many things for which we may be neither blamed nor praised. There is no single reason for, or explanation of this, but an example may make it clearer. We are responsible for all the results of our failure to do things, but we are only liable where we had a positive duty to do them. Many philosophy students will have unmarked essays this evening because of my failure to mark them. The only students to whom I am answerable, however, are those whose essays I have a duty to mark. I am not to blame for the rest.

It is important to realize that doing and not doing is not the same as acting or omitting to act. There are things I may do just as effectively by failing to act or refraining from acting as by acting. One significant example of this is the duty I have to take care in my dealings with others not to harm or injure them unjustifiably. Thus, though there may be many harms which people suffer through my failure to prevent them, I am only liable for those I had a duty of care to try and prevent. And here, a failure to act may amount to doing something – being negligent – for which I am to blame.[18] I can, therefore, be responsible not just for the accidents which happen to others which I have caused, but also for those which I both failed to prevent and might, reasonably, have been able to prevent. The concept of negligence is, therefore, of first importance in the consideration of the 'accidental'. For the deliberately brought about is, by definition, non-accidental. That for which no one is responsible or liable *might* be accidental, but is more likely to be an act of God – an event with no human contribution at all. Nonetheless, the locus of interest in most cases ties the accident to related notions of blame, compensation and prevention and it is, therefore, the negligently caused accident which is in question.

Contracts and Accidents

In his seminal paper on the history of the concept of an accident, Figlio[19] defines an accident as 'an unforeseen event which is also expected'. It must be said, however, that Figlio's paper, though challenging and interesting, is not a model of clarity. For he also says that accidents can only be formulated as 'distinct events' once social relations become contractually based and a 'field of natural expectation is ... invaded by retrospectively predictable but unforeseen events' (181). So are accidents 'expected' or do they *invade* – that is, presumably, *violate* ? – 'a field of natural expectation' (that is '*un*expected')? Later he adds that in traditional cultures 'Nothing could happen by accident, when every event is scrutinized for its place in the dense fabric of expectation' (i.e. *everything* is expected, so nothing can be accidental?) (184). The truth is that accidents are both expected and unexpected. There is the statistical regularity of *kinds* of accidents within given populations and time-frames together with the unforeseeable – or, at least, unforeseen – nature of particular *accident instances.*

What Figlio seems to be concerned with is this. The world is not static but it is in flux. Its history is constituted of sequences of events which change the state of things through time. Countless such events occur but not all of them are, or are accounted, accidents. A leaf falls from a tree and lands on the ground. A cat leaps to catch a bird. Someone at a bus stop flags down a bus and catches it. All of these events change the world in a very minor way and none of them is an accident. They simply happen. Accidents occur, according to Figlio, when we have expectations, formed or inchoate and unexplicit, which are then violated by the unforeseen but, probably, foreseeable.

It follows from this that the idea of an accident only gets off the ground in formal, legal terms once the legal notion of a contract becomes the normal way of regulating relations between individuals. This is because only with a contract can we have a set of expectations about how things ought to be, in the normal way, which forms the background for the specific agreement – the set of duties and rights – which forms the contract itself. Why is this so? To answer that question, we must step back a little way and ask what a contract is.

Legally, the concept of a contract is very complicated, but basically it is a formal promise which is intended to have legal consequences. A promise is, usually, made by virtue of a *speech-act* [20] – a form of words which does not describe or, necessarily, accompany an action, but is, itself, an action of a kind. To say 'I declare you man and wife' is not to *describe* an act of marrying someone, but to *perform* it. Likewise, to say to A 'I promise to X', is all that one need do for it to be the case that one has made a promise to A. However, there may be many occasions when saying 'I declare you man and wife' is not sufficient for a legal marriage to have taken place. There are also a number of *background conditions* which need to hold. The words need to be uttered by the right person – a minister of the Church of England, for example, or a registrar – in the right place, the persons concerned must be free to marry, a licence must have been obtained, and so on. In the same way, *saying* 'I promise to X' only amounts to making a promise where the right context exists – both parties must understand what the words mean, the promisor must not be coerced or in any other way not fully consenting, and so on. In the case of what we might call a 'moral' promise, these conditions are a little vague and the limiting cases undefined. A 'legal' promise, or contract, on the other hand is much more tightly specified – the promisee must offer the promisor a *consideration* in return for the promise, for example, and both promisor and promisee must intend to create not just mutual rights and responsibilities, as in any promise, but legally enforceable ones.

A characteristic of all speech-acts is that, although it may be possible to give a complete specification of the *positive* conditions necessary for the act in question to have been performed, there are also *negative* conditions not possible to specify completely. This is because the negative conditions can be summed up by saying that the background conditions must be normal for the act in question. What this means, in effect, is that things must be, more or less, as those involved take them to be. If I promise to lend you £50 next week, not knowing that next week I shall be bankrupted by the unexpected collapse of the stock market, or you promise to collect my dry cleaning next Tuesday not knowing, because I also did not know, that someone else has already collected it for me, then those promises do not hold. Whether we would say that they are 'negated', 'compromised' or simply laid aside – whether, that is, we would say they were never actually made, though they seemed to be, or whether, though made, they no longer hold good – ordinarily is left unclear because it does not matter: the effect is the same. In legal cases this may not be so, and it may be vital to decide whether a contract is 'void', 'illegal', 'voidable' or simply 'unenforceable'.[21] Much of the 'law of contract' is devoted to the examination of masses of case-law in order to determine what the 'normal' background to the making of a contract is and what the legal consequences might be of it being violated in particular kinds of ways.

Thus the notion of a 'contract' implies acceptance of a correlative notion of what constitutes the 'normal', the background against which it is possible to make *any* contract and the background against which *this* particular contract is made. It is against this background that the notion of an 'accident' can be delineated by contrast, for an 'accident' is precisely what a violation of that background is.

As Figlio notes without commenting on it, the move towards contract as a framework for regulating human relations dates from the Enlightenment with the development of individualism as an ideology of human nature. Before that point, what we might now call 'accidents' were seen as 'symbolically important indicators of social integrity and disruption'. As such, they are expected:

> Something like that was just about to happen and not necessarily to anyone in particular, though 'just deserts' might frequently be commented upon. An injury, an illness, or some other misfortune, brings relief from the rising community temperature. Nothing could happen by accident, when every event is scrutinized for its place in the dense fabric of expectation.[22]

The shift from this communitarian perspective to the individualistic one, which the dominance of contract presupposes, was an improvement only for those strong individuals whose situation allowed them to take full advantage of it. The ideology of contract assumes, in other words, an equality of power between contractors which is notably absent in most employment contracts now as then. Thus the law of tort, developing alongside contract, assumed that, unless fault could be demonstrated, 'the loss lies where it falls'. In a society of equals, where else should it fall? Accidents, no longer incorporated into the fabric of communal life, are hazards which befall individuals who must remain uncompensated unless an author of their misfortune can be found. It would not, therefore, be possible for an employee to sue an employer for an injury incurred in the course of employment unless malice or gross negligence could be proved. Since, in addition, it was routinely assumed that workers undertaking risky employments voluntarily undertook to run those risks, it is not surprising that, in Figlio's words, 'the relationship with respect to compensation for injury between employer and employee was skewed in the employer's favour'.[23]

Figlio would seem, then, to be asserting the claim that it is with the development of the contractual relationship that the possibility of an accident was created.[24] It would have been clearer had he maintained that what it makes possible is the legal idea of an accident, of something that is, though an accident, still legally actionable. This was not straightforward simply because of the need to provide a legal remedy whilst at the same time preserving the idea that an accident was nobody's fault. What this did, in Figlio's own words, was to legitimate the notion of 'accountability without culpability',[25] that is, liability without responsibility. This was a radical departure from the governing principle of tort law – that without fault, the loss must lie where it falls, and it represents a significant moment in the historical evolution of the ideology of law, which Figlio does not comment on.

What, in effect, happened in the historical period that Figlio refers to, was a move towards creating employer responsibility for terms and conditions of work by writing the assumption of a safe working environment into the implied terms and conditions of the employment contract. This represents a shift in what is seen as the proper scope of law: a shift from law as the arbitrator of disputes between free and equal individuals, to law as an agent of society, engineering and improving social conditions.[26] We have, in other words, moved on from the ideology of individualism which created contract law, to a social conception of law which, far from *creating* the idea of an accident, as Figlio claims, actually *abrogates* it. For if an accident is something which happens in the space between cause and motive, something for which a human agent is responsible but not, necessarily, liable, then the panoply of legislative instruments and legal devices which constitutes current public and employment law, fills that space. Everything which happens is someone's liability, even if no one's fault. This notion is, at present, imperfectly realized. But the law is working towards its realization and the pressures exist for it to continue. Atiyah has argued that the case for 'no-fault' compensation is unanswerable on moral and logical grounds and that even on policy and economic grounds it is exceedingly plausible.[27] Brazier makes a similar case for the field of medical compensation.[28] The reaction to the Zeebrugge accident was to campaign for a corporate manslaughter charge against the owners for the first time in English law, because it was clear that no *individual* was liable for the harm caused.

It would seem that the circle is closing and the social conception of the accident as no accident at all is returning.[29] It is not precisely the same, of course. No return ever is. We do not now see injury and illness as symbolic of the health of the community, but as signs of the justice of the state. If no one else is liable, then the state is. And if nothing can happen for which no one is liable, then there are no true accidents any more. As Rawls put it:

> The natural distribution is neither just nor unjust. ... What is just and unjust is the way that institutions deal with these facts. ... The social system is not an unchangeable order beyond human control but a pattern of human action.[30]

Conclusion

Accidents, then, are interventions – *slippages* – in the control we attempt to exert over the course of lives. As such, they feel random, unpredictable and threatening and we, inevitably, try and minimize their impact as far as we are able. That they are not as random as they appear is shown by the fact that they exhibit a pattern which matches certain social profiles, namely age and class. Accidents are more prevalent amongst the young and the poor than among the old and the rich. They are, therefore, socially rather than randomly distributed and are, thus, an inescapably social phenomenon. Though accidents feel unpredictable, there is no reason in theory to think that this is so. Indeed, statistically speaking, we know it to be false. Accidents are not *unforeseeable*, but only *unforeseen*, and then, only unforeseen in the particular, not the general case. In 1990 4,898 people died in motor vehicle accidents. In 1991 the figure was 4,408.[31] It seems entirely predictable that the equivalent figures for 1992 and 1993 (when they become available) will show only minor variations. What we do not and cannot know is to whom, exactly, these accidents will happen.

The ability to foresee accidents, though it may make us *responsible* (in the sense that we are in a position to do something, however little, about them), does not necessarily make us *liable*. Liability is incurred only when there is also a duty of care, when there is, in other words, the possibility of negligence. What has been noted above is a shift in the conception of who has that duty. Whereas, from the Enlightenment to comparatively recent times, that duty has been conceived of only in terms of the individual, from the nineteenth century there has been a growing tendency, reflected in the quotation from John Rawls, to think of that duty as belonging to society through the medium of the state. Increasingly, the state is being held liable both for policies designed to reduce the incidence of accidental death and injury and also for compensating those who suffer it. The state is, in other words, being held liable for attempting to reduce the impact that the 'accidental' has on people's lives. It will be interesting to see whether the emergence of neoliberal conservatism in both the UK and the USA since the early 1980s proves to be a temporary deflection of this movement or whether it leads to a radical and significant change in its direction.

Notes

1. In what follows figures cited relating to death rates and accidents, unless otherwise indicated, are drawn from UK data for illustrative purposes only. Margaret Whitehead, in 'The Health Divide', in Peter Townsend and Nick Davidson (eds), *Inequalities in Health* (Harmondsworth: Penguin, 1988), ch. 5, reveals that such data for western European countries and the USA show variations that are

marginal and insignificant for these purposes. For example, the death rate per thousand population for children under 1 year is 10.2 for England and Wales, 11.5 for USA, 8.4 for the Netherlands, but 123.9 for Bangladesh. Age expectancy at birth is 74.3 for England and Wales, 74.6 for USA, 76.2 for the Netherlands, but 54.9 for Bangladesh. (All figures are the mean of male and female rates.)

2. See the *New Law Journal*, 25 September 1987, 16 October 1987, 26 October 1990 and 3 May 1991 and, also, J. Cook, *An Accident Waiting to Happen* (London: Unwin, 1989).
3. Office of Population and Census Studies (hereafter OPCS) 1987: 3.
4. OPCS, *Monitor*, DH2 1992: 2. See also *Who Cares if I Live or Die?: Suicide in Great Britain* (Slough: The Samaritans, 1990).
5. OPCS, *Monitor*, 1992: 2.
6. A perception reinforced in English law by the decriminalization of suicide by the Suicide Act of 1961.
7. OPCS, *Monitor*, DH2 1992: 2, 7 July 1992.
8. *Ibid.*
9. *Ibid.*
10. 'The Black Report', in Peter Townsend and Nick Davidson (eds), *Inequalities in Health* (Harmondsworth: Penguin, 1988), 44–8 and ch. 6.
11. *Ibid.*, 119–20.
12. *Ibid.*, 123–40.
13. *Ibid.*, 119.
14. OPCS, *Monitor*, DH2 1992: 2.
15. L.A. Selby-Bigge (ed.), *Hume's Enquiries* (Oxford: Clarendon Press, 1962, 2nd edn), 23–33.
16. See, for example, James Gleick, *Chaos: Making a New Science* (London: Heinemann, 1988).
17. H.L.A. Hart and A.M. Honoré, *Causation in the Law* (Oxford: Clarendon Press, 1959), 33–4.
18. Karl Figlio, 'What is an Accident?', in P. Weindling (ed.), *The Social History of Occupational Health* (London: Croom Helm, 1985), 183.
19. *Ibid.*, 180.
20. The classic text on speech-acts is J.L. Austin, *How to Do Things With Words* (Oxford: Oxford University Press, 1962).
21. A.G. Guest (ed.), *Anson's Law of Contract* (Oxford: Clarendon Press, 1969, 23rd edn), 7.
22. Figlio, *op.cit.* (ref. 18), 184.
23. *Ibid.*, 182.
24. 'My argument is that the growing prominence of contract relationships and contract law, mainly from the sixteenth century for the general case, and the nineteenth century for master/servant relationships, established the possibility of an accident.' *Ibid.*, 183.
25. *Ibid.*, 181.

26. See, for example, Roscoe Pound, *Social Control Through Law* (New Haven: Yale University Press, 1942).
27. P.S. Atiyah and P. Cane, *Accidents, Compensation and the Law* (London: Weidenfeld and Nicolson, 1987, 4th edn).
28. Margaret Brazier, *Medicine, Patients and the Law* (Harmondsworth: Penguin, 1992, 2nd edn).
29. See Figlio, *op.cit.* (ref. 18), 184.
30. John Rawls, *A Theory of Justice* (Oxford: Oxford University Press, 1972), 102. See, also, Mary Midgley, 'The Flight from Blame', *Philosophy*, lxii (1987), 271–92.
31. OPCS, *Monitor*, DH2 1992: 2.

3

Accidents: The Remnants of a Modern Classificatory System

Judith Green

Milk is spilt, a car crashes, a woman unintentionally becomes pregnant, a small boy wets himself. Accidents will happen, and presumably the misfortunes and, occasionally, happy events which we label accidents always have happened. Although such misfortunes are probably universal to human society, ways of classifying them, understanding them and dealing with them are not. In contemporary cultures, accidents are an important category of misfortunes. They are found to be the third leading cause of death in Europe,[1] a major cause of disability and the object of social intervention. However, more mundane, everyday misfortunes are also described as 'accidents': the scraped knees of childhood or crockery broken in a slip in the kitchen. Indeed, accidents cover a seemingly infinite range of possible misfortunes. As a description, accident is used synonymously with 'injury' ('an industrial accident'), as a term denoting lack of intent ('it happened by accident') and as a sign of the ultimately uncontrollable nature of the material world ('accidents will happen'). Given the importance of accidents, as both cause of and explanation for misfortune, it is perhaps surprising that there have been few attempts by sociologists to account for their social construction:[2] how, and why, some misfortunes come to be classified specifically as 'accidental'. This chapter is an exploration of how the accident emerged in modern discourse.

What is an Accident?

What connects the disparate events that do get classified as accidents is not their outcome but their cause. Accidents come to be defined through their ascribed cause or, more specifically, lack of cause. We do not decide that an accident has occurred by observing what happened, but by investigating how it happened. There are two factors which apparently characterize the process by which accidents are seen to occur. The first is that an accident should be an unmotivated event. Neither the victim nor any other agency, human or divine, willed it to happen. Modern ironic usage clearly illustrates this, as in Fo's *The Accidental Death of an Anarchist*[3] or the gangster's threat 'we could arrange for you to have an accident'. In general, though, nobody can be blamed for an accident. It is this feature which distinguishes accidents from wilful damage and neglect. The arrangement of physical objects and temporal sequences that precede an accident must be seen to be purely coincidental: they cannot have been willed. The causation of accidents is arbitrary and not logical.

Second, and following from this, an accident is unpredictable as a unique event. Although the epidemiology of accidents can be mapped through aggregation and examination of their incidence, the occurrence of a particular accident cannot be foreseen. The victim, in an 'ideal' accident, has no previous knowledge of the misfortune and therefore cannot be held responsible.

It is soon apparent, though, that this working definition applies only to an 'ideal type' of accident. In practice, not all accidents are held to be unwilled and unpredicted and there are many events which are defined as 'accidental' in which some blame is apportioned: road traffic accidents caused by a driver over the legal alcohol limit, or falls over loose paving stones which should have been maintained by a local authority. Indeed, it has been argued that as a society we are becoming less capable of accepting misfortune as 'merely accidental', and more likely to seek someone to blame for such mishaps.[4] Certainly the status of an event as accidental is often a provisional one: misfortunes are only accidental until responsibility can be apportioned. Even a brief review of media reports of disasters ('accidents' which affect many people) or coroners' verdicts demonstrates how the definition is negotiated rather than given, with different parties in open conflict over how a particular event (a workplace injury, a transport disaster) should be categorized. Folk wisdom recognizes the ambiguity in phrases like 'it was an accident waiting to happen' and from an early age we learn to negotiate claims to the accidental in order to disclaim responsibility. Anyone caring for children will recognize the bid for clemency 'I didn't do it on purpose – it was an accident'. That such negotiation can happen at all, though, implies a consensus about what does constitute an 'ideal' accident: a misfortune for which no one can be blamed, as no one meant it to happen.

This consensus first assumes that there is such a thing as an 'accident': that some misfortunes do 'just happen'. It is not, however, inevitable that some misfortunes will be classified as accidents. In 1937, Evans-Pritchard described the Azande of Sudan[5] as a people whose cosmology allowed no accidental events. His ethnography has been the subject of considerable debate, much of it centring on the legitimacy of judging the 'rationality' of other cultures from an ethnocentric Western stance.[6] Evans-Pritchard's account is of interest here, though, for two reasons; first, because it illustrates the possibility of a cosmology that has no logical place for accidents.

Azande Classifications of Misfortune

According to Evans-Pritchard, the Azande held all misfortune to be the result of witchcraft. Witchcraft was an invisible substance which could be sent flying through the night to attack others. A witch did not necessarily know that s/he was a witch, and only by consulting an oracle could the identity of a witch be discovered. Thus a belief in witches was a ubiquitous and comprehensive explanatory system which functioned to explain misfortunes which arose 'not only from miscalculation, incompetence and laziness, but also from causes from which the African, with his meagre scientific knowledge, has no control'.[7] Only misfortunes which clearly resulted from the breaking of a taboo (such as not observing appropriate restrictions on when sexual intercourse could occur) were exempt from these explanations.

While concurring with the theories of natural causation that we might describe as 'rational' (that, for instance, a leg is broken because a tree branch fell on it, or that the hunting was unsuccessful because game had been frightened away), an Azande would also have expected an explanation of why such a misfortune had happened to him or her specifically – 'why me, and why now?' Such questions are not, perhaps, amenable to rational explanation. The Azande would not only have asked the question, but would also have expected to find the answer through identifying the person who bewitched them. Accidents, like other kinds of misfortune, such as illness or lack of success in hunting, were seen to be explicable in personal and moral terms as well as those of natural cause and effect. The Azande recognized a plurality of causes, relating to different levels of explanation, and witchcraft operated at the social level of explanation. In a hunting metaphor witchcraft was 'umbaga', or 'the second spear' which had as great a part to play in the death of a hunted elephant as the first spear. Thus the 'natural' causes of a misfortune such as the immediate cause of injury or lack of foresight were accepted, but not as a complete explanation: 'It is the particular and variable conditions of an event and not the general and universal conditions that witchcraft explains'.[8]

In one case, for instance, Evans-Pritchard takes issue with a boy who has a festered wound from an injury 'caused' by stubbing his toe on a tree stump while walking in the bush:

> I always argued with the Azande and criticized their statements, and I did so on this occasion. I told the boy that he had knocked his foot against the stump of wood because he had been careless, and that witchcraft had not placed it in the path, for it had grown there naturally. He agreed that witchcraft had nothing to do with the stump of wood being in his path but added that he had kept his eyes open for stumps, as indeed every Azande does most carefully, and that if he had not been bewitched he would have seen the stump.[9]

Evans-Pritchard could not really begin to engage with this boy's need to know why this stump surprised him in the bush, and why the cut was taking so long to heal. Witchcraft, in this example, has rather more explanatory power than a rational belief in cause, effect and coincidence as it can explain the local and personal aspects of misfortune, as well as the causes of foot injuries in general. As the Azande put it: 'Death has always a cause, and no man dies without a reason'.[10] Such an all-embracing explanatory system has no need of the 'mere' accident to describe those misfortunes which 'just happen', for nothing 'just happens'.

Ethnography and Child Development: The Accident Defining 'Modernity'

The second reason why Evans-Pritchard's account is of interest here lies in how accidents function within it. For him, a belief that accidents can happen apparently defines a rational and, by implication, modern conception of misfortune and how it is to be understood. In 1923 Levy-Bruhl had argued that 'primitive mentality' was essentially irrational,[11] in that it was governed by ideas, such as belief in supernatural forces, which would be held as illogical and contradictory by modern western standards. It was the 'primitive's' attitude to the events which we might label accidental that Levy-Bruhl saw as particularly indicative of this irrationality. The 'primitive' had no conception of chance, or coincidence, because all events were invested with meaning:

> From disease and death to mere accident is an almost imperceptible transition ... primitives as a rule do not perceive any difference between a death which is the result of old age or disease and a violent

> death.... Therefore every death is an accidental one, even death from illness. Or to put it more precisely, no death is, since to the primitive mind nothing ever happens by accident, properly speaking.[12]

It was not only the colonial anthropologists of the early twentieth century who used a belief in accidents as an indicator of superior mental abilities. Piaget, writing in 1930 on the development of children's causal logic, describes children's views of physical causality in terms similar to those used by Levy-Bruhl of the 'primitive':

> The child fills the world with spontaneous movements and living 'forces'; the heavenly bodies may rest and move as they please ... trees swing their branches spontaneously to make a breeze, water flows by virtue of a force residing in it.[13]

For Piaget, the child attributes animistic motives to physical objects and even in later stages of development, when mechanical cause and effect are understood, feels 'a very definite repugnance for the ideas of physical necessity and chance'.[14] Until seven or eight years old, he or she feels that there are no chance events in the world. For the child, as for Levy-Bruhl's 'primitive', everything has a reason, has been willed and is entirely moral. Only after this stage do they admit that 'there are things which serve no useful purpose and [are] due solely to chance encounters'.[15] In Piaget's developmental model, a belief in coincidence marks the move towards a mature understanding of rational cause and effect.

In these accounts of the early twentieth century, accidents are unproblematic. That some misfortunes 'just happen', and that there can be no profit in seeking explanations for them, is so obvious as to need no explanation. Accidents become noteworthy only in their absence, when explicanda exist without them. Only the primitive or the child, it seems, would seek an explanation for mere coincidence as the modern adult merely accepts that the laws of chance and rationality imply that from time to time misfortunes will occur.

Rationality and Probability

There are two, connected, explanatory models which render the accidental misfortune as 'obvious' and 'natural' in these writings from the early twentieth century. One is rationality, a set of beliefs about cause and effect, which holds some effects to be the inevitable and natural outcomes of certain causes. The other is probability, a set of beliefs about the predictability of events on an aggregated scale. In the accounts of Levy-Bruhl, Evans-Pritchard and Piaget a belief in accidents characterized the developed mind, for which some misfortunes 'just happen'. They are unproblematic because rationality was at this time itself relatively unproblematic.

An accident appears in the gaps left by a rationalist cosmology, at the limit of deterministic laws, but where superstition no longer has a legitimate part to play. These gaps in rationalist explanations emerge between what is known for sure – that which is subject to deterministic laws, such as those describing the motions of planets around the sun, or gravity on the earth – and what is known statistically – that which is subject to the laws of probability, such as the chance of reaching a certain age or of dying of a certain disease. At a local, or individual, level there is little that can be known for sure. Rationalist laws governing most of the areas of life in which misfortunes are likely to occur are statistical, not determinist. The probability of various life events and kinds of death can be known, and thus also the 'chance' of them happening to any individual in a population, but this is of little use in predicting personal misfortunes. Such misfortunes are 'merely' accidental; coincidences of time and space.

The Emergence of the Accident: Rational Cause and Probability

If the accident is made possible through the interplay of beliefs in probability and determinism, we can perhaps identify the point at which it became possible to 'have an accident' in the West. The development of concepts of probability has been variously traced by Hacking,[16] Porter[17] and, from a rather different standpoint, Foucault.[18] Hacking,[19] for instance, linked the emergence of statistics, the science of probability, to changing concepts of cause and evidence. He regarded John Graunt's 1662 publication of his *Natural and Political Observations on the Bills of Mortality* [20] as the first extensive set of statistical inferences made in the west. These observations on the bills of mortality were an attempt to define the risk of dying from various causes and they laid the foundations of the modern science of population statistics. Hacking situated Graunt's work in the context of emerging ideas about probability, evidenced by Pascal's use of probabilistic reasoning to establish a pragmatic rationale for the belief in God; Leibniz's application of probability to legal problems and Huygens' publication of the first textbook on probability. That a science of probability became possible in the West at this point in European history was, claimed Hacking, to do with the dual nature of the emergent concept of probability; it referred both to stable frequencies (an event is 'probable' because such events have a statistically calculable chance of occurring) and to degrees of belief (an event is possible because we know that such an event can occur). This concept replaced the 'probabilism' of the sixteenth century, which referred to the 'approvability' of an opinion: a probable happening or opinion was one attested to by eminent or respected authorities. To explain why a new concept of probability entered European discourse towards the end of the seventeenth century, making possible the science of statistics, Hacking examines shifts in scientific thought, and emergent concepts of evidence and deduction.

Evidence, as we now understand it, argues Hacking, appeared only by the end of the seventeenth century. Previously, 'evidence' was rooted in authority: the testimony of learned authorities. The distinction between such testimony and empirical evidence is a relatively recent one. In 1662 the *Port Royal Logic* described the distinction as being one of external evidence (the testimony of authorities) and internal evidence, from the existence of things. This idea of internal evidence was a novel one, rooted in the idea of causal inference: that one could infer one thing from another. Such internal evidence was different from the 'signs' of the Renaissance period, which were based on verisimilitude. Although signs were 'things' and not written testimony, claims Hacking, and were utilized as evidence, this was on the basis of their similarities, or correspondences with what they signified. Thus nature – in the signs of the stars, or the climate, or the symptoms of disease – could be 'read' in the same way as the testimony of learned authorities. The relationship of a bodily sign with a corresponding disease, for instance, was not conceptualized as a causal one: the disease did not 'cause' the sign, but was merely signified by it. Probability, argued Hacking, only became possible once signs were seen as internal evidence, from which causal chains could be inferred, rather than as merely the testimony of the natural world.

In 1603 Thomas Lodge, a poet and author who went on to study medicine late in life, published his *Treatise of the Plague.*[21] It illustrates both the testimony of authorities and the evidence of signs in its advice on avoiding and curing the plague. For instance, Lodge first claims to have:

> faithfully gathered out of the most approved Authors, (especially out of certaine notes which I received from Valenolaeus sonne, now Doctor of Phisique in Arles in Province) a true Methode how to know and cure the Plague.[22]

As well as such authority, though, he also cites the signs of the plague in nature, which can be 'read' to predict the arrival of a new epidemic:

> If the Winter be hot and moist, and observe not his natural temperature and when the Spring time is dry without rain.... Moreover, if at that time there appears any increase of such creatures as engendered of putrification, as worms of the earth, flies, gnattes, eales, serpents, toads, frogs and such like foretelling corruption and putrification on the earth and waters, and when the aire the same day changes from faire to foule, and from clear to cloudy....[23]

This notion of the 'sign' included the idea that it could be believed because it could be trusted: the appearance of toads and frogs heralding the arrival of a plague epidemic was to be believed because this had happened before in nature. However, such signs are not causes and, Hacking suggests, it only becomes possible to argue deductively, from observed effects to hypothetical causes, when internal evidence, the basis of new probabilistic reasoning, could be distinguished from the kind of natural signs cited here by Lodge.

Once this had happened, the modern notion of probability became possible. Hacking cites the City of London's weekly tally of christenings and burials, which were kept to detail the current state of the plague. When these could be examined as direct effects of the plague, rather than merely another natural sign of it, it became possible for statistical reasoning to emerge: the scientific study of quantitative facts about the state and its population. Although these bills of mortality were collected from 1603, it was not until John Graunt's notes on the bills of mortality were published in 1662 that anyone made such use of them. 'Once it became possible for a Graunt or a Petty to look at the data as data, and not as a "signature" of the plague, it was possible to draw a great many inferences'.[24]

Hacking's argument is important for an understanding of the emergence of accidents because these new ways of conceptualizing evidence and probability also provided new ways of thinking about cause and how it was to be attributed. It might, then, be useful to revisit some of the seventeenth-century writings of Thomas Lodge, John Graunt and William Petty examined by Hacking, together with a sermon by the preacher Samuel Ward (1577–1640) to trace how this new discourse of probability, together with the emergent consensus around rationality, could also produce the 'accident' as a marginal category of misfortune.

First, the word 'accident' itself does not occur in these writings. Most often the word accident referred simply to a happening, undistinguished in cause from any other. In 1603, Thomas Lodge used the word in an 'obsolete' sense (*OED*), that of an 'occurring symptom': 'The most troublesome or dangerous accidents in this

Sickness are weakness of vertue, faintings of the heart, soundings, raving or frenzie....'[25]

Accidents were here the deteriorations or 'events' in the course of the illness and nothing more. So what were happenings with no discernable motivation or will, those we would categorize as 'accidents', called in the early seventeenth century? It appears that there was simply no need to distinguish them from those more culpable acts or those with some definable motivation. Samuel Ward, for instance, in a sermon entitled *Woe to Drunkards,*[26] described the many misfortunes that befall those who drink. These were attributed to the direct judgment of God, to whom drunkenness is an odious sin, punished by all manner of untimely ends. He listed numerous examples of such misfortunes, including deaths from diseases we would describe as arising from alcohol abuse, such as a man who 'having surcharged his stomacke with drinke, hee fell vommiting, broke a Veyne, lay two days in extreme paine of body & distresse of mind, till in the end recovering a little comfort, he died'.[27] Other misfortunes included injuries sustained while drunk, including

> [a] man 85 yeares old, or thereabout, in Suffolk, overtaken with Wine [who] going downe a paire of staires ... fell, and was so dangerously hurt, as hee dyed soone after, not being able to speake from the time of his fall to the time of his death.[28]

Although drunkenness was seen to be an apparent cause of this and other fatalities, it was not the ultimate cause – this was God's retribution. Misfortunes which were not associated with the victim's own drunkenness were therefore also subsumed under the same explanatory framework. Thus a woman who had persuaded three men to stay to drink some more was 'suddenly taken speechlesse and sicke, her tongue swolne in her mouth, never recovered speech, the third day after dyed'.[29] Her misfortune, though not 'caused' directly by the action of alcohol, was attributed to the moral culpability incurred by encouraging others.

We would now perhaps divide such misfortunes into three distinct categories with very different moral content: effects of disease as a result of alcohol use, injuries arising from drunkenness (both of which are seen as somewhat blameworthy) and true 'accidents' – that is, injuries sustained by people who may be drinkers but who were not inebriated at the time. Those injuries not attributable to the causal effects of alcohol use we would have no ready explanation for, but within the moral universe of Ward's God there was no need for such a category since the judgment of God (rather like witchcraft for the Azande) was an all-embracing explanation. The sin of drunkenness is the ultimate cause of all the misfortunes to which drinkers are prone, through the intervention of a righteous God. There was no need, within such a universal explanatory framework, for a category of events for which no cause was known.

By the 1660s, though, this explanatory framework no longer sufficed. In tandem with the 'new' approach to evidence documented by Hacking, we find the beginnings of the concept of a category of events which are not explicable within a comprehensive cosmology. At this point, which Hacking links with the emergence of probabilistic thinking, what we would today recognize as 'rational' ways of thinking are beginning to gain precedence, and the study of disease and mortality was no exception. Graunt, writing on the bills of mortality in the second half of the seventeenth century, had an approach to investigating causality that is 'rational' in that it uses empirical evidence to examine the distribution of causes of death:

> among the several casualties some bear a constant proportion unto the whole number of Burials; such are the chronic diseases, and the diseases whereunto the City is most subject; as for example Consumption, Dropsies, Jaundice, Gowt, Stone, Palsie, Scurvy, rising of the Lights, rickets, aged, agues, Feavers, Blood Flux, and Scowring: nay, from Accidents, as Grief, Drowning, Mens' making away themselves and being killed by several accidents &c do the like, whereas Epidemical and Malignant diseases, as the Plagues, Purples, spotted Feaver, Small Pox and Measles do not keep that equality, so in some Years or Months there died ten times as many as in others.[30]

Using the new possibilities of probabilistic reasoning, Graunt differentiated a certain group of diseases (consumption, dropsies, and so on) as being perhaps unpredictable in their effect on individuals, yet predictable in their effect on the population of London as a whole. There were also, though, diseases which have no such apparent pattern: the 'epidemical' and 'malignant' diseases. So here, although 'accident' still referred to a group of happenings distinguished by the suddenness of their effect or the externality of the cause of death, rather than their exclusion from a pattern, there was the notion of happenings which do not 'bear a constant proportion to the whole'. Graunt brings accidents into that pattern: they are made predictable on a magnified scale, yet there is also the notion, equivalent to ours, of cases which don't fit *yet*. This notion is perhaps a vital condition for the possibility of an 'accident' as we know it to occur, as a temporary categorization of a lack of cause. The events which did not fit into

Graunt's scheme are the epidemics, for which he had not established a predictable pattern from his study of the Bills of Mortality. Graunt later listed some of the events which we might now label as accidents, claiming that it is not worth examining them too closely as they are not amenable to the discovery of regular patterns:

> We shall say nothing of the numbers of these that have been Drowned, Killed by falls from Scaffolds, or by carts running over them &c, because the same depends on careful Trade, and Employment of men and upon matters which are but circumstantial to the Seasons, and Regions we live in; and affords little of that Science and Certainty we aim at.[31]

Graunt's project in the *Observations* was in some senses emblematic of the beginnings of the process of rationality, although tentative in that it excludes cases which will not exhibit 'science and certainty'. It was an attempt to calculate the risk of various kinds of death in an 'objective' way, untainted by the subjective fears people have of different risks. He appealed directly to empirical evidence to calculate the exact chance of death from various causes:

> whereas many persons live in great fear, and apprehension of some of the more formidable and notorious diseases following; I shall only set down how many died of each: that the respective numbers, being compared to the total 229250, those persons may the better understand the Hazard they are in....[32]

This use of empirical evidence (the essential substance of this new rationality, as well as probability) contrasts neatly with Lodge's appeal to medieval 'proof' quoted above: that of learned authority. It is not merely that Graunt's 'science' was true whereas Lodge's was not, but that between 1603 and 1662 it became possible to frame an argument in terms which became recognized as having a rational appeal to logic and evidence. By the end of the seventeenth century Petty,[33] also writing on mortality statistics, could confidently dismiss arbitrary or non-rational causes as having no relevance to his scientific project. Reviewing changes in the population of London, he wrote:

> what reason to assign the like increase from 1604 to 1642 I know not, unless I should pick out some Remarkable Accident happening in each part of the said period and make that to be the Cause of this Increase (as vulgar People make the cause of Man's Sickness to be what he did last eat).[34]

If Graunt had merely excluded accidents from the field of fruitful objects of scientific study, Petty completely dismissed 'Remarkable

Accidents' as causes of misfortune worthy of serious consideration. Using the new-found rationality in political statistics, Petty could then separate what had for Graunt been irregular features, such as plague years, and place them neatly into the larger pattern of population shifts. He predicted, for instance, the time it will take for London's population to double by calculating population increases based on the bills of mortality and:

> including some allowance for Wars, Plagues and Famines, the effects whereof, though they may be Terrible at the Times and Places where they happen, yet in a period of 360 years is no great matter in the whole Nation.[35]

When Ward and Lodge were writing at the beginning of the seventeenth century they had no need to appeal to the 'accidental' as a cause of misfortune. By the end of the century, Petty's 'remarkable accident' was not only a necessary part of the rational world view, to explain that which did not fit a pattern, but also a despised one which could be dismissed as irrelevant to the emerging scheme. Accidents were essentially the remnants of an emerging classificatory system: left-overs that demonstrated its boundaries.

The limits to this new cosmology, in which death rates and the behaviour of populations were as worthy of study as the physical laws which were seen to govern the universe, necessitated a category of events which could not be explained. These were the random, unimportant events that could be concealed by the aggregation of vital statistics or dismissed as simply unimportant as single events. Misfortunes such as death and disease gained a new meaning beyond that of individual tragedy: they could now be interrogated as evidence for the predictable and patterned behaviour of populations. Some misfortunes, however, could not be so neatly described by the predictions of the mortality reports, as a universe governed by natural laws is inevitably unpredictable at the level of the local and the particular.

Medicine and Morality

Medicine is one arena in which growing faith in statistics and rational explanation constructed accidents as a necessary, but rather despised, category of misfortune. In Britain, cause of death first had to be registered in 1838. The first *Report* of the Registrar-General in 1839 began with the hope that it 'will not disappoint the expectations of those who hope to derive, eventually, from that source, materials of vast improvements to the advancement of the Science of Vital Statistics'.[36] In turning its attention to an exhaustive classification of all deaths, medicine was faced with a challenge in imposing order on deaths from violence, with their seemingly disparate set of causes and outcomes. The first *Report*, for instance, listed the following causes among the 4,845 deaths which were classified as 'Deaths by Violence': choking on blackberries; being struck by lightning; drinking boiling water; bites by a ferret, a lion and a donkey; pit explosions; emphysema following a fall and inflammation following a prick from a thorn.

Given the stated aim, this very heterogeneity constituted a problem: that of presenting causes of death as facts as scientific in their arrangement as any other which 'admit of numerical analysis'.[37] In an appendix to this first *Report*, William Farr wrote:

> Medicine, like other natural sciences, is beginning to abandon vague conjecture where facts can be accurately determined by observation; and to substitute numerical expressions for uncertain assertions ... the physicians of this century will be saved from the fallacies of partial generalisation.[38]

His concern was that the classification system would itself produce the kind of data that were amenable to interrogation for patterns and meaningful generalization. There should not, claimed Farr, be too much refinement in the classes used, because if they were too exactly defined 'no general principles can be deduced from small numbers; accidental irregularities destroying the results, according to the well known doctrines of probability'.[39] The causes of death that were to become classified as accidental, like other 'external' causes of death, were merely to be grouped together, with no attempt to classify them further. These 'violent deaths' were those left over from other, more homogenous categories, grouped merely by the fact that death was caused by what Farr called 'impressive external causes',[40] rather than by any biological category. Farr noted that the lack of any analysis of sudden death was a shortcoming:

> The violent deaths are extremely numerous and will perhaps lead to a general enquiry into their causes, – drownings, fires, accidents with machinery, the bursting of steam-boilers, explosions in mines, and poisons, which can be procured of the most destructive and subtle nature, with extraordinary facility.[41]

In the same vein, Farr also listed particular causes of death from want of food and from cold, noting that these were 'in some instances the effect of accident, but more frequently of destitution'.[42] Further analysis and classification, he implied, would render even this group of random, individual misfortunes as 'scientific facts'. If the disparate causes of violent deaths posed a problem for such analysis, then moral enquiry provided a partial solution. In the 1854 *Report,* Farr's appendix pioneered the analysis of the moral content of the accidental category. Noting that in England there had been a long tradition of referring deaths 'likely to be caused by wilful, careless or accidental violence' [43] to the coroner's court he went on to suggest that:

> Some of the external causes that in too many instances are fatal are wilfully or negligently set in motion by men, and the act is homicide or suicide. This subject deserves to be fully investigated, for the mental states appear to admit to a large extent of moral and physical control.[44]

In the absence of any apparent anatomical or pathological pattern, this moral content of the class of 'violent' causes of death provided a possible organizing principle, for now they too could be classified into discrete groups. Deaths from injuries and poisoning did not fit well into the now well-established nosology based on anatomy and function, but could be ordered around an examination of the intentions of the victim or others. The fatal medical sequelae of external causes were thus classified initially neither by the part of body affected, nor by the responsible pathogen, but by a moral judgement. In the early 1850s Farr introduced a new classification which divided deaths into five orders:[45]

1. Epidemic, endemic and contagious
2. Constitutional
3. Local
4. Developmental
5. Violent

He later expanded on the division of violent deaths into separate classes of 'accident', 'homicide', 'suicide' and 'legal execution':

> Human agency plays so important a part in this class, that it might be made into the basis for orders. Thus a man may die 1. a glorious death in battle (*pro patria mori*); he may die 2. by an act of homicide (murder, manslaughter); he may die 3. ignominiously on the scaffold (execution); or 4. abandoning the post where God has placed him, he may take away his own life (suicide); 5. he may die by a surgical operation 6. he may die by accident.
>
> If this grouping be adopted, the mode in which the death is produced by wounds, chemical injuries, poisons, asphyxias, and mechanical forces, would form secondary heads.[46]

These distinctions for violent deaths were based purely on the moral meaning of the death: whether glorious or ignominious; whether the victim or another was culpable. Those with no discernable moral content were the 'left-overs', the accidents. The medical sequelae of accidents were now classified by specifying their immediate cause, but the category itself was constituted as merely the remnant of a classificatory system, created through moral inquiry. An accident was an event for which there was no motivation, but which lay on a boundary between the need for a cause, as all fatalities must now be accounted for, and the lack of a 'real' cause as defined by the new scientific principles of statistics. From the unrefined category of external causes of death when annual statistics were first published by the Registrar-General in 1839, accidents had become the residual category of medical classifications of causes of death: those which occurred with no known medical cause, or at least none that fitted into the rational system of medical knowledge.

Rationalizing the Accident: The Growth of Epidemiology

Farr's suggestion in 1840 that a 'general enquiry' into the causes of violent death would prove fruitful was adopted. The analysis of causes of accidental demise became more detailed once they had been distinguished from other forms of violent death. The class of accidents became more internally differentiated in official sources, and the last order of causes of death underwent more revision than any other. The original grouping of external causes of death used by Farr in 1839 included an undifferentiated catalogue of injuries and accidents. The introduction of an internationally agreed system of classification brought a division of violent deaths along lines of culpability. From then on, the circumstances surrounding accidental injuries resulting in death were the subject of ever more sophisticated classificatory techniques, beginning with the separation of accidents that occurred in mines and on the railways in 1863. By the middle of the twentieth century tables detailing poisoning by place of occurrence, age and sex; accidents according to the nature of the injury and accidents by external cause; road accidents; accidental falls; accidents in the home and residential institutions – all were now routinely abstracted from the *Reports* of the Registrar-General.

The problems posed by the heterogeneity of the class of accidents, however, continued to be of concern to epidemiologists. In 1941, for instance, a report by Greenwood, Martin and Russell[47] on deaths by violence cited changes in classification as a deterrent to analysing trends over time. One respondent to the paper noted that:

> until recent years violent deaths have been nobody's business in the official sense, apart from industrial accidents and homicide ... the

> Registrar-General's analyses of accidental deaths have suffered from obscurities in classification and ... have failed to provide much material for those who may have wished to study these deaths in relation to social factors.[48]

Today accidents still reside at the margins of a classification system that cannot adequately describe them without reference to external causes. The current International Classification of Diseases[49] organizes accidental deaths primarily by the consequences of external causes, but still maintains a supplementary classification which describes those external causes. The anomalous status of accidents within nosology has led to several demands from within the profession over the last two decades that 'accident' be abandoned altogether as a useful medical category. It was argued in 1993 that:

> 'Accident' conveys a sense that the losses incurred are due to fate and are therefore devoid of rational explanation or predictability. Yet the motivation to study subjects like traffic safety is to discover factors that influence the likelihood of occurrence of, and resulting harm from, 'crashes', the preferred term.[50]

The objection to the term 'accident' was that it was somehow 'contaminated' by lay associations with an unwilled and unknowable process; it 'suggest[s] in addition a general explanation of why it occurred without any evidence to support such an explanation ... the word accident [should be replaced] by a more objective and crisp word'.[51] In the United States, as well, there have been calls for 'medicine to dispose of the "accident" and "accidental injury"', given that it is an 'ambivalent, misleading anachronism'.[52] In Britain, there have been some small successes in abandoning the word most notably through the retitling of the OPCS series that reports on deaths from external causes. Until 1991, it was titled *Accidents and Violence*. In 1992, it was renamed *Injury and Poisoning*.[53]

Given these persuasive arguments for medicine to abandon the 'accident', there is perhaps a need to explain why it persists in medical discourse as well as lay accounts of misfortune and its causes. One possible function the class of accidents performs is that of a still necessary marginal category. However well epidemiology may map the causes of death and the various risk factors associated, there are inevitably events which are 'left over' in that they cannot be explained by motivated cause. The category itself is constituted specifically from misfortunes that have not (yet) been defined as anything else, such as non-accidental injury, suicide, or deliberate poisoning. It may be that the space such events occupy will diminish as an increasing number of misfortunes are seen as potentially blameworthy, or as rationally explicable (in the case of sudden infant death syndrome, for instance) but the very logic of the classificatory system, produced explicitly through an interrogation of the precursors of a death, requires a residual category to account for what still remains unexplained.

The End of Marginality: The Preventable Accident

The persistence of the term 'accident' obscures, though, a rather different understanding of what constitutes the 'accidental' in the late twentieth century. From the inevitable yet inexplicable misfortunes implied by the accounts of Evans-Pritchard and Piaget, the coincidental events that we should all expect from time to time but cannot predict, accidents have become very specifically constructed as preventable events, which should not ever, in an ideal world, have happened.[54] With an increasing sophistication in the epidemiological mapping of risk factors for accidents and the correlations between them, it appears that the knowledge exists to predict all 'accidental' events. Ultimately, as one recent report suggests, accidents *can* be prevented:

> RoSPA recommends that all health authorities adopt a positive approach to accident prevention based on the premise that the majority of serious accidents could be avoided or prevented and that the risks of serious injuries can also be reduced.[55]

Medical discourse about accidents is now largely a discourse about prevention, rather than classification or treatment. In Britain, this shift in focus is enshrined in policy, in which accidents have been targeted as a priority in terms of the health of the nation. 'Most accidents', claimed the Department of Health, rather starkly, 'are preventable'.[56] Despite the ambiguity of the term, then, the accident persists within medicine: not as a random and individual misfortune, but as a predictable coalition of known risk factors manifested by the regular rates of road traffic accidents, home accidents or factory accidents. Accidents may be remnants of a rational classification of misfortune, but they are also central to the late twentieth-century discourse of risk factors and responsibility.

Sociology's 'Neglect' of the Accident

The apparent 'neglect' of accidents by sociology now seems less puzzling. The roots of traditional sociology lie in attempts to understand modern industrial society of the nineteenth century, and to build a discipline based on rational enquiry. If emergent rational explanatory systems opened up a logical, or at least a possible, space for the accident at the end of the seventeenth century, they also opened a socially denigrated one: the accident was, by definition, at the very margins of explanation and, as such, unworthy of further study. It was visible only when absent – in the cosmologies of those considered 'irrational', such as children or 'primitive' peoples. A brief review of two of the major traditions in sociological thought indicates the problematic status accidents, as constructed in the late nineteenth and early twentieth centuries, would have as a potential object of enquiry.

To begin with the classic example of Durkheim's more positivistic writings, it is difficult to see what part the 'accidental' could play. Part of the Durkheimian project, for instance, was explicitly concerned with uncovering social laws to make sense of social behaviour. Although Durkheim was concerned with 'irrational' facets of social behaviour such as religion and suicide, his aim was to demonstrate regularities at the social level which rendered individual irrationality comprehensible. His methodological premises leave no room for the 'accidental'. Durkheim claimed that:

> our principal objective is to extend scientific rationalism to human behaviour. It can be shown that the behaviour of the past, when analysed, can be reduced to relationships of cause and effect.[57]

The capricious accident can furnish no useful data for such a project. Although *The Rules of Sociological Method* represent only a small, and perhaps atypical, part of Durkheim's work, the sentiments expressed there have had an enduring impact on the positivistic tradition in social theory. Durkheim's sociology here and in *Suicide*[58] relied on the kind of vital statistics that were well established by the end of the nineteenth century. Such statistics were the basis for uncovering 'social facts' which, Durkheim claimed, were:

> represented with considerable exactness by the rates of births, marriages and suicides, that is by the number obtained by dividing the average annual total of marriages, births and suicides by the number of persons whose ages lie in the range in which births, marriages and suicides occur. Since each of these figures contains all the individual cases indiscriminately, the individual circumstances which might have had a share in the production of the phenomena are neutralized and, consequently, do not contribute to its determination. The average, then, expresses a certain state of the group mind.[59]

In such aggregations the 'accidental' is neutralized. Some apparently 'accidental' events will only reveal their structured causes after appropriate investigation: 'facts most arbitrary in appearances will come to present, after more attentive observation, qualities of consistency and regularity that are symptomatic of their objectivity'.[60] Those that do not reveal such consistency and regularity are presumably not worthy of further investigation. The vital statistics available to Durkheim did not include the sophisticated analyses of accident rates that were produced from the middle of the twentieth century, but since then there has of course been considerable scope for a positivist sociological analysis of accidental injuries in terms of such social division as class, gender and ethnicity. These studies, though, have fallen largely within the domain of epidemiologists, rather than sociologists, and accidents have attracted little of the interest and academic debate that surrounds Durkheim's analysis of suicide rates. The few exceptions have explicitly challenged the concept of accidents as random, morally neutral misfortunes. In the debate about how far workplace accident rates can be seen as indicators of economic recession, for instance, such events have been referred to as 'industrial injuries', to indicate that there is nothing 'accidental' about their causation.[61] The accident, by definition, has to be reconceptualized as something other before it can be used in positivistic sociological enquiry. As soon as accidents are analysed, they disappear.

If the concern is with an exploration of the meaning of accidents and with how they are constructed as a category of misfortune, then the Weberian tradition in sociology could perhaps more reasonably be expected to provide a theoretical starting-point, as Weber is the theorist associated with an approach which centred on understanding meaning as it is constructed by social actors. Given the suggestion that accidents are somehow defined outside the bounds of rational behaviour and understanding, Weber's problematization of rationality may also be helpful. However, a major legacy of Weber's work has been a prioritization of the rational as an essential feature of the modern world and a conceptualization of non-rational behaviour or belief as characteristic of 'pre-modern' society, or as simply uninteresting as a subject of social enquiry. Giddens, for instance, quotes Weber on the comparison of modern capitalist society which is 'rationalised on the basis of rigorous calculation, directed with foresight and caution', with traditional peasant economy which is 'orientated to the exploitation of political opportunities and irrational speculation'.[62] Belief in accidental cause appears as anachronistic within a modern rational cosmology, an example of ritual, that does not constitute proper social action. Action is only properly social, Weber claims, 'in so far as its subjective meaning takes account of the behaviour of others, and is thereby orientated in its course'.[63] Only action so orientated is seen as a fruitful object of sociological enquiry. As accidents do not result from this kind of motivated behaviour, describing a misfortune as an 'accident' rules it outside the bounds of rational calculation. Characterizing modernity as rational once again renders the accident a left-over; an event of little interest.

As a specific category of misfortune, the accident has apparently, then, been neglected. Early twentieth-century accounts, as we have seen, constructed the accident as a self-evident given, unworthy of attention except when absent.

Recent Sociological Theory: Post-modernity and the Accident

If sociology has neglected the accident, how has it now become possible to speak of it? In the last quarter of the twentieth century there have been attempts to accommodate chance, and by implication accidents, as a legitimate area for enquiry in sociological theory. Smith,[64] for instance, reviews the major traditions in social theory, particularly Weberian ones, and concludes that chance has, until recently, been treated as a residual category. From the 1980s onwards, though, he claims, the work of writers such as Foucault and Giddens have recognized the potential importance of chance as an explanatory concept. He attributes the shift in focus to the undermining of the structural functionalist consensus in sociology in the 1960s and to a renewed interest in the mechanisms of change rather than stability. From the middle of the 1970s 'late modernity' provided an added incentive, in terms of both the cultural environment and methodologies developed to understand that environment. The cultural factors are those of fragmentation, with an attendant focus on difference and ambiguity. Smith argues that chance itself becomes a more significant feature when there are fewer certainties to describe social life. Furthermore, sociologists, in reacting to these new 'conditions for chance', have developed more flexible approaches which must encompass the fragmentary and arbitrary in social life, as well as the patterned and structured elements that were reviewed above. Foucault,[65] for instance, is cited as elaborating a conceptual framework within which chance holds a dominant place.

Smith's outline of what could be called the rehabilitation of chance in sociology is an interesting one, which suggests accidents as a significant set of what we choose to define as 'chance' events. However, it does raise the question of how certain events or outcomes come to be defined as characterized by 'chance'. To argue that chance events are somehow a more central feature of our cultural life in late modernity and that therefore sociological theory must, if it is to be useful and relevant, encompass it, risks a rather circular argument, for it is impossible to test empirically whether chance has become more significant or whether by theorizing it, we make it so. Sociology is one discourse that helps produce 'late modernity', with its fragmentation and ambiguity, and can logically have no privileged position in accounting for how it is constituted. To account for sociology's neglect of the 'accidental' is, then, to answer the wrong question, as it presumes there was some natural pre-existing category of 'accidental' event, produced by some other discourse. Here it has been argued that accidents, like any other category, are socially constructed and that sociology, of course, helps produce such conceptual spaces as well as merely describing them. Specifically, accidents were made possible as a category of misfortune by rational and probabilistic conceptions of causality which had their roots in the late seventeenth century, made necessary by early twentieth-century attempts to define the 'modern', and constructed as a marginal and despised category by such scientific discourses as nosology. In the late twentieth century, the consensus about rationality has perhaps fractured, and the shifting space occupied by accidents, as preventable rather than random misfortunes, is one aspect of this. The 'ideal' accident of our original working definition may soon, perhaps, become merely the remnant of an earlier age.

Acknowledgements

I am grateful to David Armstrong for advice on earlier versions of this paper.

Notes

1. *Targets for Health for All 2000* (Copenhagen: World Health Organization, 1985).
2. For a notable exception, see Karl Figlio, 'What is an Accident?' in P. Weindling (ed.), *The Social History of Occupational Health* (London: Croom Helm, 1985), who argues that the emergence of the concept of the 'accidental' is tied to the development of contractual working relations of production, in which it becomes possible to cause harm through 'negligence' as well as motivation. See also the Introduction to this volume, and the chapter by Robert Campbell for an account of Figlio's argument.
3. D. Fo, *The Accidental Death of an Anarchist: A Farce*, adapted by G. Richards (London: Pluto Press, 1980).
4. See, for instance, the arguments of Mary Douglas and Aaron

Wildavsky, *Risk and Culture* (Berkeley and Los Angeles: University of California Press, 1983) and R. Fox, 'The Evolution of Medical Uncertainty', *Milbank Memorial Fund Quarterly/Health and Society*, lviii (1980), 1–49.

5. E.E. Evans-Pritchard, *Witchcraft, Oracles and Magic Among the Azande* (Oxford: Clarendon Press, 1937).
6. See, for instance, the debates in M. Hollis and S. Lukes (eds), *Rationality and Relativism* (Oxford: Basil Blackwell, 1982); B. Wilson (ed.), *Rationality* (Oxford: Basil Blackwell, 1970), and J. Overing (ed.), *Reason and Morality* (London: Tavistock, 1985).
7. Evans-Pritchard, *op.cit.* (ref. 5), 64.
8. *Ibid.*, 69.
9. *Ibid.*, 65–6.
10. *Ibid.*, 111.
11. L. Levy-Bruhl, *Primitive Mentality* (London: George Allen and Unwin, 1923).
12. *Ibid.*, 43.
13. J. Piaget, *The Child's Conception of Physical Causality*, trs. M. Gabain (London: Kegan Paul, Trench, Trubner and Co., 1930), 114.
14. *Ibid.*, 117.
15. *Ibid.*, 227.
16. See Ian Hacking, *The Emergence of Probability* (Cambridge: Cambridge University Press, 1975); Ian Hacking, 'Was There a Probabilistic Revolution 1800–1930?' in L. Krüger, L. Daston and M. Heidelberger (eds), *The Probabilistic Revolution*: vol 1: *Ideas in History* (Cambridge, MA: MIT Press, 1987) and Ian Hacking, *The Taming of Chance* (Cambridge: Cambridge University Press, 1990), 16.
17. Theodore M. Porter, *The Rise of Statistical Thinking 1820–1900* (Princeton: Princeton University Press, 1980).
18. Michel Foucault, *The Order of Things: An Archaeology of the Human Sciences* (London: Routledge, 1989).
19. Hacking, *Probability* (ref. 16).
20. John Graunt, *Natural and Political Observations Mentioned in a Following Index, and Made upon the Bills of Mortality* (London, 1662).
21. Thomas Lodge, *A Treatise of the Plague, Containing the Nature, Signes and Accidents of the Same* (London: E. White, 1603).
22. *Ibid.*, A4.
23. *Ibid.*, C2.
24. Hacking, *Taming of Chance* (ref. 16), 106.
25. Lodge, *op. cit.* (ref. 21), K2.
26. Samuel Ward, *Woe to Drunkards: a Sermon* (London: John Marriott and John Grismand, 1622).
27. *Ibid.*, 24–5.
28. *Ibid.*, 29.

29. *Ibid.*, 20.
30. Graunt, *op.cit.* (ref. 20), 18.
31. *Ibid.*, 23.
32. *Ibid.*, 16.
33. William Petty, *Several Essays in Political Arithmetic* (London: R. Clavel and H. Mortlock, 1699).
34. *Ibid.*, 27.
35. *Ibid.*, 18.
36. Registrar-General, *Annual Report of Births, Marriages and Deaths* (London: HMSO, 1839), 8.
37. *Ibid.*, 63.
38. *Ibid.*, 64.
39. *Ibid.*, 70.
40. Registrar-General, *Annual Report of Births, Marriages and Deaths* (London: HMSO, 1840), 7.
41. *Ibid.*, 7–8.
42. *Ibid.*, 7.
43. Registrar-General, *Annual Report of Births, Marriages and Deaths* (London: HMSO, 1854), 129.
44. *Ibid.*, 136.
45. *Ibid.*, 129.
46. Registrar-General, *Annual Report of Births, Marriages and Deaths* (London: HMSO, 1862), 78.
47. M. Greenwood, W.J. Martin and W.T. Russell, 'Deaths by Violence, 1837–1937', *Journal of the Royal Statistical Society*, civ (1941), 146–71.
48. *Ibid.*, 147.
49. *International Statistical Classification of Diseases and Related Health Problems* (Geneva: World Health Organization, 1992).
50. L. Evans, 'Medical Accidents: No Such Thing?', *British Medical Journal*, cccvii (1993), 1438–9.
51. *Ibid.*
52. T.C. Doege, 'An Injury is No Accident', *New England Journal of Medicine*, ccxcviii (1978), 509–10.
53. These are reported in the Office of Population and Census Studies: Series DH4 (London: HMSO).
54. For a fuller account of the reconstruction of the accident as a preventable account see Judith Green, 'Accidents and the risk society' in Roger Burrows, Robin Bunton and Sarah Nettleton (eds), *A Sociology of Health Promotion and the New Public Health* (London: Routledge, 1995).
55. M. Henwood, *Accident Prevention and Public Health: A Study of the Annual Reports of Directors of Public Health* (Birmingham: Royal Society for the Prevention of Accidents, 1992), 26.
56. Department of Health, *The Health of the Nation Key Area Handbook: Accidents* (Leeds: Department of Health, 1993).

57. Emile Durkheim, *The Rules of Sociological Method*, trs. S.A. Solouay and J.M. Mueller (Glencoe: Free Press, 1950), xxxix.
58. Emile Durkheim, *Suicide: a Study in Sociology*, trs. J. Spaulding and G. Simpson (London: Routledge and Kegan Paul, 1963).
59. Durkheim, *Rules*, 8.
60. *Ibid.*, 28.
61. See, for instance, the debate between Nichols and Tombs on the 'meaning' of accident rates: Theo Nichols, 'On the Analysis of Size Effects and "Accidents"', *Industrial Relations Journal*, xx (1989), 62–5; T. Nichols, 'Industrial Injuries in British Manufacturing Industry and Cyclical Effects: Continuities and Discontinuities in Industrial Injury Research', *The Sociological Review*, xxxix (1991), 131–9; S. Tombs, 'Industrial Injuries in British Manufacturing', *The Sociological Review*, xxxviii (1990), 324–45; S. Tombs, 'Safety, Statistics and Business Cycles: A Response to Nichols', *The Sociological Review*, xl (1992), 132–45.
62. Anthony Giddens, *Capitalism and Modern Social Theory: an Analysis of the Writings of Marx, Durkheim and Weber* (Cambridge: Cambridge University Press, 1971), 127.
63. Max Weber, *Economy and Society: An Outline of Interpretive Sociology*, Vol. 1, edited by G. Roth and C. Wittich (New York: Bedminster Press, 1968), 4.
64. M. Smith, 'Changing Sociological Perspectives on Chance', *Sociology*, xxvii (1993), 513–31.
65. Michel Foucault, *The Archaeology of Knowledge* (London: Tavistock Publications, 1974).

4

Working Environments: An Ecological Approach to Industrial Health and Safety

Arthur F. McEvoy

One of the many changes that environmentalism has brought to modern historiography is an emphasis on context and contingency. For historians, ecology offers both an object and a method of study. As a subject, it encompasses not only natural objects – plants, animals, the planet itself – but the many different ways in which human and natural systems interact with each other. As a mode of analysis, or what William Cronon called a 'habit of thought', environmental history describes change in terms of that interaction, paying attention to the simultaneous and reciprocal influences that work between the natural and the social orders.[1] In both of its guises, ecology highlights the dynamic interrelatedness of things and undermines our efforts to order them neatly. It focuses our attention on the complex interactions between subjects and contexts, on the systemic effects of obscure relationships and unforeseen events.

A penchant for interdisciplinarity is one manifestation of this tendency, as environmental historians harvest other disciplines for ideas and methods to help them highlight connections between the natural and the cultural. 'More than most of the other "new" histories', Cronon recently observed, 'environmental history erodes the boundaries among traditional historical subfields … and suggests new ways of building bridges among them'.[2] Ecologically-inclined historians in other areas, meanwhile, have lately infused their work with the same kind of attention to context and interdependence that has distinguished environmental historiography for some years now.[3] Inevitably, new methods and new points of view bring into focus new objects of study that earlier works passed by.

In technological history, as in a number of other subfields, environmentalism has reinforced the tendency of recent scholarship to unsettle the systematicity and teleology that characterized earlier work. In David Landes's landmark study *The Unbound Prometheus*, for example, technological innovation proceeds according to its own logic, in rational response to impersonal market forces.[4] The same is true of *Prometheus*'s US counterpart, Nathan Rosenberg's *Technology and American Economic Growth*.[5] Innovation in these works tends to be linear, orderly, and bloodless. More recent treatments, in contrast, have emphasized the roles of context and contingency in technological change. Joel Mokyr has criticized the Whiggishness of the literature in the field and emphasized the social and cultural environments from which innovations emerge. Following Eric Jones, Mokyr emphasizes the accidental or improbable character of technological progress; following Stephen Jay Gould, he highlights its spasmodic character.[6] A recent dissertation by Ken Alder epitomizes the field's new direction in its analysis of how the Revolutionary-era French military experimented with and then discarded interchangeable parts manufacture in artillery. Here, technology did not determine its own history but took second seat to political, social, and professional considerations.[7]

A particularly significant locus of contingency in the history of technology is industrial health and safety. Like pollution, occupational injury and disease are unwanted, unintended consequences of industrial development. They are part of development's social cost, typically falling at random to a diffuse body of victims and figuring only marginally, if at all, in the management decisions that prepare the ground for them.[8]

For this reason, perhaps, injuries to workers figure not at all in the field's classic works. Some works that treat technology from the perspective of cultural or intellectual history have dealt at length with the perceived dangers of mechanization, but the danger about which their subjects worry is usually a metaphorical one, not the far more tangible danger of injury and death that machines posed to the historically inarticulate people whose lives they most thoroughly transformed.[9]

A number of studies have lately looked at industrial health and safety from several different perspectives, all of them emphasizing the centrality of danger and mishap to the social experience of technology and technological change.[10] Kai Erikson's *Everything in its Path*, which details the destruction of a West Virginia town in a mine accident, and Martin Cherniak's study of the Hawk's Nest tunnel incident in the 1930s are exemplary works in sociology and public health, respectively.[11] Focusing on the development of public health policy, David Rosner's and Gerald Markowitz's *Deadly Dust* examines changing political and scientific responses to silicosis during the first half of the nineteenth century.[12] Walter Licht devoted a chapter of his history of railroad labour to safety problems, making clear that physical danger was 'an integral part of the work': 'If many men ultimately escaped accidental injuries and death, the fear and threat of such happenings were inescapable and hung over everyone working on the line'.[13] In legal history, a number of recent works analyse safety regulation and accident compensation with varying degrees of sophistication; most notable among these is Christopher Tomlins's study of early nineteenth-century industrial safety law, which shows how accident liability figured centrally in the construction of capital–labour relations in industrializing America.[14]

Industrial health and safety issues mark out a promising, though as yet largely undeveloped, site at which complementary developments in a great many historical fields come into focus. Environmentally-inclined historians of technology have moved into the field by way of a substantial body of work on pollution, both as a product of and as a stimulus to technological change.[15] For their part, environmental historians have lately paid increasing attention to cities and other, so-called 'built' environments although, as Martin Melosi recently observed, urban environmental studies still lack the broad, synthetic focus and theoretical depth of the field's mainstream.[16]

Making occupational safety into an environmental subject would mean attending to relationships between technology and the bodies of people who work with it. Workers' bodies are, after all, biological entities no less than trees or fish and wildlife. Recent work in cultural history that discusses changing attitudes toward the human body is suggestive in this regard, although thinking about the body in ecological rather than cultural terms would underscore not the plasticity of our attitudes but rather the constancy of the body's vulnerability to injury even as technology changes.[17] As a method, ecology points to an analysis of industrial health and safety in terms of the interactions between a number of systems: the worker's body and its maintenance, the productive processes that draw on the worker's energy, and the law and ideology that guide them. The relationship between people who work and the technologies they operate is a complex, dynamic, ecological one that entails elements of sociology and ideology as well as the more direct impacts of technology on worker health. The same political and conceptual barriers that obstruct our understanding of well-recognized environmental problems like pollution and deforestation, however, tend also to obscure the systematic relationships between industrial technology and industrial accidents and make them difficult to describe. The key to the approach is to treat the workplace as an ecological system, of which the worker's body is the biological core.

An Ecological Approach to Technology

Environmental history is a relatively new field, though one of its lines of descent reaches into a distinguished history-of-science literature.[18] Thomas Kuhn's germinal essay, *The Structure of Scientific Revolutions*, was an important catalyst to a contextual study of ecology because it uncovered the contingency of scientific thought, albeit from the internalist perspective.[19] Environmental history portrays non-human nature as an active player in human history. Its fundamental insight is that nothing that people do is without causes and consequences in non-human nature. The interaction between the two works ecologically, through the medium of biology and adaptation, whether the human protagonists are aware of it or not. Technology is what distinguishes human activity in nature from that of other animals; because technology is a means of interacting with nature, however, it should be amenable to ecological analysis.

Environmental historians for a long time avoided what they call 'built' environments such as cities, much less factories. Early studies focused on 'natural' subjects such as parks or frontier areas inhabited by hunting-gathering people with low-tech, low-intensity economies.[20] Later work began to analyse the ways in which commercial development has disrupted and degraded natural systems. Several works in this group treat the ecological history of extractive industries, typically in non-urban environments where the ecological impacts of development are relatively easy to trace.[21] Fully-developed, industrial-urban environments are dauntingly complex, ecologically, and received much less attention at first, although the logic of the field's methods and the energy of its practitioners inevitably brought cities into view.[22] William Cronon's *Nature's Metropolis*, for example, analysed the ways in which interactions between Chicago and its hinterland changed each of them over time.[23] Taking their cue from Cronon, environmental historians took as the theme for their 1993 conference 'City and Country: Contrasting and Interacting Environments'.

Environmentalists have traditionally preferred 'natural' subjects, partly because they are easier to work with but also, doubtless, because of their political interest in nature protection. Beneath the preference, however, lies a distinction between Nature and humankind that is fundamental to our culture and whose pervasive influence on our thinking is difficult to escape.[24] According to this view, the terms 'nature' and 'ecology' refer to that which is not human: the more 'artificial' a thing is, the less it is part of nature and the less fit an object of ecological study. Artefacts like cities and factories, conversely, are somehow removed from Nature, the creatures solely of human planning and artifice.[25]

One of the few recent studies to bring ecological methods to bear on an industrial subject is Andrew Hurley's history of post-World War II Gary, Indiana, which relates changing technology in steel production to changes in anti-pollution laws and the varying impact of environmental determination on different racial, occupational, and neighbourhood groups with changes in the technology of control. What distinguishes the study as ecological is the way in which industry, politics, and pollution all interact with each other to shape the environment in which people in different parts of the city lived.[26] Another is Christopher Sellers's work on early twentieth-century occupational health, which skilfully analyses the interaction between law, technology, and the professional politics of experts in a number of fields that touched on the problem of occupational health. Bringing an industrial subject squarely into the mainstream of environmental history, Sellers concludes that Progressive-era developments in industrial hygiene 'figured crucially into the evolution of post-World War II environmental policy'.[27]

In terms of method, environmental history looks to the ways in which ecology, political economy, and consciousness interact with each other over time, each continually adapting to a dynamic environment made up of the other two. Nature is an active party to this interaction. Resource endowments influence the development of production and thus of productive technology in particular environments. Local ecologies respond in characteristic ways to human impact and, in turn, present new challenges to production and social organization. People's consciousness of themselves and their place in the world, finally, both guides their activity in the world and changes itself as it confronts environmental changes that that activity inevitably calls forth from a responsive nature.[28] Technology is the tangible instrument of the process: it is the point of interaction between the human and the natural.

Modern environmentalism has made it clear that complex social and ecological relations pervade the use of any technology. The biological reproduction of the workforce on a daily and intergenerational basis is as central to human ecology as is the productivity of 'natural' resources.[29] Our experience with toxic chemicals and radiation since 1950, certainly, has made it clear that a workplace is a biological environment no less than a national park. That some hazards work physically on the body rather than biochemically on its processes does not alter the fact.

Technology does not develop autonomously, according to its own logic; it has roots in and impacts on its environment.[30] Every technology entails a politics. Rachel Carson showed how chemical-intensive farming both fed on and, in turn, nurtured a political system dominated by research universities, agribusiness, and chemical companies.[31] Amory Lovins demonstrated the links between nuclear power and corporate giantism, the arms race, and the security state.[32] Every technology entails a particular ecology, moreover, as *Silent Spring* showed most powerfully. Alfred Crosby and other environmental historians have shown that European agriculture brought with it to frontier areas not only ploughs, pigs and honeybees, but coherent assemblages of tools, techniques, plants, animals, diseases, and property relations. It was the aggregate working as a system, more than any single part of it, that utterly transformed the ecology of colonized areas and just as utterly displaced the economies of the existing population.[33]

The relationship between technology and its natural and social environments is not only reciprocal but dynamic as well. Esther Boserup made the point that producing communities always have a large repertoire of techniques available to them; which ones they choose depends on demography, local resource endowments, and other contingencies.[34] Technological innovation, moreover, inevitably changes a community's ecology and social structure. My own work on the California fisheries showed that fishing technology evolved in a dynamic, recursive relationship with the progressive, anthropogenic transformation of entire ecosystems, as well as by strictly 'human' market forces and strictly 'environmental' changes in climate, currents, and so on.[35] Technology, then, is anything but an autonomous force in history; it develops in continual, reciprocal adaptation with the natural and social environments in which people use it. A healthy respect for the capricious and the chaotic is a final 'habit of thought' that students of biological systems can bring to the historical study of technology. Modern evolutionary theorists, notably Stephen Jay Gould and Niles Eldredge, emphasize the accidental, discontinuous, and above all the historical nature of evolution in contrast to the orderly, progressive picture drawn by Darwin and his immediate successors. Life may exfoliate according to pattern, in this view, but it is the occasional, unpredictable catastrophe that winnows out some lines of development and spurs others, essentially at random. Evolution is thus path-dependent, that is to say historical: it may have an internal logic, but the form it actually takes depends on particular sequences of discrete events.[36] Similar interest in non-linear, non-progressive explanation has taken hold in physics and chemistry as well as biology; the new orientation has focused scientists' attention on the kinds of accidents, anomalies, and discontinuities that only fifteen or twenty years ago they would have ignored as errors in perception or experimentation.[37] Economists and other social scientists have applied the new insights to their own work.[38] Mokyr worked with Gould's discontinuous model of evolution in his essay on technological history, though he cautioned his readers not to press the analogy too far.[39]

In many fields, it seems, accidental events and unforeseen consequences of planned activities have taken on new importance in our understanding of the world. The factories and other workplaces that industrial engineers portray as models of order and rationality may, instead, be precisely the kinds of high-energy, non-equilibrium environments in which the chaotic and the unpredictable are the norm rather than the exception.[40] Tomlins noted that historians have too often taken the word of nineteenth-century writers that the industrial workplace was an orderly, rational place and suggested, instead, that 'industrial "order" was, to an important extent a mask for arbitrariness and confusion, a facade behind which employees daily confronted an unpredictable terrain'.[41] Tomlins showed, on the contrary, that work injuries were a critical problem in industrializing America and that allocating liability for them was a crucial step in the development of the modern legal system.

Technological accidents, of course, take place in people's homes as well as at work. Domestic injuries are no less crucial to the social experience of industrial technology than are ones that take place at work, although the common perception is that they are less systematic, less preventable, and thus rest even more firmly in the natural order of things.[42] The modern law of products liability, for example, owes as much to suits brought by plaintiffs injured at home as by those hurt at the workplace.[43] The workplace, however, is where exposure to technological risk is most immediate, concentrated, and sustained, and thus where it comes into focus most sharply as a political issue and as a catalyst for social change, as both Tomlins and Sellers have shown.[44]

Technology and Industrial Accidents

What, then, can we learn about the social history of technology from an ecologically-minded study of occupational safety and health? Given that the issue has received little sustained attention from labour historians or historians of technology, occupational safety may be a useful perspective from which to view the development of industrial technology.[45] Cherniak's study of the Hawk's Nest incident, in which miners working on a West Virginia hydroelectric project suffered cruelly from silicosis and were abandoned to their fates by employers and government alike, took this approach to the end of making a statement about government regulation of public health. It may be counter-intuitive to discuss the broad sweep of technological development in terms of work accidents; we call them 'accidents', after all, because we perceive them as isolated events, unconnected to larger systems or long-term trends.[46] Particular accidents, however, may offer useful texts from which to interpret the role of mayhem in industrial development.[47]

An ecological approach to the problem suggests, further, that we look at the interaction between injuries to workers' bodies – the biological core of the workplace environment – and the technology, organization, and ideology of production. The industrial revolution, as Karl Polanyi showed, is a revolution in social organization as much as or more than a revolution in productive technology.[48] Accidents and disease are an ecological consequence of that organization no less than soil erosion is a consequence of the economics of agriculture or fishery depletion has its roots in the regulatory structure of fishing. Technology, in addition, plays an important role in shaping people's consciousness of occupational hazard, just as it does in the awareness of other social problems, by laying out the boundaries between injuries that society perceives as preventable, as inevitable costs of economic life or, indeed, as no injury at all. Technology, then, structures the ecology of the workplace in three ways: by posing hazards directly, by shaping the social organization that exposes workers to risk, and by influencing society's awareness of danger to its working population.

Sometimes an individual injury assumes historical significance all by itself, by way of its legal or political repercussions. Christopher Tomlins's study of employer-liability law in Massachusetts uses the case of *Farwell* v. *Boston and Worcester Railroad*, which came down from the Massachusetts Court of Appeals in 1842.[49] The railroad was an entirely new phenomenon in the early nineteenth-century

United States; never before had so many workers been brought together in close company with heavy machinery. Economic depression and increased competition in the late 1830s led the railroads to intensify operations and generated what Tomlins called a 'quickening flood' of derailments, collisions, and injuries.[50] One of those injured was Nicholas Farwell, who lost his arm when a negligent co-worker caused a locomotive to derail.

Dismissing the suit in favour of the defendant railroad, Massachusetts Chief Justice Shaw ruled that engineer Farwell had assumed the risk of injury – even at the hands of negligent fellow-workers – when he agreed to work on the railroad at a bargained-for wage. *Farwell* thus stood for two of the three great common-law defences available to defendant employers in work injury cases: 'assumption of risk', the 'fellow-servant' rule, and the rule that any contributory negligence on the part of the injured plaintiff was an absolute bar to recovery. Together, the three defences shielded employers from nearly all liability for worker injuries, thus granting them near-plenary authority to control the pace and conditions of work. As Tomlins put it, Shaw's ruling 'endorsed the structure of disciplinary power that permeated the employment relationship and yoked the public interest in industrial safety to its perpetuation'.[51]

The decision controlled the law of employer's liability until the advent of workers' compensation in the early twentieth century: Tomlins called it '*the* case in the common law of employer liability, treated not only in Massachusetts but throughout the Anglo-American jurisprudential world as the requisite authoritative statement of the limits to an employer's responsibilities, the point of departure in all subsequent litigation in any industrial situation'.[52] Another historian, Eric Tucker, wrote that *Farwell* 'effectively banished from legal consideration the most important transformation that was taking place in the labor process under industrial capitalism: the shift of control over the labor process from workers to capitalists'.[53] One of the very earliest injuries involving industrial machinery was thus pivotal for subsequent development. *Farwell* not only encouraged rapid technological development by allocating the costs of accidents to workers rather than to entrepreneurs but did much to structure relations between labour, business, and the state under industrial capitalism.[54]

Another work accident, the Triangle Shirtwaist fire of 1911, was as critical to the evolution of American political economy in the twentieth century as engineer Farwell's had been in the nineteenth. The Triangle fire took place in a New York City garment factory and claimed the lives of 146 workers, many of whom leapt nine storeys to their deaths before crowds of horrified onlookers. Neither criminal prosecutors nor civil plaintiffs, however, were able to secure judgments against the factory's owners because at the time the law did not allow them to argue that the employers had been so careless of fire hazard as to make such a tragedy inevitable. Anything more than a misdemeanour conviction under local fire ordinances would have required proof of some act by which the employers directly caused the deaths of their workers. Because prosecutors and plaintiffs were unable to demonstrate such an act, the Triangle employers collected their insurance and were soon back in business.[55]

The fire did expose, however, the deadly consequences of employers' licence to maintain unsafe working environments. So great was public outrage over the fire and the employers' escape from liability that within three years of the disaster New York enacted comprehensive changes in factory safety and accident compensation law, changes for which reformers had been struggling with little success for decades.[56] Frances Perkins later wrote that 'the extent to which this legislation in New York marked a change in American political attitudes and policies toward social responsibility can scarcely be overrated. It was, I am convinced, a turning point ...'.[57] The fire made clear the ecology of the turn-of-the-century workplace and the law's active role in sustaining it. In so doing, it catalysed the formation of a modern regulatory state in a key jurisdiction.

Other examples might be found of particular industrial accidents either that contributed directly to changes in the political economy of the workplace or that provide opportunity for 'thick description' of ways in which machines transformed the ecology of the workplace.[58] Erikson's study of the Buffalo Creek disaster is a model for this kind of enquiry, though the focus of his interest was on the community surrounding the mine rather than on the organization of production *per se*. One spectacular railway accident in Ontario in 1854 both focused public attention on railroad safety at the time and left a detailed record for historians to interpret.[59] Workers frequently come first and most intensively into contact with new technological hazards; their stories tell of technology's social significance not only to later historians but to contemporaries who learn about them as they happen.

In relatively few cases, however – spectacular incidents like the Triangle fire or the odd injuries whose victims give their names to legal precedents – do industrial accidents have much direct impact on historical struggles over the social control of industrial technology.

This may be one reason why they so seldom figure in technological historiography. So closely did safety issues cut to the employer's prerogative in the workplace, as Tomlins showed, that legal authorities decided very early on that workers would have to fend for themselves for the time being.[60] Eric Tucker concluded that what safety regulation did emerge in nineteenth-century Ontario did so mainly where public concern over accidents reinforced paternalistic attitudes about the special vulnerability of women and children. It is not clear that late nineteenth-century factory legislation improved the workers' situation at all.[61] It is by now notorious that Upton Sinclair wrote his exposé of the meat-packing industry out of a concern for industrial safety rather than for the quality of the product, which is what seized public attention: 'I aimed for the public's heart', he wrote later, 'and by accident I hit it in the stomach'.[62] Economically, the damage that industrial accidents and disease do to workers' bodies is very much like the damage that industry does to the natural environment: both pollution and work injuries are social costs, so broadly diffused over large numbers of politically inarticulate victims that employers are rarely called to account for them.[63] Ecologically, thus, the two are close cousins working on opposite sides of the factory gate: one destroys the productivity of air, water, and other natural systems while the other destroys a human body's biological capacity to work.

Work accidents are less typically the result of new technologies than they are of more mundane hazards that befall people by way of the political and sociological organization of their workplaces. One might describe the history of machines, for that matter, as much as a political process as a narrowly technical one: machinery, in this view, is the means by which owners and representatives of capital take control over the workplace away from those who do the work.[64] Work accidents, by the same token, are at once the manifestation and the method of that domination. Workers themselves know this: health and safety issues have historically been an important cause of labour unrest, although they are so crucial to employers' authority that workers are seldom able to bring them into serious question. Modern surveys show that union members tend to give higher priority to health and safety issues than to wages and benefits, while the reverse obtains among management and union leadership.[65]

Tomlins and Tucker both noted that nineteenth-century industry not only exposed people to new hazards but also subjected them to new ways of organizing and controlling production that new techniques brought with them. It was the combination of the two, especially, that put worker health and safety at risk.[66] Workers given the choice of producing faster or facing the wrath of their superiors have always circumvented safety devices and procedures and thus, in the eyes of employers, the law, and the general public, brought their injuries on themselves.[67] Work accidents, then, are often the result of employer decisions to intensify production and reduce investment in safety, thus increasing the danger to workers. Complicit in these decisions, of course, is the legal system that entitles employers to make such decisions.[68] Law, business, technology, and the worker's body thus come together in the issue of occupational safety and health. Every work injury is a text laden with meaning about technology, society, and the law.

Technological change affects the ecology of the workplace in yet a third way, which has to do with people's awareness of the chains of cause-and-effect that link technology with its impacts on worker health and safety. As a cognitive activity, causal attribution is as much a social process as it is an objective, 'scientific' one: it takes different patterns in different social/cultural environments according to prevailing standards of judgement and what Foucault called 'the architecture of knowledge' in a culture.[69] The process is thus, necessarily, an historical one, though it has been little studied.[70] Spectacular accidents teach people about the meaning of technology in their lives. Technology itself, however, is an important engine of change in people's understanding of the world because it influences their ability to manipulate reality and thus to grasp cause-and-effect relationships in the world around them: 'the notion of causation', a philosopher wrote, 'is essentially connected with our manipulative techniques for producing results'.[71] Social experience, and work experience in particular, is a key source of heuristics and paradigms for attributing causality not only in social life but in the natural world as well.[72]

A number of historians have dealt with the relationship between causal attribution and social change. Chief among these is Thomas Haskell, whose study of the professionalization of social science showed how the increasing complexity and interrelatedness of late nineteenth-century US society encouraged people to attribute the causes of social phenomena to remote, impersonal social forces rather than to individuals.[73] In another work, Haskell attributed the rise of anti-slavery humanitarianism in the early nineteenth century to merchants' ability, through business contracts, to manipulate events at greater removes of time and space. Such merchants increasingly understood that their dealings with the slave industry contributed to human suffering in Africa and the slave states.

Boycotting the trade, conversely, became a means to end it.[74] Calvin Woodard showed how the growing power of the industrial economy to produce goods transformed poverty from an 'inevitable' fact of social life to a social ill with identifiable causes and attainable cures.[75] My own work on the California fishing industry related changes in prevailing theories of fishery depletion in the 1960s to public familiarity with computer technology, sampling theory and stochastic analysis, and the public health effects of radioactive and chemical pollution.[76] In each case, new technologies enhanced people's ability to influence the course of events and helped to shift the boundaries between what they categorized as preventable evil and what they chalked up to the natural order of things.

Like poverty in the pre-industrial era, industrial injuries frequently offer themselves to view as an inevitable part of life in a technologically advanced society, a necessary cost of innovation. Observers frequently attribute accidents to poor equipment or, more typically, the carelessness of the injured worker him/herself, but seldom to the technologies themselves and the social relations that surround their use.[77] Even late twentieth-century observers often attribute accidents to 'operator error' when they are, in fact, necessary complements to working with highly complex, dangerous technologies under legal arrangements that guarantee employer prerogative to determine the conditions under which they are to be used.[78] Legal doctrines that shield employers from liability for accidents play a major role in narrowing the available scope of causal attribution.[79] Work accidents are powerful indicators of maladjustment in the ecology of production, although it takes more than the mere knowledge that suffering exists to motivate social action. People must first recognize the suffering as systematic rather than random, 'caused' by something and thus preventable. It is people's social experience, of which both law and technology are a part, that enables that recognition.[80] *Laissez-faire* in industrial safety came to an end at the turn of the twentieth century as people recognized the systemic causes of accidents and conceived political remedies for them. In the words of J. Willard Hurst, 'sharper perception of cause-effect relations, developed out of increasing science-and-technology-based manipulation of affairs, generated political pressures for more rational and humane arrangements, given form, however inadequately, in factory safety laws and workmen's compensation'.[81] What Hurst did not mention was the fact that public outrage over the enormous toll that work accidents took at the turn of the century, as well as the litigation crisis they spawned, was a significant impetus to industrial reform in the Progressive Era.[82] The relationship between technology and injury was recursive: life in an advanced, interdependent industrial society taught people to look for the systemic causes of industrial mayhem, while the mounting toll of accidents generated political pressure for controlling industrial hazards. Economic life also provided a repertoire of remedies for social ills: experience with the executory contract suggested the boycott; casualty insurance suggested worker's compensation; work on the assembly line suggested the sit-down strike.[83]

Technology, then, structures the ecology of the workplace in a number of ways. Particular machines and processes may pose direct hazards to worker health and safety. A more subtle, pervasive threat to workers may stem from the social organization of the workplace, which is a product not only of the labour requirements of particular technologies but of the legal arrangements under which employers hire and control their workers. By conditioning social awareness of the causes of industrial health and safety problems, finally, technology plays a role in motivating public action to control those hazards that appear controllable. Like all environments in which humans are active, the workplace is the product of ongoing, reciprocal interaction between biology, political economy, and consciousness. What distinguishes a workplace from a forest or a fishery is that its biological heart is the worker's body itself.

De-Naturalizing Industrial Accidents

Occupational injury, then, is a key aspect of life for industrial workers; the historiography of technology is seriously incomplete without it. Every technology nests in a dynamic system that includes the worker's body, the social conditions under which production takes place, and the ideology that both springs from and mediates the interaction between biology and production. As the means of production, technology structures the workplace environment by posing direct threats to the worker's body, by influencing the social relations of work, and by moulding social perception of the industrial order. For too long, as Tomlins put it, 'the maiming or death of employees at work could be treated as part of the social landscape – a routine, if regrettable occurrence' that is just part of the price we pay for progress.[84] Ironically, perhaps, highlighting the role of the human body in workplace ecology may help to 'de-naturalize' industrial accidents – remove them from the background against which technology develops and expose them as contingent phenomena, systematically related to their social and historical contexts.[85]

Scholars concerned with explaining the historical degradation of the natural environment have faced a similar task in developing their field. Nineteenth-century Americans typically thought environmental destruction a necessary companion to social progress, if only because it seemed impossible to do anything about it. To many, indeed, the extermination of Indians and wildlife, the clearing of the forests, and the fouling of city air by smoking factories signified progress and were thus to be welcomed: efforts to interfere with the process were not only pointless but positively vicious.[86] Critical to the success of modern environmentalism were the efforts of Rachel Carson and others to portray nature as an active partner in human life as opposed to a passive victim; that insight, which George Perkins Marsh had articulated in 1864 but which went unnoticed for many years, has lately enabled historians to explain the nation's progress in a different and more sophisticated way.[87]

The task of denaturalizing industrial mayhem is a difficult one, however, politically as well as historiographically. This is because, like our historical abuse of nature, industrial accidents nest in a set of social relations that we perceive as 'natural' and hence ineluctable.[88] If work accidents appear 'inevitable' to us, it may be because our habits of thought and action render their systemic causes invisible. Writing the history of industrial accidents, like the task of controlling them politically, requires bringing them into relief against that background. The problems involved in doing so are nearly identical with those of highlighting the causes of environmental destruction. They involve the voluntarism, the mechanism, and the teleology that colour our view of history and politics. These problems are, of course, interrelated.

The problem of *voluntarism* refers to our tendency to see human will as the prime mover of social change and to focus our attention narrowly on the intended consequences of human behaviour.[89] When nineteenth-century Americans thought about their use of natural resources, they looked first at the wealth they intended to create and only as an afterthought, if at all, at the devastation they left in their wake. A related tendency was to look for the causes of environmental and other social problems in the intentional acts of individuals; because pollution, species extinction, soil erosion, and so on are social problems with systemic causes, courts and legislatures were thus ill equipped to deal with such problems when they took note of them at all.[90] This reflex is still common and confounds modern efforts to fix liability for many environmental problems, particularly those involving toxic substances.[91] Historians are not immune, either: this is why environmental studies focused first on what historically articulate people have thought about nature, then on political controversies over how to use nature, and only then on how nature and society create each other.

Voluntarism suffuses our thinking about industrial accidents, as well. The persistent, reflexive tendency to blame accidents on 'operator error' is the clearest manifestation of this.[92] Inventors may make technological innovations so as to exploit the labour power of workers more efficiently, but they seldom mean to push that exploitation to the point of killing and maiming. The killing and maiming that do result are unintended and thus (we think) incidental consequences. Industrial safety regulation in Ontario, Tucker found, ran up against the background assumption of many factory inspectors that the interests of workers and employers were fundamentally compatible: their attitude, then, was that accidents reported to them were for the most part inevitable, given the fact of employer control over plant safety and work discipline.[93] Employers avoided having to account for accidents for as long as they did partly because liability depended on finding some individual directly at fault for mishaps, many of which stemmed from causes over which no individual had real control.[94]

More subtle was the law's ability to obfuscate the systemic causes of accidents by portraying working conditions as the product of the individual worker's voluntary choice. The judge in the *Farwell* case reasoned that the injured plaintiff had taken his job at a bargained-for wage and thus assumed the 'normal' risks of his job, including the negligence of co-workers. The court would not hold the defendant railroad liable for the chance consequences of Farwell's voluntary act.[95] Factory laws and workers' compensation came about around the turn of the century once a militant workforce and an outraged public became unwilling any longer to think of existing rates of injury as 'normal' and realized that choice had little to do with workers' exposure to them. Once the horrible toll of industrial accidents had systemic, articulable causes and thus imaginable cures, the *laissez-faire* regime in industrial relations began to collapse. Legal scholars have sometimes portrayed the workers' compensation regimes that supplanted it as a product of rational public choice, although it is not clear that 'rationalizing' the liability system in this way either compensated workers adequately or improved workplace safety to any great degree.[96] Here, again, the rhetoric of voluntarism rendered invisible the power of the employer to expose defenceless workers to the risk of injury and disease.[97]

The problem of *mechanism* refers to the tendency to describe both nature and society in mechanical terms: composed of interchangeable parts, rationally ordered, and manipulable through technology and experimentation.[98] This view came into being in the seventeenth century as the Scientific Revolution, the emergence of new theories of political sovereignty, and the diffusion of capitalist economic relations fundamentally altered the architecture of knowledge in Western culture, teaching people to understand themselves and the world around them in new ways.[99] As Carolyn Merchant has shown, the change in view entailed 'the death of nature': the earth, no longer perceived as an organism but as a mechanical system of inert matter in motion, could be taken apart and rearranged with impunity to serve exclusively human needs.[100] Ecological disruption on a scale hitherto unknown ensued as people assumed voluntaristic control over the planet, unable or unwilling to account for the real complexity of the natural systems they overwhelmed.[101] Americans, to whom voluntarism was an article of faith, believed that science and technology could make a more orderly, more productive nature and that any problems they might encounter would have technological solutions.[102]

A product of the seventeenth century, mechanism most thoroughly transformed the ecology of the workplace with the spread of industrialism and the division of labour in the nineteenth. The worker's personality disappeared from social view as labour became an abstract factor of production, to be bought at a price determined by impersonal market forces and combined with capital and resources at the will of the entrepreneur.[103] The worker's body became a mere appendage of the machine, subject to the impersonal discipline of employers who attended to health and safety concerns only to the extent that they entailed out-of-pocket costs.[104] Nineteenth-century writers analysed the worker's body itself as a species of machine.[105] Visiting Manchester in 1844, Engels was stunned by the manifestations of this transformation in poverty, illness, and especially in workplace injuries.[106] The law's representation of the employment relation as a voluntary, contractual agreement between equal bargainers further obscured what Foucault called the 'new mechanism of power' that allowed 'time and labor, rather than wealth and commodities, to be extracted from bodies'.[107]

One important manifestation of mechanism in modern industrial safety law is the economic approach to safety and liability issues in current vogue among judges and legal scholars. Neoclassical economics is a supremely mechanistic discipline, postulating as it does an economy made up of atomized, rational utility-maximizers moved this way and that by Newtonian market forces.[108] A substantial law-and-economics literature, then, has emerged around problems of accident liability and safety regulation, much of it taking the view that market incentives generally deter accidents by leading employers to maintain appropriate levels of safety in their plants.[109] Some scholars, echoing the argument in *Farwell* v. *Boston and Worcester Railroad*, claim that industrial wages include a premium for the risks entailed in particular jobs.[110] Just as they do in environmental areas, however, market forces over-discount the costs of industrial injuries (thus subsidizing employers at the expense of injured workers), particularly when the harms involved are long-term, hard to identify, or difficult to value in money terms.[111] Injuries to workers from asbestos and other toxic substances are the clearest example of this kind of market failure in the safety area.[112] Just as the industrial economy extracts resources from nature, it extracts labour from the bodies of workers with insufficient regard for the complexity of their ecology and thus their ability to sustain the yield.

The problem of *teleology*, finally, refers to the notion, embedded deep in our culture, that technological development is progressive, self-motivating, and benign. The idea of autonomous technological progress, of course, is a cornerstone of modern Western culture: Polanyi called it 'a mystical readiness to accept the social consequences of economic improvement, whatever they might be'.[113] Nowhere is this more evident than in the United States where, at least until the late twentieth century, private initiative in science and technology was a powerful engine of economic growth and social progress.[114] That the course of development was left to market forces made it look autonomous and inevitable. The size and natural wealth of the country, meanwhile, combined with chronic shortages of labour and capital to place a premium on the rapid development of resources; for a long time the environmental costs that came with headlong development were simply not noticed. As Hurst put it, 'we would realize the greatest present production we could from the land, though in the contemporary state of the economy this meant throwing away much that a broader future development could use'.[115] Only after the turn of the century did the law reflect any effort to slow the pace of destruction, of the country's workforce as well as its natural wealth. Only late in the twentieth century did it attempt, haltingly, to direct the course of innovation and to assess rationally the social costs and benefits of developing particular technologies. The Office of Technology Assessment is one institutional manifestation of this new concern; environmental impact statements are probably the best procedural example.[116]

One of the environmental costs of progress, of course, was the toll in industrial accidents. Because people did not recognize their systemic causes, however, accidents became a necessary evil, to be tolerated on the way to the brighter future that technology would bring. This spirit suffuses the opinion in the *Farwell* case of 1842, which makes vague but repeated references to 'considerations of policy': Shaw and his contemporaries would not let sporadic damage to individuals stand in the way of technological innovation and economic growth, in which the future of the country lay.[117] Technological change was one of the impersonal, Newtonian forces that drove social change. Its progress, moreover, was benign. Given the presumed teleology of technological development, the law's unwillingness to control it, and the instinct to blame individuals for what accidents did occur, the tendency to perceive the cost as 'inevitable' – like taxes, paid in blood and bone – seems only natural.

Conclusion

The fact that industrial health and safety has so seldom figured in analyses of technological change is remarkable, given the pervasive influence of injury on the lives of the people who work most closely with industrial technology and the significance of accident liability in allocating the social costs of industrial production. Treating the workplace as an ecological system, however, taking into account the dynamic, reciprocal interaction between the worker's body, the political economy of technological development, and changing perceptions of the role of machines in social life, may offer a broader perspective on the problem of industrial safety and thus highlight its importance in a way that other approaches to technology and labour historiography cannot. Work accidents contribute to the social meaning of technology in three ways: they constitute the most dramatic and immediate social cost of mechanization; they catalyse the construction of power relations in the workplace; and they contribute to public consciousness of the industrial order. Highlighting that role is as difficult an intellectual process as it has been historically because the habits of mind that condition our thinking about technology and industrial accidents – voluntarism, mechanism, and teleology – obscure the systemic relationships between them. That we call workplace injuries 'accidents' rather than, say, 'production costs', illustrates the tendency to think of them as somehow peripheral and not central to the role of technology in our lives.

The fact that we can now talk about industrial safety in this new way is itself a product of a significant shift in the architecture of our knowledge of the world, a shift that has gathered momentum since the middle of this century.[118] Late twentieth-century environmentalism, itself catalysed by qualitatively new hazards posed by post-1950 developments in chemical and nuclear technology, as well as by developments in information sciences that have made those hazards comprehensible, is both symptom and cause of the current, ongoing change in our understanding. Industrial health and safety have come into sharper relief with the gathering scholarly emphasis on the role of accident, of unforeseen consequences, and of complex interaction in history and social life as well as in the natural world. Re-emphasizing the significance of industrial accidents in the ecology of the workplace may perhaps highlight the hidden truth that labour is more than just an economic activity controlled by impersonal market forces: it is the manifestation of the worker's life force, the expression of which makes human life distinctively human.

Acknowledgements

This paper was first prepared for the Conference on Critical Problems and Research Frontiers in History of Technology and History of Science, Madison, Wisconsin, 30 October – 3 November 1991. Research was supported in part by the American Bar Foundation, National Endowment for the Humanities Grant #FT-34785, and National Science Foundation Grant #SES-9223512. Able research assistance was provided by Greg Lind and Ricki Shine; helpful comments by Robert Friedel, Chris Sellers, Peter Siegelman.

Notes

1. William Cronon, 'The Uses of Environmental History', *Environmental History Review,* xvii (1993), 1–22, at 12–16.
2. *Ibid.*, 5.
3. For recent surveys of environmental historiography, see Donald Worster (ed.), *The Ends of The Earth: Perspectives on Modern Environmental History* (Cambridge: Cambridge University Press, 1988), and *idem* (ed.), 'A Round Table: Environmental History', *Journal of American History,* lxxvi (1990), 1087–1147. Recent environmental symposia published in other subfields include Christine Meisner Rosen and Joel A. Tarr (eds), 'The Environment and The City', *Journal of Urban History,* xx (1994), 299–434.
4. David Landes, *The Unbound Prometheus: Technological Change and Industrial Development in Western Europe from 1750 to the Present* (Cambridge: Cambridge University Press, 1969).
5. Nathan Rosenberg, *Technology and American Economic Growth* (New York: Harper & Row, 1972).
6. Joel Mokyr, *The Lever of Riches: Technological Creativity and Economic Progress* (Oxford: Oxford University Press, 1990); E. L. Jones, *The European Miracle: Environments, Economies, and Geopolitics in the*

History of Europe and Asia (Cambridge: Cambridge University Press, 1987); Stephen Jay Gould, *Wonderful Life: The Burgess Shale and the Nature of History* (Harmondsworth: Penguin, 1991); Gould, 'Evolution and the Triumph of Homology, or Why History Matters', *American Scientist*, lxxiv (1986), 60–9.

7. Ken Alder, 'Forging the New Order: The Origins of French Mass Production and Two Languages of the Machine Age, 1763–1815' (unpublished Ph.D. diss., Harvard University, 1991).
8. On social cost, see R. H. Coase, 'The Problem of Social Cost', *Journal of Law and Economics*, iii (1960), 1–44; Jan G. Laitos, 'Legal Institutions and Pollution: Some Intersections Between Law and History', *Natural Resources Journal*, xv (1975), 423–51; James Willard Hurst, *Law and Markets in United States History: Different Modes of Bargaining Among Interests* (Madison: University of Wisconsin Press, 1982), ch. 3.
9. See, for example, John F. Kasson, *Civilizing the Machine: Technology and Republican Values in America, 1776–1900* (New York: Grossman, 1976), 164–6; Leo Marx, *The Machine in the Garden: Technology and the Pastoral Ideal in America* (Oxford: Oxford University Press, 1964), 169–79.
10. Two noteworthy anthologies are David Rosner and Gerald Markowitz, *Dying For Work: Workers' Safety and Health in Twentieth-Century America* (Bloomington: University of Indiana Press, 1987), and Paul Weindling (ed.), *The Social History of Occupational Health* (London: Croom Helm, 1985).
11. Kai T. Erikson, *Everything in Its Path: Destruction of Community in the Buffalo Creek Flood* (New York: Simon & Schuster, 1976); see also Gerald M. Stern, *The Buffalo Creek Disaster* (New York: Vintage Books, 1976); Martin Cherniak, *The Hawk's Nest Incident: America's Worst Industrial Disaster* (New Haven: Yale University Press, 1986). A useful source in the history of industrial health safety is the autobiography of one of the field's pioneers, Alice Hamilton, *Exploring the Dangerous Trades: The Autobiography of Alice Hamilton, M.D.* (Boston: Little Brown & Co., 1943).
12. David Rosner and Gerald Markowitz, *Deadly Dust: Silicosis and the Politics of Occupational Disease in Twentieth-Century America* (Princeton: Princeton University Press, 1991).
13. Walter Licht, *Working For the Railroad: The Organization of Work in the Nineteenth Century* (Princeton: Princeton University Press, 1987), 181.
14. Christopher L. Tomlins, 'A Mysterious Power: Industrial Accidents and the Legal Construction of Employment Relations in Massachusetts, 1800–1850', *Law and History Review*, vi (1988), 375–438. See also Tomlins, *Law, Labor, and Ideology in the Early American Republic* (Cambridge: Cambridge University Press, 1993), ch. 10. Jonathon Simon built on Tomlins's work in his study of late nineteenth-century accident law in 'For the Government of Its Servants: Law and Disciplinary Power in the Work Place, 1870–1906', *Studies in Law, Politics, and Society*, xiii (1993), 105–36. See also Eric Tucker,

Administering Danger in the Workplace: The Law and Politics of Occupational Health and Safety in Ontario, 1850–1914 (Toronto: University of Toronto Press, 1990), 231, n.3; Barbara Ellen Smith, *Digging Our Own Graves: Coal Miners and the Struggle over Black Lung Disease* (Philadelphia: Temple University Press, 1987); Edward H. Beardsley, *A History of Neglect: Health Care for Blacks and Mill Workers in the Twentieth-Century South* (Knoxville, Tenn.: University of Tennessee Press, 1987); and James Whiteside, *Regulating Danger: The Struggle for Mine Safety in the Rocky Mountain Coal Industry* (Lincoln, Neb.: University of Nebraska Press, 1990).

15. See Jeffrey K. Stine and Joel A. Tarr (eds), 'Special Issue on Technology and The Environment', *Environmental History Review*, xviii (1994), 1–140.
16. Martin V. Melosi, 'The Place of the City in Environmental History', *Environmental History Review*, xvii (1993), 1–24, at 2.
17. See Catherine Gallagher and Thomas Laqueur (eds), *The Making of The Modern Body: Sexuality and Society in the Nineteenth Century* (Berkeley: University of California Press, 1987); Laqueur, *Making Sex: Body and Gender from the Greeks to Freud* (Cambridge, Mass.: Harvard University Press, 1990). Elaine Scarry discusses work in *The Body in Pain: The Making and Unmaking of the World* (Oxford: Oxford University Press, 1985), 169–72, 243–56.
18. Good introductions to the field may be found in Donald Worster (ed.), 'A Round Table', *op.cit.* (ref. 3); and Richard White, 'American Environmental History: The Development of a New Historical Field', *Pacific Historical Review*, liv (1985), 297–335. Exemplars of the history-of-science strain of environmental history are Ronald C. Tobey, *Saving the Prairies: The Life Cycle of the Founding School of American Plant Ecology, 1895–1955* (Berkeley: University of California Press, 1981); Donald Worster, *Nature's Economy: A History of Ecological Ideas* (Cambridge: Cambridge University Press, 1977); and especially Carolyn Merchant, *The Death of Nature: Women, Ecology, and the Scientific Revolution* (New York: Harper & Row, 1980).
19. Thomas Kuhn, *The Structure of Scientific Revolutions* (Chicago: University of Chicago Press, 1962). See also Carolyn Merchant, *Ecological Revolutions: Nature, Gender, and Science in New England* (Chapel Hill: University of North Carolina Press, 1989), 3.
20. The earliest efforts in the field were intellectual treatments of 'wilderness' issues such as Roderick Nash, *Wilderness and the American Mind* (New Haven: Yale University Press, 1967), or analyses of conservation such as Samuel P. Hays, *Conservation and the Gospel of Efficiency: The Progressive Conservation Movement, 1890–1920* (Cambridge, Mass.: Harvard University Press, 1959). Amongst the best exemplars of an ecological approach to hunter-gatherer economies are Richard White, *The Roots of Dependency: Subsistence, Environment, and Social Change Among the Choctaws,*

Pawnees, and Navajos (Lincoln, Neb.: University of Nebraska Press, 1983); and Robert Harms, *Games Against Nature: An Eco-Cultural History of the Nunu of Equatorial Africa* (Cambridge: Cambridge University Press, 1987).

21. Donald Worster, *Dust Bowl: The Southern Plains in the 1930s* (Oxford: Oxford University Press, 1979); Theodore Steinberg, *Nature Incorporated: Industrialization and the Waters of New England* (Cambridge: Cambridge University Press, 1991); Arthur F. McEvoy, *The Fisherman's Problem: Ecology and Law in the California Fisheries, 1850–1980* (Cambridge: Cambridge University Press, 1986).
22. A recent survey of the field is Martin V. Melosi, 'The Place of The City in Environmental History', *Environmental History Review,* xvii (1993), 1–24. See also Christine M. Rosen and Joel A. Tarr (eds), 'The Importance of an Urban Perspective in Environmental History', *Journal of Urban History,* xx (1994), 299–310.
23. William Cronon, *Nature's Metropolis: Chicago and the Great West* (New York: Norton, 1991).
24. Cronon, *op.cit.* (ref. 1), 10–11.
25. The dichotomy between nature and culture is a fundamental problem in environmental historiography – indeed, in western thought generally: Roberto Mangabeira Unger, *Knowledge and Politics* (New York: Free Press, 1984), 205–13. One school of thought traces the dichotomy to the deepest roots of Western culture. See, in this respect, Lynne White, Jr, 'The Historical Roots of Our Ecologic Crisis', *Science,* clv (1967), 1203–7. Another school finds its origin in the early modern period; Carolyn Merchant's *The Death of Nature* (ref. 18) is a good exemplar of this group. Still another group finds the schism rooted in basic human nature; see Garrett Hardin, 'The Tragedy of the Commons', *Science,* clxii (1968), 1243–8. An excellent discussion of the problem is Lawrence Tribe, 'Ways Not To Think About Plastic Trees: New Foundations for Environmental Law', *Yale Law Journal,* lxxxiii (1974), 1315–48.

    The converse of the preference for confining ecological study to undeveloped environments is the reluctance of those concerned with work accidents (whether as an object of study or of regulation) to concentrate on 'heavy' industry at the expense of agriculture. See, for example, Peter Kendall, 'Friends Make Sure Death Can't Deprive Farmer of Final Harvest', *Chicago Tribune,* 7 October 1991, pt 1, 1, 9.
26. Andrew J. Hurley, 'Environmental and Social Change in Gary, Indiana, 1945–1980' (unpublished Ph.D. diss., Northwestern University, 1988). See also Hurley, 'Creating Ecological Wastelands: Oil Pollution in New York City, 1870–1900', *Journal of Urban History,* xx (1994), 340–64.
27. Christopher Sellers, 'Factory as Environment: Industrial Hygiene, Professional Collaboration and the Modern Sciences of Pollution', *Environmental History Review,* xviii (1994), 55–83, at 58. See also Sellers, 'Manufacturing Disease: Experts and the Ailing American

Worker' (unpublished Ph.D. diss., Yale University, 1991).

28. Cronon, *op.cit.* (ref. 1), 12–14. Other theoretical discussions of the method are Barbara Leibhardt, 'Interpretation and Causal Analysis: Theories in Environmental History', *Environmental Review*, xii (1988), 23–36; Arthur F. McEvoy, 'Toward an Interactive Theory of Nature and Culture: Ecology, Production, and Cognition in the California Fishing Industry', in Worster, *Ends of the Earth* (ref. 3), 228–9; and Merchant, *op.cit.* (ref. 19), ch. 1.
29. I thank Barbara Leibhardt and Carolyn Merchant for pointing this out to me. See also Merchant, *op.cit.* (ref. 19), 14–19.
30. Charles F. Sabel, *Work and Politics: The Division of Labor in Industry* (Cambridge: Cambridge University Press, 1982), 37–49.
31. Rachel Carson, *Silent Spring* (New York: Fawcett Crest, 1962). See also John H. Perkins, *Insects, Experts, and the Insecticide Crisis: The Quest for New Pest Management Strategies* (New York: Plenum, 1982).
32. Amory B. Lovins, 'Energy Strategy: The Road Not Taken?', *Foreign Affairs*, 55 (1976), 65–96; Amory B. Lovins, L. Hunter Lovins, and Leonard Ross, 'Nuclear Power and Nuclear Bombs', *Foreign Affairs*, lviii (1980), 1137–77. See also Charles Perrow, *Normal Accidents: Living with High-Risk Technologies* (New York: Basic Books, 1984), 305.
33. Alfred W. Crosby, *Ecological Imperialism: The Biological Expansion of Europe, 900–1900* (Cambridge: Cambridge University Press, 1985), 188–90; William Cronon, *Changes in the Land: Indians, Colonists, and the Ecology of New England* (New York: Hill & Wang, 1983), 135–40; McEvoy, *op.cit.* (ref. 21), 41–51.
34. Esther Boserup, *The Conditions of Agricultural Growth: The Economics of Agrarian Change Under Population Pressure* (Chicago: Chicago University Press, 1965), 117–18. See Mokyr, *op.cit.* (ref. 6), 190–2.
35. McEvoy, *op.cit.* (ref. 21), 91 and 125–32.
36. Stephen Jay Gould, *Wonderful Life* (ref. 6), 50–2 and 283–5; Gould, *Ontogeny and Phylogeny* (Cambridge, Mass.: Harvard University Press, 1977); Gould, 'Evolution and the Triumph of Homology' (ref. 6).
37. James Gleick, *Chaos: The Making of A New Science* (New York: Penguin, 1987), 41; Robert M. May, 'Simple Mathematical Models with Very Complicated Dynamics', *Nature*, cclxi (1976), 459–67; Ilya Prigogine and Isabelle Stengers, *Order Out of Chaos: Man's New Dialogue With Nature* (London: Flamingo, 1984); Daniel B. Botkin, *Discordant Harmonies: A New Ecology for the Twenty-First Century* (Oxford: Oxford University Press, 1990), 8–13.
38. See here William J. Baumol and Jess Benhabib, 'Chaos: Significance, Mechanism, and Economic Applications', *Journal of Economic Perspectives*, iii (1989), 77–105; Richard H. Day, 'The Emergence of Chaos from Classical Economic Growth', *Quarterly Journal of Economics*, xcviii (1983), 201–13.
39. Mokyr, *op.cit.* (ref. 6), 279.

40. Lindy Biggs, 'The Engineered Factory', paper read at joint History of Science Society/Society for the History of Technology annual meeting, Madison, Wisconsin, 1 November, 1991; and Perrow, *op.cit.* (ref. 32), 5–8.
41. Tomlins, *op.cit.* (ref. 14), 385–386.
42. Bill Luckin, 'Accidents, Disasters, and Cities', *Urban History*, xx (1993), 5–18.
43. Compare *Greenman* v. *Yuba Power Products, Inc.*, 59 Cal.2d 57, 377 P.2d 897, 27 Cal. Rptr. 697 (1963), a case involving a home power saw in which the California Supreme Court made manufacturers strictly liable for defects in their products, with *Beshada* v. *Johns-Manville Products Corp.*, 90 N.J. 191, 447 A.2d 539 (1982), in which the New Jersey Supreme Court made an asbestos manufacturer strictly liable for injuries to employees of an electric utility even though the dangers were not fully known until after the injuries in question had taken place. Toxic torts, which are of particular interest to environmentalists, are also as likely to emerge from the home as from the workplace. Here, compare *Beshada*, the asbestos case, with *Sindell* v. *Abbott Laboratories*, 26 Cal. 3d 588, 607 P.2d 924, 163 Cal. Rptr. 132, *cert. denied*, 449 U.S. 912 (1980), which concerned the Dalkon Shield. See, generally, Robert L. Rabin, 'Environmental Liability and the Tort System', *Houston Law Review*, xxiv (1987), 27–63; Jean Macchiaroli Eggen, 'Toxic Reproductive and Genetic Hazards in the Workplace: Challenging the Myths of the Tort and Workers' Compensation Systems', *Fordham Law Review*, lx (1992), 843–912.
44. Tomlins, *op.cit.* (ref. 14), 421 and Sellers, *op.cit.* (ref. 27), 57.
45. Labour historians have, surprisingly, paid little attention to safety issues: one finds occasional mention of industrial accidents in their work, but only as one aspect of the 'working conditions' their subjects faced rather than as a central feature of working-class life. Herbert Gutman, *Work, Culture, and Society in Industrializing America: Essays in American Working-Class and Social History* (New York: Knopf, 1976), 249 and 270. This inattention to safety issues was a general failing of the 'new' labour history of the 1960s and 1970s. Allan M. Brandt, 'Exploring the Dangerous Trades', *Reviews in American History*, xvii (1989), 101–7, at 101.
46. See Karl Figlio, 'What is an Accident?', in Weindling, *op.cit.* (ref. 10), 180–206.
47. I take as a model of this kind of interpretation the 'thick description' of Clifford Geertz. See, for example, his essay, 'Deep Play: Notes on the Balinese Cockfight', in *The Interpretation of Cultures: Selected Essays* (New York: Basic Books, 1973), 412–54.
48. Karl Polanyi, *The Great Transformation: The Political and Economic Origins of Our Time* (New York: Farrar & Rinehart, 1944), 40–1.
49. *Farwell* v. *Boston and Worcester Railroad*, 45 Mass. (4 Met.) 49 (1842); and Tomlins, *Law, Labor, and Ideology* (ref. 14), 347 and 352–63.

50. Tomlins, 'A Mysterious Power' (ref. 14), 391–2.
51. *Ibid.*, 415.
52. Tomlins, *Law, Labour, and Ideology*, 303.
53. Tucker, *op.cit.* (ref. 14), 44.
54. The literature on nineteenth-century employers' liability is vast. Noteworthy examples are Lawrence M. Friedman and Jack Ladinsky, 'Social Change and the Law of Industrial Accidents', *Columbia Law Review*, lxvii (1967), 50–82; Morton Horwitz, *The Transformation of American Law, 1780–1860* (Cambridge, Mass.: Harvard University Press, 1977), 209–10; Jonathon Simon, 'For the Government of Its Servants: Law and Disciplinary Power in the Workplace, 1870–1906', *Studies in Law, Politics, and Society*, xiii (1993), 105–36. A good review of the historiography may be found in Tucker, *op.cit.* (ref. 14), 52–66. See, also, Tucker, 'Law of Employers' Liability in Ontario, 1861–1900: The Search for a Theory', *Osgoode Hall Law Journal*, xxii (1984), 257–79.
55. The story of the fire and its aftermath is well told in Leon Stein, *The Triangle Fire* (Philadelphia: J.B. Lippincott Company, 1962). The role of the fire and its aftermath in catalysing changes in contemporary law and social thought is discussed in Arthur F. McEvoy, 'The Triangle Shirtwaist Factory Fire of 1911: Social Change, Industrial Accidents, and the Evolution of Common-Sense Causality', *American Bar Foundation Working Paper* #9315 (Chicago, 1994), *Law and Social Inquiry*, xx (1995).
56. A number of writers have pointed to the Triangle Fire's signal importance in catalysing Progressive reform. See Robert F. Wesser, *A Response to Progressivism: The Democratic Party and New York Politics, 1902–1918* (New York: New York University Press, 1986), 71; Stephen Bokat and Horace A. Thompson III (eds), *Occupational Safety and Health Law* (Washington: Bureau of National Affairs, 1988), 20; Joseph Huthmacher, *Senator Robert F. Wagner and the Rise of Urban Liberalism* (New York: Atheneum, 1968), 7–9 and 10–11.
57. Frances Perkins, *The Roosevelt I Knew* (New York: Viking, 1946), 23.
58. The phrase, again, is Geertz's. See Geertz, 'Thick Description: Toward an Interpretive Theory of Culture', in Geertz, *op.cit.* (ref. 47), 3–30. Friedman and Percival devoted a chapter of their book on criminal justice in Alameda County, California, to 'Sensations in the Courtroom': criminal trials (usually for murder) that were particularly noteworthy at the time. Their point is that 'what people knew about criminal justice they learned mostly from these show trials, and from nowhere else': Lawrence M. Friedman and Robert Percival, *The Roots of Justice: Crime and Punishment in Alameda County, California, 1870–1910* (Chapel Hill: University of North Carolina Press, 1981), 260.
59. Paul Craven, 'The Meaning of Misadventure: The Baptiste Creek Railway Disaster of 1854 and Its Aftermath', in Roger Hall *et al.* (eds), *Patterns of the Past: Interpreting Ontario's History* (Toronto: Dundurn Press, 1988), 108–29.

60. Tomlins, 'A Mysterious Power', (ref. 14), 421; Michel Foucault, *Discipline and Punish: The Birth of The Prison* (New York: Penguin, 1979), 137–8; Robert W. Gordon, 'Critical Legal Histories', *Stanford Law Review*, xxxvi (1984), 57–126, at 122.
61. Tucker, *op.cit.* (ref. 14), 122–9 and 209.
62. Gabriel Kolko, *The Triumph of Conservatism: A Reinterpretation of American History, 1900–1916* (New York: Free Press, 1963), 103.
63. Hurst, *op.cit.* (ref. 8); Jan G. Laitos, 'Legal Institutions and Pollution' (ref. 8); Joel Franklin Brenner, 'Nuisance Law and the Industrial Revolution', *Journal of Legal Studies*, iii (1974), 403–33.
64. Harry Braverman, *Labor and Monopoly Capital: The Degradation of Work in the Twentieth Century* (New York: Monthly Review Press, 1974), 184–93.
65. David Rosner and Gerald Markowitz, 'Introduction: Workers' Health and Safety – Some Historical Notes', in Rosner and Markowitz, *op.cit.* (ref. 12), xx. Other sources that point to the centrality of health and safety concerns are Rosner and Markowitz, *'Slaves of the Depression': Workers' Letters About Life on the Job* (Ithaca: Cornell University Press, 1987), 108–49; Daniel M. Berman, *Death on the Job: Occupational Health and Safety Struggles in the United States* (New York: Monthly Review Press, 1978); Dorothy Nelkin and Michael S. Brown, *Workers At Risk: Voices from the Workplace* (Chicago: University of Chicago Press, 1984); Nicholas A. Ashford, *Crisis in the Workplace: Occupational Disease and Injury* (Cambridge, Mass.: MIT Press, 1976).
66. Tucker, *op.cit.* (ref. 14), 15.
67. Perrow, *op.cit.* (ref. 32), 67 and Tucker, *op.cit.* (ref. 14).
68. Tucker, *op.cit.* (ref. 14), 19–22 and Tomlins, 'A Mysterious Power' (ref. 14), 386–7.
69. Michel Foucault, *The Order of Things: An Archaeology of the Human Sciences* (London: Tavistock, 1970), xx; Fritz Heider, 'Social Perception and Phenomenal Causality', *Psychological Review*, li (1941), 358–74, at 359; Susan Fiske and Shelley Taylor, *Social Cognition* (Reading, Mass.: Addison-Wesley, 1984), 34–5; Geertz, *op.cit.* (ref. 47), 83; and John C. Burnham, 'The Quest for Health as the History of Modernization', *Reviews in American History*, xvii (1989), 357–63, at 357–8.
70. H.L.A. Hart and Tony Honoré, *Causation in the Law* (Oxford: Oxford University Press, 1985), 16; Thomas Haskell, *The Emergence of Professional Social Science: The American Social Science Association and the Nineteenth-Century Crisis of Authority* (Urbana: University of Illinois Press, 1977), 249; Arthur F. McEvoy, 'The Triangle Shirtwaist Factory Fire' (ref. 55).
71. Douglas Gasking, 'Causation and Recipes', *Mind*, lxiv (1955), 479–87, at 483; Thomas Haskell, 'Capitalism and the Origins of the Humanitarian Sensibility', *American Historical Review*, 90 (1985), 339–61, at 357; and J. Willard Hurst, *Law and Social Order in the*

United States (Ithaca: Cornell University Press, 1977), 157–8.

72. Merchant, *op.cit.* (ref. 19), 23; Elizabeth Ann R. Bird, 'The Social Construction of Nature: Theoretical Approaches to the History of Environmental Problems', *Environmental Review*, 11 (1987), 255–64. On the politics of causal attribution see Deborah Stone, *Policy Paradox and Political Reason* (New York: Harper Collins, 1988), ch. 8.
73. Haskell, *op.cit.* (ref. 70), 15–17.
74. Haskell, *op.cit.* (ref. 71), 563. The cultural historian Thomas Laqueur, likewise, showed how narratives of worker suffering relayed in nineteenth-century Parliamentary inquiries educated the British public about the causes of work accidents and generated pressure for factory reform: Thomas W. Laqueur, 'Bodies, Details, and the Humanitarian Narrative', in Lynn Hunt (ed.), *The New Cultural History* (Berkeley: University of California Press, 1989), 190–5.
75. Calvin Woodard, 'Reality and Social Reform: The Transition from Laissez-Faire to the Welfare State', *Yale Law Journal*, lxxii (1962), 286–328. Lord Bryce observed that the more people learned how to manipulate their natural and social worlds, the less willing they were to tolerate the continued existence of preventable evil: James Bryce, *American Commonwealth* (New York: 1889), Vol. 2, 407. J. Willard Hurst, *Law and the Conditions of Freedom in the Nineteenth-Century United States* (Madison: University of Wisconsin Press, 1956), 73.
76. McEvoy, *op.cit.* (ref. 21), 215–16, 227 and 233; *idem*, *op.cit.* (ref. 28), 222–3.
77. Perrow, *op.cit.* (ref. 32), 67; Laqueur, *op.cit.* (ref. 74), 192–3; Tucker, *op.cit.* (ref. 14), 160; Crystal Eastman, *Work Accidents and the Law* (New York: Charities Publication Committee, 1910), 5, 95; Berman, *op.cit.* (ref. 65), 23–4.
78. Perrow, *op.cit.* (ref. 32), 233 and 246–9.
79. Craven, *op.cit.* (ref. 59), 126; Tucker, *op.cit.* (ref. 14), 63; Tomlins, 'A Mysterious Power' (ref. 14), 421; McEvoy, *op.cit.* (ref. 55).
80. Robert W. Gordon, 'Law and Ideology', *Tikkun*, iii (1985), 14–18, and 83–6, at 15; Robert L. Rabin, 'Federal Regulation in Historical Perspective', *Stanford Law Review*, xxxviii (1986), 1189–1326, at 1280–3.
81. Hurst, *op.cit.* (ref. 8), 198.
82. McEvoy, *op.cit.* (ref. 55); William Hard *et al.*, *Injured in the Course of Duty* (New York: Ridway Co., 1910); Morton Keller, *Affairs of State: Public Life in Nineteenth-Century America* (Cambridge, Mass.: Harvard University Press, 1977), 401–4; Friedman and Ladinsky, *op.cit.* (ref. 54), 65–9.
83. Haskell, *op.cit.* (ref. 70), 565; Jeremy Brecher, *Strike!* (San Francisco: Straight Arrow Books, 1972), 177–85.
84. Tomlins, 'A Mysterious Power' (ref. 14), 421. See also Figlio, *op.cit.* (ref. 46), 197–201.

85. Ecology, indeed, is a way of thinking about otherwise disaggregated phenomena in systematic ways. Describing things from a higher level of integration – species rather than individual organisms, say, or communities rather than populations – makes it possible to perceive otherwise invisible relationships between them and to discern characteristics of the system that contains them. Such elements as stability, diversity, trophic structure, entropy, would disappear from view at a lower level of integration. Arnold M. Schultz, 'The Ecosystem as a Conceptual Tool in the Management of Natural Resources', in S. V. Ciriacy-Wantrup and James J. Parsons (eds), *Natural Resources: Quality and Quantity* (Berkeley: University of California Press, 1967). See also J. K. Feibleman, 'Theory of Integrative Levels', *British Journal of the Philosophy of Science*, v (1954), 59–66.
86. McEvoy, *op.cit.* (ref. 21), 93–5 and 104; Woodard, *op.cit.* (ref. 75), 292–6; Jan G. Laitos, 'Continuities from the Past Affecting Resource Use and Conservation Patterns', *Oklahoma Law Review*, xxviii (1975), 60–96, at 66.
87. Samuel P. Hays, *Beauty, Health, and Permanence: Environmental Politics in the United States, 1955–1985* (Cambridge: Cambridge University Press, 1987), 14–41; Donald Fleming, 'Roots of the New Conservation Movement', *Perspectives in American History*, v (1971), 7–91; George Perkins Marsh, *Man and Nature: Or, Physical Geography as Modified by Human Action*, edited by David Lowenthal (1864, reprinted Cambridge, Mass.: Harvard University Press, 1965), xxii.
88. Unger, *op.cit.* (ref. 25), 9; Antonio Gramsci, *Selections from the Prison Notebooks* (London: Lawrence & Wishart, 1971), 157–8, 195–6; Foucault, *Power/Knowledge: Selected Interviews and Other Writings, 1972–1977* (New York: Pantheon Books, 1980), 104–7.
89. There is a very pertinent statement of this tendency, its roots in contemporary social organization, and its effects on the natural environment in Frederick Engels, 'The Part Played By Labor in the Transition from Ape to Man', in *The Origin of the Family, Private Property, and the State* (New York: Lawrence & Wishart, 1972), 262–4.
90. Laitos, *op.cit.* (ref. 86), 76–8; McEvoy, *op.cit.* (ref. 28), 213 and 218.
91. Robert L. Rabin, 'Environmental Liability and the Tort System', *Houston Law Review*, xxiv (1987), 27–63, at 29; Robert A. Baruch Bush, 'Between Two Worlds: The Shift From Individual to Group Responsibility in the Law of Causation of Injury', *UCLA Law Review*, xxxiii (1986), 1473–1563.
92. Tucker, *op.cit.* (ref. 14), 160; Edison L. Bowers, *Is It Safe to Work?: A Study of Industrial Accidents* (Boston: Houghton Mifflin Co., 1930), 6; and Perrow, *op.cit.* (ref. 32), 9.
93. Tucker, *op.cit.* (ref. 14), 161 and 173.
94. Craven, *op.cit.* (ref. 59), 119; and Tucker, *op.cit.* (ref. 14), 160.
95. *Farwell* v. *Boston and Worcester Railroad*, 45 Mass. at 57.

96. Hurst, *op.cit.* (ref. 71), 198; and Philippe Nonet, *Administrative Justice: Advocacy and Change in a Government Agency* (New York: Russell Sage Foundation, 1969) implicitly take the 'rationalization' perspective. The 'co-optation' view is that of Gabriel Kolko, *op.cit.* (ref. 62), 301–3, though he did not deal with worker's compensation *per se*. For the mixed results of industrial reform, see Tucker, *op.cit.* (ref.14), 209; and Price V. Fishback, 'Liability Rules and Accident Prevention in the Workplace: Empirical Evidence From the Early Twentieth Century', *Journal of Legal Studies*, lvi (1987), 305–28.
97. Tomlins, 'A Mysterious Power' (ref. 14), 411–15.
98. Worster, *op.cit.* (ref. 18), 39–44; Marx, *op.cit.* (ref. 9), 161–2; Botkin, *op.cit.* (ref. 37), 12–13; Prigogine and Stengers, *op.cit.* (ref. 37), 27–55 and 111.
99. Unger, *op.cit.* (ref. 25), 230; Polanyi, *op.cit.* (ref. 48), 56–67.
100. Merchant, *Death of Nature* (ref. 18), 216, 227–35 and 290–3.
101. Donald Worster, 'Toward an Agroecological Perspective in History', *Journal of American History*, lxxvi (1990), 1087–1106, at 1097.
102. McEvoy, *op.cit.* (ref. 21), 104; Clarence J. Glacken, *Traces on the Rhodian Shore: Nature and Culture in Western Thought from Ancient Times to the End of the Eighteenth Century* (Berkeley: University of California Press, 1967), 685–93; Hurst, *op.cit.* (ref. 75), 67–70 and 96–100.
103. Polanyi, *op.cit.* (ref. 48), 68–76 and 163–5.
104. Foucault, *op.cit.* (ref. 60), 150–1; Marx, *op.cit.* (ref. 9), 176–7; and Tomlins, 'A Mysterious Power' (ref. 14), 210.
105. See Mark Seltzer, *Bodies and Machines* (New York: Routledge, 1992); and Anson Rabinbach, *The Human Motor: Energy, Fatigue, and the Origins of Modernity* (Berkeley: University of California Press, 1990).
106. Friedrich Engels, *The Condition of the Working Class in England* (Stanford: Stanford University Press, 1968), 185–8.
107. Foucault, *op.cit.* (ref. 88), 104.
108. Foucault, *op.cit.* (ref. 69), 253–63.
109. See, for example, William M. Landes and Richard A. Posner, 'Causation in Tort Law: An Economic Approach', *Journal of Legal Studies*, xii (1983), 109–34; Guido Calabresi, *The Costs of Accidents: A Legal and Economic Analysis* (New Haven: Yale University Press, 1970); and Steven Shavell, *Economic Analysis of Accident Law* (Cambridge, Mass.: Harvard University Press, 1987). An intelligent discussion of the interaction between regulation, compensation, and tort law is W. Kip Viscusi, 'Toward a Diminished Role for Tort Liability: Social Insurance, Government Regulation, and Contemporary Risks to Health and Safety', *Yale Journal on Regulation*, vi (1989), 65–107.
110. Sherwin Rosen, 'The Theory of Equalizing Differences', in *Handbook of Labor Economics*, Vol. 1 (Amsterdam, 1986), 641–92. For a review of the empirical literature on the problem, see R. S. Smith, 'Compensating Wage Differentials and Public Policy: A Review', *Industrial and Labor Relations Review*, xxxii (1979), 339–52.

111. Smith, *op.cit.* (ref. 110), 350; W. L. F. Felstiner and Peter Siegelman, 'Neoclassical Difficulties: Tort Deterrence for Latent Injuries', *Law and Policy*, xi (1989), 309–29; Richard L. Abel, 'A Critique of American Tort Law', *British Journal of Law and Society*, viii (1981), 199–231, at 200 and 203–6.
112. William L. F. Felstiner and Robert Dingwall, *Asbestos Litigation in the United Kingdom: An Interim Report* (Oxford: Oxford University Press, 1988); Rabin, 'Federal Regulation in Historical Perspective' (ref. 80), 1304; and *idem*, 'Environmental Liability and the Tort System' (ref. 91), 28–33.
113. Polanyi, *op.cit.* (ref. 48), 33.
114. Hurst, *op.cit.* (ref. 71), 160–5.
115. *Ibid.*, 70.
116. *Ibid.*, 203; Lawrence H. Tribe, 'Technology Assessment and the Fourth Discontinuity: The Limits of Instrumental Rationality', *Southern California Law Review*, xlvi (1973), 617–60.
117. *Farwell* v. *Boston and Worcester Railroad*, 45 Mass. at 57, 58, 61; Friedman and Ladinsky, *op.cit.* (ref. 54), 57–8; Hurst, *op.cit.* (ref. 75), 5–6. A nice statement of the faith in the technological future is the opinion of Chief Justice Taney in *Charles River Bridge* v. *Warren Bridge*, 36 U.S. (11 Peters) 420, 552–3 (1837).
118. Foucault, *op.cit.* (ref. 69), xxiv; Unger, *op.cit.* (ref. 25), 185–8; Merchant, *op.cit.* (ref. 19), 261–70.

5

Accidents in the Eighteenth Century

Roy Porter

> A gentleman and lady travelling from Tonbridge towards that part of the Sussex coast which lies between Hastings and Eastbourne, being induced by business to quit the high road, and attempt a very rough lane, were overturned in toiling up its long ascent, half rock, half sand. The accident happened just beyond the only gentleman's house near the lane.

Thus, the first sentences of *Sanditon*, Jane Austen's final, unfinished, novel. Mr Parker has a 'sprained foot'; he begs the handy gentleman to summon the surgeon. '"The surgeon, sir!" – replied Mr Heywood – "I am afraid you will find no surgeon at hand here, but I dare say we shall do very well without him"'; for, he adds, 'we are always well stocked with all the common remedies for sprains and bruises'.[1]

Jane Austen opened her story with an accident. Laurence Sterne filled his masterpiece with them; indeed, the hero of *Tristram Shandy* is the 'sport of small accidents'.[2] 'Begot and born to misfortune', 'a child of interruption', the homunculus Tristram is dogged by 'disgrazias' right from his mis-conception.[3] Dragged into 'this scurvy and disastrous world'[4] by the forceps of the *accoucheur*, Dr Slop, Tristram's nose is 'squeezed as flat to my face as if the destinies had actually spun me without one'.[5] Having lost his name, he later loses his foreskin, when, urged by his lazy nurse to piss out of the window, the sash gives way ('nothing was well hung in our family').[6] In short, Tristram concludes, that 'ungracious Duchess', Fortune, 'has pelted me with a set of as pitiful misadventures and cross accidents as ever small HERO sustained'. Alas poor Yorick![7]

Drama in Austen? Comedy in Sterne? Of course. Yet realism too. *Modern* society, we assume, is uniquely accident-ridden (perhaps, with the fate of Huskisson in mind, the railway appears the watershed:

'shocking accidents reported in almost every day's newspapers happening on the railways', diarized Dick Dyott in 1840).[8] But was not the pre-industrial environment equally hazardous? Roads were abominations, work was performed with unruly beasts of burden and under the heavens, there were the hazards of open fires, naked lights, or universal darkness, and everywhere hordes of infants ('what a many such scrapes from death doth a boys headless [sic!] life meet with', remembered John Clare).[9] Small wonder newspapers, diaries and other sources for the 'long eighteenth century' tell so many sad stories of tragic falls, fires, drownings, firearms explosions, mishaps with tools and knives, potions and poisons, and of ubiquitous traffic spills ('I shall begin to think from my frequent overturns', rued Elizabeth Montagu, 'a bone-setter a necessary part of my equipage for country visiting').[10]

From its opening issue in 1731, the *Gentleman's Magazine* carried a column headed 'Casualties', meaning by that strokes of fate. Most items recorded deaths. Strong-minded readers of the February number encountered one man dropping dead of an apoplectic fit; two murdered in their beds; a pair suffocated while digging a pit; someone drowned in Islington ponds; a coal dealer falling out of a lighter, an attorney tumbling into a fire, a man drowned in the Thames, another in Queenhythe dock, a city butler, just sacked, who slit his throat, a servant's arm broken after a granary collapsed, a house-fire by the River Medway, another in a Stratford corn-mill, a silk-weaver who cut his throat, a drunken clock-maker likewise, a labourer slaying his children, a man gored by an ox in Cheapside, and, completing the carnage, an Oxonian who lurched off Bottley Bridge and met a watery end.[11] Fast-forward to the March number and you find an Eton scholar stabbing his chum to death with a penknife (on the playing field, one wonders?), and the burning of the Duke of Beaufort's seat.[12]

Accidents often stemmed from dangers at work, as with the 'poor man employed at Mr Elliot's brew house, Pimlico' who 'fell into the copper of boiling liquor, and was scalded to death'.[13] Others were endemic in a rickety world of wood, leather and thatch that was always falling apart, as when, in 1765, the floor of the Radcliffe Infirmary gave way, killing six workmen.[14] 'On thursday last', a Norwich newspaper reported, twenty-five years later:[15]

> a fine boy, about five years of age, fell thro' the seat of the necessary belonging to Mr Mapes, in the Hay-market, the reservoir to which is not less than 40 feet deep; in this shocking situation he remained from a quarter past ten till three o'clock in the afternoon, before he was discovered by his cries. A person immediately went down to his

> relief [!], and when he had raised him halfway up, the bucket in which the child was, striking against a timber that had not been perceived, he was again precipitated to the bottom, head forward.

The kid survived. These days he would be further subjected to 'counselling'.

Many had mishaps in liquor, especially through the pre-industrial equivalent of drunken driving: the third Cambridge Professor of Modern History, the immortal Brocket, died of a drunken decline and fall from his horse; and, then as now, what Lawrence Stone dubbed 'affective individualism' made death through misadventure a family event. 'A man working in his vineyard at Argenteuil in France, Aug. 15', the *Gentleman's Magazine* informed its readers,[16]

> bid his son fetch him a vineprop. The boy refused; upon which his father struck him a blow on the temples, whereof he instantly died. The father, stunned with grief, went to throw himself into the well; which the mother seeing, laid down her young child to prevent him, but was drawn with him into the well; and a hog came and killed the child; so that the whole family perished at once.

Little things could be lethal. The Queen of Portugal died of sepsis after having her ear pierced, Erasmus Darwin's son, a medical student, succumbed to septicaemia after cutting his finger while dissecting. Pepys evidently got off light: 'up and to the office (having a mighty pain in my forefinger of my left hand, from a strain that it received last night in struggling avec la femme que je mentioned yesterday)'.[17]

It is too early to graph the varying frequency of calamities – historians cannot even agree whether something as relatively well documented as criminal violence rose or fell over the centuries.[18] What seems indisputable, however, is that the changes and chances of this our mortal life were experienced as ever-lurking threats to life. They could come in battalions. 'We have been very much at leisure for several days past till Sunday last', wrote old Richard Weekes, the Sussex general practitioner to his son, Hampton, in 1802; but then it was all Keystone Cops:[19]

> I was sent for to Pollards wife at Poynings, who has an Infln of the Plura while I was bleeding her Godly's Wife at Ditchg sent out the man came to Poynings after me when I got to Grainger's Gate met Mrs Bridgers Man with his horse sweating profusely said Mrs lay dead & had been near an hour as he had been to my home when I got there she was recoverd from a strong Convulsion fit has had two before I think them of serious consequence rode home very fast, there was Godley teasing me when I got into the shop there was Dr

> Dick with Woolven's Son a lad abt 15 or 16 years of age with his hand shatterd all to pieces by the Bursting of a Gun, he had put a Tourniquet on his Arm & layd him flat on his back, just at this instant, one of Chandler's Girls set her clothes on fire & is most terribly burnt while the man and his wife where at the Church....

Accidents were definitionally unpredictable, but they were taken to heart as moral fables about the human condition, the tragicomedy of the homunculus man, so proud, so vulnerable. An accident was a *memento mori.* And as Mary Fissell has emphasized, when people represented their sicknesses to themselves and their doctors, they often cast their minds far back, locating their troubles in some memorable accident. 'Mr Justinian Pagit's wife fell from her Horse', Elias Ashmole noted on 11 October, 1638, 'which was the cause of all her future sickness'.[20]

Of course, accidents concentrated the mind because they carried deeper significance to Protestant thinking. They were the fingerposts of Providence and divine portents, punishments and reprieves. It was no accident (no *mere* accident, we would say), thought partisans of the Stuarts, that William III's usurping interlude closed after his horse stumbled over a molehill (Jacobites toasted the 'little gentleman in velvet'); that Jacobitical High Tory, Thomas Hearne, reflected likewise when collapsing scaffolding killed dozens watching George I's coronation.[21] 'At Redruth in Cornwall, a miner', noted the *Gentleman's Magazine* obituary column in 1795, 'he was drinking at the Three Compasses in that town, and, in a fit of inebriety, blasphemed the Evangelists, wished perdition to all the kings of the earth, and drank Tom Paine's health; when, on a sudden, his jaw became locked, and he died on the spot in the most excruciating torments'.[22]

Protestant Dissenters had the best X-ray eyes for plotting the paths of Providence, and none was more brimming with malignant *Schadenfreude* than the Revd Oliver Heywood. 'Thursday night Octob 15 1668 was James Duhurst of Newhav, found dead huddling by the church gate at Ratchdale', gloated the Presbyterian, 'his armes over the gate, they found no wound onely his arme hurt with a glasse he had broken being very drunk, tis thought he bled to death, not being able to help himself he was lately turned papist, but indeed an atheist, being an exceeding vile person arrived at a great height of wickedness'.[23]

But if Providence slew, it also saved, averting seemingly unavoidable accidents. Claver Morris, the Wells physician, was ambling home. 'At Weary-All Hill my Mare was so frighted at a Young Bear that was lead along, that she ran down a very Steep and

High place into the Hollow Way, But by the favourable Providence of Almighty God I was not thrown down'.[24] The Lancashire practitioner, Richard Kay, was equally sure of the Divine safety-belt: 'Had we not been preserved by a special Hand of Providence we cou'd not have escaped being much bruised or taken up dead', he wrote after his horse careered off a bridge at night, 'I do believe the Guardianship of Holy Angels, and that a Divine Providence frequently interposeth both for our Safety and Comfort'.[25] Guardian angels also protected the Revd William Jones. Another riding accident: 'that I had not dashed out my brains, by the extreme violence of my fall, was amazing', Jones reflected, ''Twas because angels had charge of me. Providentially [my horse] fell on even, dusty ground. Had it happened 3 or 4 yds onward, where the ground became very stony, falling, as I did, on my left temple, (to speak after the manner of men) my skull, if not composed of steel, must have been fractured'.[26]

Faith in personal Providence was ubiquitous in early modern times, a way of coping with an environment difficult to master. But Enlightenment minds, as Keith Thomas and others have argued, newly tempered Providence with probability, precautions and prudence. The insurance industry grew. In the 1790s, John Byng noted that even wagons could now be seen emblazoned with the Phoenix Insurance emblem, 'which is a novel safeguard, many having taken fire'.[27]

Alongside insurance, the Enlightenment spirit of pragmatic improvement also devised self-help against disaster. Fire-fighting became better organized. 'The wind being very high on Sunday night last Nov 2', noted Thomas Hearne in 1733, 'there had like to have been a very dismal fire, the wind being south west, at Crabtre corner by Smith gate in Oxford.' Calamity was, however, averted: 'The engine was sent for, and good assistance coming, it was happily stopp'd'.[28] In that clubbable age, one of the more useful voluntary associations was the amateur fire brigade. Tirelessly practical, Ben Franklin penned a 'paper ... on the different accidents and carelessnesses by which houses were set on fire, with cautions against them, and the means proposed of avoiding them', before founding a fire-fighting society in Philadelphia, that required its members to provide 'a certain number of leather buckets, with strong bags and baskets ... which were to be brought to every fire; and we agreed to meet once a month and spend a social evening together, in discoursing and communicating such ideas as occurred to us upon the subject of fires, as might be useful in our conduct on such occasions'. Franklin helped set up the Union Fire Company, with its own 'fire-engines, ladders, fire-hooks'.[29]

Alas, neither Providence nor prudence always prevented personal injury. In the days before ambulances, hi-tech casualty wards, X-rays, and operating theatres the medical profession was rarely able to make a decisive contribution, even when (unlike in *Sanditon*) a surgeon was to hand. In early Victorian times, the Quaker, Isabella Harris, was sitting in her gig outside a Yorkshire inn. A commotion blew up; the horse bolted:[30]

> I felt the gig turn, (which I suppose would be when the horse reached the palings), and from that time I have no recollection, till I found myself laid in a room on some chairs, with my dear E. [her husband] and a stranger watching over me. My situation was one of great suffering, feeling so much pain down my left side, that I could not ascertain whether my bones were sound or not; scarcely had I power to lift my hand to my head, which was also severely bruised, my eye being closed without power to open it. They immediately sent for a medical man, who lived three miles distant: when he came he attempted to bleed me, but this he found impracticable, as from my extreme faintness the blood would not flow. He had a further call [to make], and returned to us in about an hour, when he was able to effect his purpose.

That was all the physician did. Next day she was moved to her mother's at Scarborough, where a doctor administered a purge and leeches, and she hovered between life and death for many days. There was no medical examination, however, or further treatment.

Assailed by everyday accidents, people applied first-aid. 'Cut off the top of my thumb', lamented Robert Hooke, 'but cured it in 4 days by Balsamum Peruvianum'.[31] They aided others. 'In shearing Wheat this Afternoon', reported Parson Woodforde, 'Briton cut of part of his left hand Thumb with the Sickle, owing in a great measure to his making too free with Liquor at Norwich to day ... It bled very much. I put some Friar's Balsam to it and had it bound up, he almost fainted'.[32]

First-aid was nothing new. Indeed, Norman Gevitz has traced the genre of first-aid manuals back as far as Stephen Bradwell's *Helps for Suddain Accidents* (1633). But it was Enlightenment practicality and consumerism that got first-aid organized, not least through the sale of ready-made medicine chests (Richard Rees marketed three sorts, one for gentlemen, one for ladies, one for horses).[33]

Domestic self-help in a crisis left doctors in two minds. They worried about silly folk-saws which could prove fatal. In his best-selling *Domestic Medicine* (1769), William Buchan condemned the

> horrid custom immediately to consign over to death every person who has the misfortune by a fall, or the like, to be deprived of the

> appearance of life. The unhappy person, instead of being carried into a warm house, and laid by the fire, or put in a warm bed, is generally hurried away to a church, or barn, or some other cold damp house, where, after a fruitless attempt has been made to bleed him ... he is given over for dead, and no further notice taken of him.

This folly was the result of 'ignorance', 'supported by an ancient superstitious notion, which forbids the body of any person supposed to be killed by an accident to be laid in an house that is inhabited' – a view 'contrary to all the principles of reason, humanity and common sense'.[34]

Like the Genevan Tissot, Buchan was one of many Enlightenment popularizers who set great store by lay first-aid. It was requisite: often no practitioner was available. But it was also perfectly adequate. Experienced and careful lay people could handle most accidents, even serious-sounding conditions such as fractures or dislocated necks ('I have known instances of its being happily performed even by women, and often by men of no medical education').[35] At bottom, Buchan argued, 'every man is in some measure a surgeon whether he will or not'.[36]

Of vital importance, however, Buchan argued, was proper instruction in accident management. The desire to help was rarely matched by skill. Though the villager 'feels an inclination to assist his fellow-creatures in distress, and accidents happen every hour which give occasion to exercise this feeling', ignorance might be fatal, leading to paralysed inaction or rash intervention.[37] For instance, 'Midwives, Gardeners, Blacksmiths, &c.' commonly let blood in accident cases, but 'we have reason to believe that very few know when it is necessary'.[38] In any case, they were misled by various vulgar errors (e.g., that bleeding an extremity drew the disorder in that direction). Not that 'physicians' were any better, Buchan typically insisted, being 'so much the dupes of fashion in this article, as to render it the subject of satire and ridicule'.[39] Yet, at bottom, he commended popular first-aid, being generally optimistic about the healing power of Nature. With wounds, cuts and bruises, best let be, and take plenty of rest: 'It is Nature alone that cures were wounds'.[40] No mysterious expertise was needed, no miracle cures to be expected. He would give no elaborate details about bandaging, Buchan told readers, because 'common sense will generally suggest the most commodious method of applying a bandage'.[41] Doubtless Buchan would have judged Mr Parker's sprained ankle in safe hands with Mr Heywood.

A flood of kitchen physic and 'Every Man His Own Doctor' books gave similar advice. James Parkinson's *The Village's Friend and*

Physician (1804), taught labourers how to cope with high-risk environments, and his *Dangerous Sports. A Tale Addressed to Children* (1808) warned naughty boys not to climb trees or fool around in toolsheds.[42]

For Enlightenment optimism held that hazards lay within human power. Accidents could be avoided, or damage limitation put in hand. Be careful with candles! warned *A Present for a Servant Maid* and dozens of other advice books for domestics.[43] Newspapers campaigned to remedy dangers. On 11 November, 1784, the *Morning Chronicle* protested against the 'frequent accidents that happen from the overflow of outside travellers upon stage coaches', which, it emphasized, is 'a very great nuisance'.[44]

Collective action sometimes followed. In particular, the Society for the Recovery of Persons Apparently Drowned was founded in 1774 – in 1776 it changed its name to the Humane Society and in 1785 to the Royal Humane Society – seeking to spread skills in rescue techniques, especially in accidents with water, though in other sorts of apparent sudden death too. Based on a Dutch predecessor, the Society supplied equipment, awarded prizes, and published pamphlets, advocating mouth-to-mouth resuscitation, tobacco clysters, electric stimulation and the importance of rubbing and keeping warm. Supported by eminent London physicians like William Heberden and John Coakley Lettsom, and blessed by fashionable society, it promoted its views in periodicals such as the *Gentleman's Magazine.*[45]

But public activism went beyond the drowned. Take the *Gentleman's Magazine* itself. It is full of practical tips, contributed by medical men and laymen alike, for countering domestic emergencies – crises caused by eating toadstools,[46] swallowing arsenick,[47] snake bites,[48] farm injuries,[49] mad-dog bites,[50] and the like.

Households were tooling up to cope with crises. But precisely at this time, another solution seems to have become available: the hospital. Here we will be skating on thin historiographical ice till we possess fuller research into Georgian hospitals. But the story may run somewhat as follows. The new charity hospital that loomed so large on the Enlightenment medical map was not initially intended (so far as may be judged from pulpit and press publicity) to be a casualty depot. It was to serve medically useful and morally uplifting purposes in succouring the labouring poor.

Nevertheless, as Mary Fissell has shown,[51] the role of lay governors in hospital business tended to wane, physicians too were not specially assertive, and, as a result, surgeons succeeded in seizing the lion's share in the day-to-day running of the infirmary. Surgeons freely admitted casualty cases, thereby acquiring plenty of patients upon whom to practise and a greater share of the hospital population itself. This liberality with admitting casualties proved self-fulfilling. Increasingly, sick people seeking admission would present themselves as casualty patients. In time, the public came to view hospital as the site for casualties to go, and, perhaps, to die.

In mid-eighteenth-century London, John Baker's man, Jem Kinsett, was thrown off his horse and mangled by a chaise. He was (Baker recorded in his diary)

> brought into house and Mr Nursham [a surgeon] bled him; sent for Dr Hill, who came, and then for Mr Martin, surgeon St Thomas's, lives near Alderman Oliver's, but Mr Nursham, being still there, bled his left arm (he being put on George's bed in back room and clothes pulled off); came Mr Martin out of bed and bled him in right arm - very low – no outward hurt but dreadful pains across his side. At last Mr Martin said it might be a long business and advised to send him to St Thomas's Hospital of which he Surgeon, and a chair was getting for that purpose when I came away at above half past eleven, so it took a full hour.

Baker later visited St Thomas's, bringing the man's clothes (he later died).[52]

By the close of the century, urban accident victims, it seems, were typically being taken to hospital. A speeding carman ran over three women by Blackfriars Bridge, reported the *Gentleman's Magazine* in 1795: 'one woman was killed on the spot, and the other two so much bruised, that they were taken to St Bartholomew's hospital, without hopes of recovery'.[53] Another instance: 'this morning, in Soho Square, a fine boy was fastened on by a large dog, which tore him from the shoulder to the hip, in a manner too shocking to describe. The child was humanely taken into Sir Joseph Banks's house, where fortunately a surgeon happened to be at breakfast, who gave him temporary relief, previous to his being taken to the Middlesex Hospital'.[54]

Hospitals had their own general admission day, but casualties could be admitted at any time, and without a governor's letter. What was the hospital's procedure? The patient was taken to a ward with a spare bed, and the duty dresser called; he was allowed to dress wounds and to do simple operations like 'putting up fractures', 'opening abscesses, or cutting off a finger'. In serious cases, he had to decide whether to send for the duty surgeon or physician; and the patient would be seen in any case by the apothecary next morning.[55]

Waiting to treat him at St Thomas's, a patient around 1800 might have found Weekes, none other than the recipient of the frenzied letter from the Sussex practitioner mentioned above. 'I am taking ye cases of two bad fractures from Wheels passing over', Hampton wrote his father on 2 January, 1802, 'one ye elbow ye other ye ancle & in both ye capsular ligament was compleatly toren thro: but in neither was ye extremity amputated, but I fear they will not do quite well'.[56] Casualties made up much of his workload: 'we have as many accidents now as in winter time', he wrote home that summer, 'ye other day we had a Mason brought in, who had fallen 40 or 50 feet from a scaffolding upon ye left Parietal bone, wh. however was not fractured, but ye integuments lacerated, & some of his brain forced out of ye Ear on that side ... he died in 24 hours'.[57]

The mason fell from the scaffolding. His fall may be symbolic. Originally accidents were subsumed within Providence. In the age of Enlightenment, secularization and self-help spurred first-aid. But the eighteenth century closed, I suggest, with accident cases falling out of lay hands, and into the clutches of a modernizing medical profession with its modernizing institutions.

Notes

1. Jane Austen, *Sanditon*, ed. Margaret Drabble (Harmondsworth: Penguin, 1974), 155. There is of course another and even more significant accident in *Persuasion*. It is a sad irony that Jane Austen did not live to complete *Sanditon*, dying of Addison's disease.
2. Laurence Sterne, *The Life and Opinions of Tristram Shandy*, ed. C. Ricks (Harmondsworth: Penguin, 1967), 179. For discussion see Roy Porter, '"The Whole Secret of Health": Mind, Body and Medicine in *Tristram Shandy*', in John Christie and Sally Shuttleworth (eds), *Nature Transfigured* (Manchester: Manchester University Press, 1989), 61–84, which has extensive bibliography of the theme of medical accidents in the novel.
3. Sterne, *Tristram Shandy*, 68, 295.
4. Sterne, *Tristram Shandy*, 236.
5. Sterne, *Tristram Shandy*, 69.
6. Sterne, *Tristram Shandy*, 369.
7. Sterne, *Tristram Shandy*, 7.
8. Reginald W. Jeffery (ed.), *Dyott's Diary: 1781–1845*, 2 vols (London: Archibald Constable, 1907), ii, 329 (6 December 1840). Discussing the death of Huskisson, George Greville relates: 'I had for days before a strong presentiment that some terrible accident would occur at this ceremony': H. Reeve (ed.), *The Greville Memoirs: a Journal of the Reigns of King George IV and King William IV by the Late Charles C. F. Greville*, 3 vols (London: Longmans, Green, 1875), ii, 48.

9. E. Robinson (ed.), *John Clare's Autobiographical Writings* (Oxford: Oxford University Press, 1983), 35.
10. E. J. Climenson (ed.), *Elizabeth Montagu, The Queen of the Blue Stockings: Her Correspondence from 1720–1761* (London: John Murray, 1906), i, 33. Drownings were exceptionally common. Apparently, surprisingly few people knew how to swim. See N. Orme, *Early British Swimming, 55BC – AD1719* (Exeter: University of Exeter, 1983). For some discussion of a seventeenth-century surgeon's encounters with urban injuries, see Lucinda McCray Beier, 'Seventeenth-Century English Surgery: The Casebook of Joseph Binns', in Christopher Lawrence (ed.), *Medical Theory, Surgical Practice: Studies in the History of Surgery* (London and New York: Routledge, 1992), 48–84, esp. 58–61. Binns's casebooks reveal 14 patients injured in industrial accidents and 19 hurt by horses or carriages, as well as 41 wounded by personal violence.
11. *Gentleman's Magazine* i (1731), 81. Clearly, the *Gentleman's Magazine* was chiefly interested in the news value of violent and sudden deaths, not all of them being what we might call 'accidental'. For discussion see Karl Figlio, 'What is an Accident?', in Paul Weindling (ed.), *The Social History of Occupational Health* (London: Croom Helm, 1985), 180–208; and Paul Weindling, 'Linking Self Help and Medical Science: The Social History of Occupational Health', in Paul Weindling (ed.), *ibid.*, 2–31. For suicides, see O. Anderson, *Suicide in Victorian and Edwardian England* (Oxford: Clarendon Press, 1987). For the health-information role of the magazine, see Roy Porter, 'Laymen, Doctors and Medical Knowledge in the Eighteenth Century: The Evidence of the *Gentleman's Magazine*', in Roy Porter (ed.), *Patients and Practitioners: Lay Perceptions of Medicine in Pre-Industrial Society* (Cambridge: Cambridge University Press, 1985), 283–314; *idem*, 'Lay Medical Knowledge in the Eighteenth Century: the Case of the *Gentleman's Magazine*', *Medical History*, xxix (1985), 138–68.
12. *Gentleman's Magazine*, i (March, 1731), 128.
13. *Gentleman's Magazine*, lxxiii (1803), 1181. The first great work on occupational diseases in English is C. T. Thackrah, *The Effects of Arts, Trades, and Professions ... on Health and Longevity* (London: Longman, 1832).
14. *Gentleman's Magazine*, xxxv (1765), 196.
15. E. A. Goodwyn (ed.), *Selections from Norwich Newspapers* (Ipswich: East Anglian Magazine, 1972), 28.
16. *Gentleman's Magazine*, i (1731), 358.
17. R. Latham and W. Matthews (eds), *The Diary of Samuel Pepys*, 11 vols (London: Bell & Hyman, 1970–83), v, 40.
18. P. E. H. Hair, 'Deaths from Violence in Britain: A Tentative Secular Survey', *Population Studies*, xxv (1971), 5–24; John M. Beattie, *Crime and the Courts in England, 1600–1800* (Oxford: Clarendon Press,

1986); John Styles, 'Crime in Eighteenth Century England', *History Today*, xxxviii (1988), 36–42; J. A. Sharpe, *Crime in Early Modern England 1550–1750* (London: Longman, 1984); P. E. H. Hair, 'Accidental Death and Suicide in Shropshire, 1780–1809', *Transactions of the Shropshire Archaeological Society*, lix (1972), 63–75; Alan Macfarlane, *The Justice and the Mare's Ale* (Oxford: Blackwell, 1981).

19. J. M. T. Ford (ed.), *A Medical Student at St Thomas's Hospital, 1801–1802: The Weekes Family Letters, Medical History*, Supplement No. 7 (London: Wellcome Institute for the History of Medicine, 1987), 57: letter 13, Richard Weekes to Hampton Weekes, 28 Oct., 1801.
20. C. H. Josten (ed.), *Elias Ashmole (1617–1692): His Autobiographical and Historical Notes, His Correspondence*, 5 vols (Oxford: Clarendon Press, 1966), ii, 322; Mary E. Fissell, *The Physic of Charity: Health and Welfare in the West Country, 1690–1810* (Cambridge: Cambridge University Press, 1990), ch. vii, 'The Patient's Perspective'.
21. C. E. Doble (ed.), *Remarks and Collections of Thomas Hearne*, 3 vols (Oxford: Clarendon Press, 1888–9), i, 432–3. For the longer history of Christian attitudes towards Providence, disease and injuries, see Eleanora C. Gordon, 'Accidents Among Medieval Children as Seen from the Miracles of Six English Saints and Martyrs', *Medical History*, xxxv (1991), 145–63. Within medieval Catholicism, the recovery of those apparently killed in accidents had often been credited to divine miracle or the intervention of saints: such attributions apparently stopped within British Protestantism.
22. *Gentleman's Magazine*, lxv (1795), 495.
23. J. H. Turner (ed.), *The Rev. Oliver Heywood B.A. 1630–1702. His Autobiographical Diaries, Anecdote and Event Books*, 4 vols (Brighouse and Bingley: T. Harrison, 1881–5), iii, 101; cf. also iii, 207.
24. E. Hobhouse, *The Diary of a West Country Physician, AD 1684–1726. Extracts from Dr Claver Morris's Diary* (London: Simpkin Marshall, 1934), 90.
25. W. Brockbank and F. Kenworthy (eds), *The Diary of Richard Kay (1716–51) of Baldingstone, near Bury* (Manchester: Chetham Society, 1968), 135.
26. O. F. Christie (ed.), *The Diary of the Rev'd William Jones, 1777–1821: Curate and Vicar of Broxbourne and the Hamlet of Hoddesdon 1781–1821* (London: Brentano's, 1929), 76.
27. C. B. Andrews (ed.), *The Torrington Diaries*, 4 vols (London: Eyre & Spottiswoode, 1954), ii, 120; Keith Thomas, *Religion and the Decline of Magic: Studies in Popular Beliefs in Sixteenth and Seventeenth-Century England* (London: Weidenfeld & Nicolson, 1971; reprinted, Harmondsworth/New York: Penguin, 1978); I. Hacking, *The Emergence of Probability* (Cambridge: Cambridge University Press, 1975); B. Supple, *The Royal Exchange Assurance* (London: Cambridge University Press, 1970).
28. P. Bliss (ed.), *Reliquiae Hearnianae: The Remains of Thomas Hearne,*

M.A. of Edmund Hall, 3 vols (London: John Russell Smith, 1869), i, 107: 13 Nov., 1733.

29. J. Bigelow (ed.), *The Life of Benjamin Franklin by Himself* (Oxford: Oxford University Press, 1924), 124.
30. I. Harris, *Family Memorials: Chiefly the Memoranda Left by Isabella Harris with Some Extracts from the Journal of Her Mother* (no publication place: privately printed, 1869), 148.
31. H. W. Robinson and W. Adams (eds), *The Diary of Robert Hooke (1672–1680)* (London: Taylor & Francis, 1935), 205. First-aid awaits its historian. See meantime J. Webb, 'The Development of First-Aid', *Physiotherapy*, lvii (1971), 365–9; 'First Aid 140 Years Ago', *British Medical Journal*, i (1944), 263.
32. J. Beresford (ed.), *The Diary of a Country Parson: The Rev. James Woodforde, 1758–1802*, 5 vols (reprinted Oxford: Oxford University Press, 1978–81) 210, 28 August, 1790.
33. For the early history of first-aid, see Norman Gevitz, '"Helps for Suddain Accidents": Stephen Bradwell and the Origin of the First Aid Guide', *Bulletin of the History of Medicine*, lxvii (1993), 51–73. The full title of Bradwell's book is *Helps for Suddain Accidents Endangering Life, by Which Those that Live Farre from Physitians or Chirurgions May Happily Preserve the Life of a Poore Friend or Neighbour, Till Such a Man May Be Had to Perfect the Cure. Collected out of the Best Authors for the Generall Good* (London: Thomas Purfoot for T. S., 1633). The medicine chest awaits its historian. But see Roy Porter, 'The Patient in the Eighteenth Century', in Andrew Wear (ed.), *The Social History of Medicine* (Cambridge: Cambridge University Press, 1992), 91–118.
34. W. Buchan, *Domestic Medicine, or a Treatise on the Prevention and Cure of Diseases by Regimen and Simple Medicines* (Edinburgh: Balfour, Auld & Smellie, 1769), 730. People often looked dead, Buchan insisted, but were recoverable. Above all, they should be kept warm, and then the likely cause of misfortune investigated. If it was something in the windpipe, one should try to remove it. If it seemed a case of drowning, victims could often be revived even after they had been under water a couple of hours. Buchan recommended 'a strong person may blow his own breath into the patient's mouth with all the force he can; or, what will generally succeed better, the smoke of tobacco may be blown into the lungs, by means of a pipe or funnel'. Volatiles should be applied to the nose, or the patient put into a warm bath, warm ashes, or hot dung. Buchan also discussed cases of apparent strangulation and of being overcome by fumes, fits, intoxication, and so forth. In all these casualties, Buchan insists on 'a steady perseverance in the use of such means as are therein pointed out'. 'Every good man must feel the strongest propensity, upon such emergencies, to do all in his power to preserve the life of an useful citizen, a beloved friend, or even of an enemy; nor can any pleasure

equal that which a generous mind experiences, when such endeavours are crowned with success': Buchan, *Domestic Medicine*, 730–58. See E. W. A., 'First Aid 140 Years Ago', *British Medical Journal*, i (1944), 262.

35. Buchan, *Domestic Medicine*, 718. For Buchan as a medical popularizer, see C. Lawrence, 'William Buchan: Medicine Laid Open', *Medical History*, xix (1975), 20–35; C. Rosenberg, 'Medical Text and Medical Context; Explaining William Buchan's *Domestic Medicine*', *Bulletin of the History of Medicine*, lvii (1983), 22–4; Roy Porter, 'Spreading Medical Enlightenment: The Popularization of Medicine in Georgian England, and its Paradoxes', in Roy Porter (ed.), *The Popularization of Medicine, 1650–1850* (London: Routledge, 1991), 215–31.

    Regarding 'broken bones', Buchan notes that 'there is in most country villages some person who pretends to the art of reducing fractures. Though in general such persons are very ignorant, yet some of them are very successful; which evidently proves, that a small degree of learning, with a sufficient share of common sense and a mechanical head, will enable a man to be useful in this way.' He concludes, however, 'we would however advise people never to trust such operators, when an expert and skilful surgeon can be had; but when that is impracticable, they must be employed': Buchan, *Domestic Medicine*, 722.

    For Buchan's Swiss equivalent, who offered very similar advice, see S.-A.-A.-D. Tissot, *Advice to People in General, With Respect to Their Health* (London: T. Becket & P. A. de Hondt, 1765; Edinburgh: A. Donaldson, 1766); Antoinette Emch-Dériaz, *Tissot: Physician of the Enlightenment* (New York: Peter Lang, 1992); Maria Szlatky, 'Tissot as Part of the Medical Enlightenment in Hungary', in Roy Porter (ed.), *The Popularization of Medicine, 1650–1850* (London: Routledge, 1992), 194–214.

36. Buchan, *Domestic Medicine*, 695.
37. Buchan, *Domestic Medicine*, 696.
38. Buchan, *Domestic Medicine*, 696. Buchan believed venesection overused.
39. Buchan, *Domestic Medicine*, 696. Buchan lists 'certain harmful prejudices with regard to bleeding [which] still prevail among the country people' – e.g. the notion that taking blood from a limb will draw the disorder in that direction (698), before proceeding to give detailed instructions as to how to carry out the operation.
40. Buchan, *Domestic Medicine*, 705.
41. Buchan, *Domestic Medicine*, 706.
42. James Parkinson's *The Villager's Friend and Physician* (London: Whittingham, 1804). Parkinson explicitly recommended the methods promoted by the Humane Society. There is a good discussion in A. D. Morris, *James Parkinson, His Life and Times* (Boston: Birkhauser, 1989), 57. On drownings, Parkinson suggests (p. 57) 'life has been restored by assiduous exertions. Fail not, therefore, of giving every possible aid,

should the distressful opportunity offer. In this case, let the wet clothes be first entirely taken off, and the body thoroughly dried by rubbing with cloths. This friction is then to be continued, for the purpose of exciting warmth, and particularly over the belly, chest and limbs; and after a little time the warmth of the body should be still farther promoted by placing it in a moderately warm bath of water, sand, ashes, or any other matter, most readily obtained.' With cases of apparent hanging, blood should be let. Those in alcoholic stupor should be vomited and given sal volatile. In the case of those who had suffered wounds from sharp instruments, 'first restrain the bleeding, then bring the parts as nearly as possible into their natural situation and retain them there by slips of sticking plaster and bandages', and apply 'Turlington's Balsam'. In all such cases, 'a life may be saved by the firmness and calmness you may be able to command, and the soundness of the principles on which you act' (p. 60).

See also L. Guthrie, 'The Lady Sedley's Receipt Book, 1686, and Other Seventeenth-Century Receipt Books', *Proceedings of the Royal Society of Medicine*, vi (1913), 150–70; and for broader discussion of medical self-help at this time, Roy Porter and Dorothy Porter, *In Sickness and in Health: The British Experience 1650–1850* (London: Fourth Estate, 1988); Dorothy Porter and Roy Porter, *Patient's Progress: Doctors and Doctoring in Eighteenth-Century England* (Cambridge: Polity Press, 1989).

43. *A Present for a Servant Maid* (Dublin: Faulkner, 1743), 18. For Enlightenment optimism, see David Spadafora, *The Idea of Progress in Eighteeenth Century Britain* (New Haven: Yale University Press, 1990).
44. The newspaper noted that the Hertford coach, which had twenty-five 'outside' passengers, had, not surprisingly, overturned on a road with a steep camber at Houndsditch.
45. P. J. Bishop, *A Short History of the Royal Humane Society* (London: The Society, 1974); Elizabeth H. Thomson, 'The Role of the Physician in Humane Societies of the Eighteenth Century', *Bulletin of the History of Medicine*, xxxvii (1963), 43–51. A scholarly history of the Humane Society would be welcome.

Carolyn Williams has demonstrated that the work of the Humane Society was effectively promoted within a framework of polite, Enlightenment, sentimental values: 'The Genteel Art of Resuscitation', *Transactions of the International Congress of Enlightenment*, viii (1982), 1887–90. This can be discerned from Alexander Johnson, *A Short Account of a Society at Amsterdam ... for the Recovery of Drowned Persons* (London: J. Nourse, 1773), the first publicity exercise on behalf of the Royal Humane Society.

Evidently inspired by the founding of the Humane Society, newspapers began to carry advice for dealing with accident victims. Thus *Jopson's Coventry Mercury*, 31 May, 1784:

> a correspondent has communicated the following directions for the recovery of persons seemingly drowned. – In the first place, strip them of all their wet cloaths; rub them and lay them in hot blankets before the fire: blow with your breath strongly, or with a pair of bellows into the mouth of the person, holding the nostrils at the same time: afterwards introduce the small end of a lighted tobacco-pipe into the fundament, putting a paper pricked full of holes near the bowl of it, through which you must blow into the bowels. Rub all the body, particularly the backbone, hands and feet, with flannels dipped in warm brandy, mixed with sal ammoniac or spirit of hartshorn: strew the flannel as you use it with a little salt. Bleed, if possible, in the jugular vein: give fourteen or fifteen drops of sal ammoniac in water, as soon as it can be swallowed; afterwards, upon recovery, give a cordial of brandy and water warm. Bathe the temples, and rub the nose with any volatile spirit, such as hartshorn or sal volatile; give a clyster or an infusion of tobacco with salt and oil.
>
> Do not easily be persuaded to give over rubbing, or using means for the recovery of the person: many having been recovered, who have shewn little or no signs of life for a great while, and who have lain under water for a considerable time. Apply stone bottles of hot water to the soles of the feet. When all other things have failed, persons have been recovered who have lain several hours under water, by being lain upon a bed of pot-ashes (or dry salt, if that is not to be had) three inches deep; sprinkle upon the person some more pot-ashes about two inches deep; put a cap upon the head containing a good quantity of the same; fill a stocking likewise, with the pot-ashes, and put it round the throat; lay the blankets of the bed over all, but so contrived as not to hinder the person from breathing. When the person begins to recover give a cordial.

For Humane Society insertions in the *Gentleman's Magazine*, see Roy Porter, 'Lay Medical Knowledge in the Eighteenth Century: the Case of the *Gentleman's Magazine*', *Medical History*, xxix (1985), 138–68, at 140, 156.

Gentleman's Magazine, xxxvii (1767), 488.

Gentleman's Magazine, xxxii (1762), 386.

Gentleman's Magazine, viii (1738), 416.

Gentleman's Magazine, xix (1749), 407.

Gentleman's Magazine, xxii (1752), 318; C. Mullett, 'Hydrophobia; its History in England to 1800', *Bulletin of the History of Medicine*, xviii (1945), 44–65.

Mary E. Fissell, *The Physic of Charity: Health and Welfare in the West Country, 1690–1810* (Cambridge: Cambridge University Press, 1990), ch. v, 'The Abdication of the Governors', and ch. vi, 'Surgeons and the

Medicalization of the Hospital'; see also J. Woodward, *To Do The Sick No Harm. A Study of the British Voluntary Hospital System to 1875* (London & Boston: Routledge & Kegan Paul, 1974). Evidence is presented of the role of hospital surgeons in treating industrial and urban accidents in Bernice Boss, 'The Bristol Infirmary (1761–1762) and the "Laborious-Industrious Poor"' (Ph.D. thesis, University of Bristol, 1995).

Of course, surgeons had always fulfilled similar roles. For a good discussion of the role in the community of the early modern surgeon, see L. M. Beier, *Sufferers and Healers: The Experience of Illness in Seventeenth-Century England* (London: Routledge & Kegan Paul, 1987). On the professional emergence of surgery in the eighteenth century see T. Gelfand, *Professionalizing Modern Medicine: Paris Surgeons and Medical Science and Institutions in the Eighteenth Century* (Westport, Conn.: Greenwood Press, 1982).

52. C. Yorke (ed.), *The Diary of John Baker, 1751–58* (London: Hutchinson, 1931), 311.
53. *Gentleman's Magazine*, lxv (1795), 787.
54. *Gentleman's Magazine*, lxix (1800), 790.
55. *Memorials of John Flint South* (London: Murray, 1884), 125. Cf. p. 19: 'cases of strangulated hernia, retention of urine, and all fractures and other accidents were admitted at the discretion of the [duty] dresser, ... who resided entirely in the hospital at his own expense ... upon the dresser in charge was also the responsibility of sending for his surgeon when he considered it necessary'.
56. J. M. T. Ford (ed.), *A Medical Student at St Thomas's Hospital, 1801–1802: The Weekes Family Letters, Medical History*, Supplement No. 7 (London: Wellcome Institute for the History of Medicine, 1987), 100: Hampton Weekes to his father, 2 Jan., 1802: letter 34.
57. Ford (ed.), *A Medical Student at St Thomas's*, 189: Hampton Weekes to his father, 10 July, 1802: letter 83.

6

The Moment of the Accident: Culture, Militarism and Modernity in Late-Victorian Britain

Roger Cooter

Before the last third of the nineteenth century accidental injuries, whether occurring randomly or routinely, were seldom a matter of much public concern. Except when a major disaster struck, attention rarely turned towards them, and collective action was hardly ever called for. A horrible railway collision, a coal pit collapse, a boiler explosion in a factory, might trigger a relief fund for the victims and their families, along with a commission of inquiry and, sometimes, the building of a hospital. Sermons on these tragedies were common; oddtimes a ballad, a tale, or a poem.[1] But all such responses did was to divert attention from the routine of fatal and non-fatal injuries – what were sometimes specified as 'bodily accidents'.[2]

In England – the principal setting for this chapter's concern with such injuries – violent deaths from accidents, according to the Registrar-General in 1846, were 'twice as frequent as in other countries of Europe'.[3] Yet they continued to be decreed 'acts of God', at the same time as they were often attributed to negligence. Their arbitrary, providential nature was reinforced by endless newspaper accounts of bizarre deaths from bolts of lightning, bites from pigs, falls from monuments and bedroom windows, slips into pits of new slaked lime and vats of ale-wort, and legendary consumptions of everything from tobacco, tartar emetic, laudanum, arsenic (mistaken for magnesia), rat poison and corrosive sublimates, to hard peas, marbles and dentures.[4] Accidents were thus conceived as individual, mostly private misfortunes, whether they occurred in the home, on the street, or in mills, mines, factories and workshops.

It is true, of course, that from early in the nineteenth century certain kinds of accident victims acquired a public political presence. Children crippled through employment in mines and factories became a potent issue in Britain in the 1830s and 1840s; revelations in the mid-1840s of the shocking conditions in which railway navvies sustained countless injuries and fatalities became a matter of public concern; and cognizance of accidents in coal mines led to the creation of a mines' inspectorate (of sorts) in 1850. But factory reform, rather than the causes of the breaking of innocent bodies, was the object of the focus on children; the concern with railway labourers concentrated on their living conditions, rather than on their accidents; and the legendary injuries and fatalities of miners mostly provided social statisticians with a resource for moral exhortation.[5]

In the 1870s and 1880s, however, the situation changed; a widespread consciousness of accidental injuries emerged together with general interest in the supply and organization of accident provision. In effect, accidents went public. Although the individualizing, sensational side of accident reportage continued in newspapers, even there qualitative and quantitative changes occurred. In *The Times* the number of reports of accidents of all kinds rose from an average of 300 per annum (from the 1830s) to well over 500 (after 1870).[6] Injuries sustained on streets and on railways, in particular, became regular newsworthy items – but now, not just as anecdotes, but as awesome statistics. A Parliamentary return in 1870 revealed that in London, over the previous four years, some 4,647 persons had been maimed or injured on the streets, of whom 343 had died.[7] In 1879 alone, the year in which a Society for Preventing Street Accidents and Dangerous Driving was established in London,[8] 3,399 persons were reported to the police as injured on the streets of the metropolis, and another 236 were reported as killed – 'a regular increase of about ten percent annually'.[9] Meanwhile, as a result of a clause inserted into the Regulation of Railways Act in 1871, railway companies were required to submit returns on 'accidents and casualties' to the Board of Trade. As the ghastly figures poured in (around a thousand persons killed annually and nearly four times that number injured),[10] publications such as *Railway Accidents: Their Principal Causes and Remedies* (1873) became increasingly common.

At the same time, ambulance transport for the victims of accidental injury became a major preoccupation. An 'ambulance movement' was first spoken of in the 1870s,[11] the concerns of which extended well beyond the hundreds of articles, books, conferences and lectures by doctors, vehicle salesmen, humanitarians, hospital managers, civic officials, local authorities, and legislators.[12] Under the auspices of the St John Ambulance Association, established in 1877, ambulance classes became so popular as to be likened to 'the contagiousness of the "Salvation Army"'.[13] In London, the classes were heavily subscribed to by the police (long responsible for the removal of the victims of accidents in public places) as well as by fashionable 'young ladies'.[14] Indeed, so extensive was the Ambulance Association's encouragement to 'playing at surgery', as the *Saturday Review* mocked the enthusiasm of the 'young ladies' in 1879, that a market was opened for popular lectures on 'accidents to life and limb', and lecturers who were not of the Order of St John felt compelled to establish their credentials.[15] By the late 1880s, by which time there were over 300 St John Ambulance Centres in England, there were already priority disputes as to who had pioneered the movement for 'first-aid'.[16] Meanwhile, the St John Ambulance Brigades (launched in 1887) were mobilized among the working class. By the First World War there were some 23,000 'brigadiers' in British factories, mines and workshops, and at the fields, grounds and pitches of the new mass sports; around a million first-aid certificates had been issued by the St John Ambulance Association; and first-aid competitions had become familiar aspects of pit villages and factory towns.[17]

Again, whereas before the 1870s the number of 'first-aid' manuals could be counted on one hand, by 1879, when the word 'first-aid' was minted,[18] the genre had proliferated, with most such publications spiralling through edition after edition (see Appendix). Much the same occurred within a related body of writing, variously called 'popular', 'household', 'practical' and 'minor' surgery, which was mainly produced by and for the medical profession. Comparatively rare before the 1870s, this literature ceased to be so thereafter when to a considerable extent it merged with the new first-aid literature and/or fed off it.[19] By then, too, there had arisen hospitals intended specifically for 'accident cases'. Although in Britain these institutions were never numerous, it is significant that it was in the 1870s that one of them became nationally and internationally famous – that at Walsall, Staffordshire, established by the Anglican 'Sister Dora'.[20] Around the same time some other hospitals which had long been preoccupied with 'casualty' cases began to style themselves 'Accident Hospitals'.[21]

The moment of the accident had 'arrived', it might be said, both in terms of a social movement and in terms of a new public discourse around accidental injury. But how is this moment – this focusing – to be explained? Like most events in history, reference needs making to a broad spectrum of interests and forces, as this chapter will seek to illustrate. As we shall see, some interests were more important than others. However, the 'moment' cannot be explained simply by reference to them, or rather, it cannot be understood only from the perspective of interests operating in a social and cultural vacuum. For the 'moment' can also be seen as linked to deeper strains and stresses in the late Victorian city, in relation, in particular, to perceptions of arbitrary violence, and to social disorder and destabilization. In various ways the historical moment of the accident aligns with the discursive shift in the representation of public landscapes (from ordered to socially disordered) so well illuminated for late nineteenth-century London by Judith Walkowitz.[22] The moment also articulated with the late nineteenth-century discourse on public health, the entry into which of infective agents violated the boundaries between the private and the public. In these and other ways this chapter seeks to historicize the late nineteenth-century interest in accident provision, treatment and avoidance. In so doing it aims to further extricate the accident from the anecdotal realms of the merely 'accidental'.

Yet it might be protested that the explanation for the growth of interest in accidents towards the end of the century reflects nothing more than their greater incidence. According to an expert on accident insurance writing in the *Journal of the Statistical Society* in 1881, a 15 per cent rise in accidents of all kinds had been detectable since the 1860s. Whereas in 1860, one person in twelve had met with an accidental injury per annum, by 1881 the odds had risen to one person in ten.[23] Such figures were based on insurance claims, however, and insurance claims in turn were based on the sale of accident insurance policies. The figures thus tell us a good deal more about changes in social behaviour and the economic regard of accidents than about their incidence. (They also tell us something about the growth of insurance companies.) But it remains an open question whether accidental injury – as opposed to its reportage – became more prevalent towards the end of the nineteenth century. The number of accidents reported increased, but whether this was an increase relative to the population as a whole is not certain. According to some contemporaries, drawing on statistics from the Registrar-General's reports for the period 1865–81, 'violent deaths' in England and Wales fell from 797 to 675 per million.[24] In 1874 it was calculated that the number of factory accidents 'is much less, in proportion to the number employed, than it was formerly'.[25] The historian John Benson has concluded on the basis of mortality statistics for coal mining in nineteenth-century Britain that the industry actually became safer in the second half of the century.[26]

As Judith Green shows in her contribution to this volume, it is not easy to draw statistically useful conclusions from the figures on fatal accidents in the Registrar-General's reports for the nineteenth century (let alone for non-fatal accidents). For one thing, the types of 'Cause or Character of Violence' referred to by the Registrar-General under the heading of 'Violent Deaths From Accident and Negligence' were, like this general heading itself, frequently changed and rearranged. At different times the list included 'accidents in childbirth', deaths from opium, cocaine, and chloroform, as well as homicides, suicides and executions. But even if the categories could be segregated and standardized, and the statistics regarded as 'accurate' there would be little point, since the meaning of an 'accident' itself has no stability. As all who have written on this subject concur, accident statistics must be treated as subjective attempts at the construction of evidence.[27] Like all statistics they are textual representations, assemblies of rhetorics. Moreover, the mere presence of high-profile statistics on accidents is no guarantee of their public interest. Today, the medical profession periodically remind us that accidents are now the largest cause of death in the age group 1–35,[28] but there is little evidence of immoderate public interest.

Similar cautions need to be extended to the extant hospital records of casualty and accident cases. While these make plain that many hospitals were increasingly inundated with accident cases in the nineteenth century (at the London Hospital, for instance, the number of such cases rose from 5,500 in 1842 to 28,500 in 1901)[29] the apparent increases may only indicate changes in the perceived function of these institutions as places to which injuries (as well as trivial 'casualties')[30] could be reliably taken. As stated in the *Annual Report* of one such hospital in 1892, the increase in accident cases

> would appear to be due, not to an actual increase in the risks of the surrounding manufactories, but to a fuller appreciation of, and confidence in, the means of relief available ... on the part of the managers and employees concerned.[31]

Possibly, too, the greater supply of hospitals in some areas by the end of the nineteenth century (around docks for instance) encouraged this hospitalizing trend. But the reclassification of some hospital patients as 'accident cases' – rather than, as formerly, cases of 'burns, scalds, fractures', etc. – mocks any attempt to use this evidence to quantify the prevalence of accidental injury. The abundance of such statistics towards the end of the century, *vis-à-vis* their earlier absence,[32] again tells us less about the actual size and scale of the problem, than about the cultural context in which it was deemed necessary to gather the statistics.

Arguably, one of the most impressive aspects of that context was the spectre and reality of railway accidents. It has been claimed of these that they were largely responsible for transforming the pre-industrial 'grammatical and philosophical' conception of an accident (as more or less synonymous with 'coincidence') to its modern meaning of a 'technological mishap'.[33] They were also responsible for the abrogation in English common law (in 1846) of the ancient principle of *deodand* requiring the forfeiture of the objects or instruments which had occasioned a person's death. The extent of railway accidents and the amount of capital bound up with them came to render deodand 'irrational'.[34] In other ways too, as negative indicators of the modernity symbolized by railways, these accidents began deeply to concern the public from before the middle of the nineteenth century. It mattered little that there were then (in England) twice as many persons killed annually by horse and horse conveyances as by railways (1000 to 500),[35] and six times as many drowned.[36] The awesome 'railway dragon' had psycho-social and economic dimensions – indeed, theological and intellectual implications – which were lacking among most other potentially large-scale and routine sources of accidents, for railway accidents involved (and continually threaten to involve) persons of status and wealth.[37] That the overwhelming majority of injuries and fatalities on railways (as in other industries) occurred to workers was overridden by this aspect of class.[38] This largely explains not only why Disraeli in 1877 declared railway accidents to be 'perhaps our greatest domestic question',[39] but also why in *Palmer's Index to 'The Times'* from the late 1830s to the 1890s the number of entries on railway accidents was consistently much greater than that on mining accidents, though the latter almost always took a higher toll of life.[40] The average ratio of reports on railway accidents compared to mining accidents was around 5:1; the most striking differential in reportage occurred in 1870 when slightly over 300 railway accidents were reported but only 35 mining accidents, a ratio of nearly 8:1.[41]

But however much railway accidents impacted on Victorian culture, it would be wrong to read the post-1870 public interest in accidental injury as either directly or entirely stemming from this source. The 4,697 trains that arrived daily into London's 22 stations by 1900[42] may have compelled a more 'technological' interpretation of accidents than before, but they were not the only, nor, I will argue, the decisive factor stimulating interest in accidents. Significantly, the *Lancet*'s concern with railways in the 1860s was in relation to public health, not accidents. In the series of articles that the journal published on the subject, the concern was especially with the harmful cerebral effects of train travel on the then 163 million lives annually entrusted to the railways.[43] A reviewer of the book that was compiled from the articles remarked that, as to the question of railway accidents 'producing death or bodily mutilations', these were 'probably very small in comparison with the fatalities arising from diseases engendered and fostered by rapid and persistent railway locomotion'.[44]

Neither was the 'moment' directly occasioned by concern over industrial injury. It is true that the very first venture into ambulance work by the Order of St John began when one of its members organized a rescue service for the ironworks, coal mines and potteries around Burslem in Staffordshire in 1873. In the following year another member, Sir Thomas Longmore, delivered to the General Assembly of the Order his 'Observations on the Preliminary Care and Attention Necessary for Accidental Bodily Injuries and Mutilations Occurring in Mines and Establishments Where Many Workpeople are Employed'. And in the 1880s St John agents undertook 'crusades' in the industrial North of England to promote and then implement those sections of the Acts for the regulation of mines and railways referring to first-aid instruction and provision at the workplace.[45] But there is little evidence to connect this activity, or that of the Brigades after 1887, with raising public consciousness to industrial injury, let alone its politicization. Trade unionists and others interested in workmen's compensation may well have benefited from the 'moment' of the accident, but the origins of the Workmen's Compensation Act of 1897 are not to be found in public demonstrations around industrial accidents, and seem, in fact, to be quite separate.[46] It needs bearing in mind that one of the objects of the St John Ambulance Association was the promotion of itself as a secular humanitarian organization. In part because of this, it soon became less interested in gesturing to the 'bodily injuries and mutilations' of workpeople (to whom first-aid was, as its leaders confessed, 'far from the site of approving witnesses'),[47] than in attending to the needs of large crowds at royal processions, military parades and the like.[48] By 1882, it was also seeking to 'extend its programme so as to place its benefits at the disposal of the sick [of all classes] as well as the injured'.[49] To the latter end, the Association established the Invalid Transport Corps in 1884 which was intended to be financially self-supporting.[50] The purpose in forming the Brigades in 1887 and placing them under the supervision of the Association centres was essentially to enable workers to fend for themselves in first-aid.

From the point of view of accounting for the 'moment of the accident', then, the facts and politics of industrial injury seem less than wholly relevant. To all intents and purposes, industrially injured adult workers remained where they had always been – beyond public gaze. In 1860 the Manchester medical practitioner, John Roberton, observed that 'if "plague, pestilence, and famine" used to be the evils most feared in bygone times, contusions, fractures, dislocations, burns, and other kinds of injury may well be regarded as the dread of the present'. But there was, he noted, one crucial difference between these dreads of past and present: 'whereas the plague and the pestilence were the terror of all ranks, the rich as well as the poor, the bodily injuries now so frequent are the lot mainly of the labouring classes'.[51] However, it was precisely this social and spatial aspect of industrial injuries that tended to keep them out of sight. The overwhelming majority of injuries occurred on building sites and docks, and in railway yards, mines and quarries – relatively private places. As Rosalind Williams has observed with regard to miners and railway tunnellers, their frequent accidents (in contrast to those sustained by railway passengers) were kept 'hidden from the day-light of public awareness'.[52] Industrial accidents did not therefore threaten the splendour of the Victorian city in the way that issues of public health manifestly did, especially once the railways had cut through and exposed the once 'hidden slums'. They were unlike accidents in public thoroughfares which, it was beginning to be commented in 1866 by the middle-class, were of interest 'to all classes'.[53]

It is, finally, no easier to account for the moment of the accident narrowly in terms of medical interests. As I have argued elsewhere, the medical profession had little market interest in the specialist treatment of accidents before the First World War.[54] Those, like Roberton, who might have raised consciousness in relation to accidents, usually did so in the course of pursuing broader agendas, such as hospital and philanthropic reform. Some members of the profession benefited from the setting up of accident hospitals and accident wards, but the principal agents behind these types of provision were not doctors, but persons motivated by religion, humanitarianism and workplace economies (such as the local industrialists who financed Sister Dora).[55]

The medical profession, moreover, rarely took the lead in generating popular interest in accident treatment or prevention. For the most part, they were forced to respond to public enthusiasm. Some undertook the teaching of St John Ambulance classes (largely for reasons of local self-promotion), though the Association's initial insouciance towards these doctors' voluntary labour led to much ill-feeling.[56] Others, perhaps seeking to undermine lay initiatives, began producing textbooks on the treatment of minor emergencies – textbooks intended for the use of general practitioners.[57] Unlike Sir Edward Sieveking, one of the Queen's Physicians and a prominent advocate and committee member of the St John Ambulance Association, most general practitioners were not enamoured of the Association. After all, persons with a grounding in first-aid would be less likely to panic and call for a doctor in the event of a minor accident; self-help was penny-wise. Not only was there good reason to *doubt* the view of the *British Medical Journal*, that first-aid would 'do much to extinguish quackery, bonesetting, and the like',[58] but 'first-aiders' who whisked broken bodies to homes or hospitals robbed doctors of their call-out fee for accidents – in 1870, 3s 6d during day-time and 7s 6d at night.[59] Furthermore, these enthusiasts often upstaged practitioners by demonstrating superior skills at the bandaging and handling of fractures. It was noted in one of the surgical handbooks for medical students and practitioners published in the 1880s that those who had taken St John Ambulance classes 'can put up a fracture better than most medical men'; it therefore behooved the medical profession 'to see that they are not out-stripped in this matter by their lay brothers'.[60] The knowledge that doctors might riot against such lay-upmanship and meddling in their trade was among the principal reasons for the promotion of the prefix 'first' in 'first-aid'. The 'first' was meant to underline that it was aid 'preliminary' to the arrival of qualified and superior medical assistance, as in the tradition of George Hope's *Till the Doctor Comes and How To Help Him*, published by the Religious Tract Society in 1870.[61] While this consideration in itself reflects a degree of medicalization around aid to the injured (absent, say, in the humanitarian provision of food and blankets), the initiation of first-aid and accident awareness and provision largely falls outside a history of medicine focused on professional interests.

Raising consciousness in relation to accidents may have fallen more within the province of the insurance industry. According to Cornelius Walford in his *Insurance Cyclopaedia* (1871–80) – its multi-volumes themselves offering considerable testimony to the contemporary interest in accidents – the modern business of accident insurance 'dates no further back than 1848' when the first fully funded insurance schemes for railway passengers were established. Thereafter – although insurance against railway accidents was to form 'but a very unimportant part of the business of Accident Insurance'[62] – the industry expanded rapidly. Interestingly, early attempts to sell insurance against 'accidents from all causes' to workers, were unsuccessful. Walford himself took credit for informing the insurance companies that 'the real field for their enterprise lay with the professional and mercantile classes' not with workers.[63] 'For the higher classes', he maintained, accident insurance would serve as 'Friendly Societies [already did] ... for the industrial classes'.[64] Here, manifestly, the class specificity of the 'public' interest in accidents is apparent.

There is British and American evidence of medically-authored works on first-aid being widely distributed by life insurance companies to policy holders.[65] But the social and cultural history of insurance in general, and accident insurance in particular – the 'public' history of the process of privatizing and protecting, as it were – has yet to be written.[66] Still largely unknown are the ideological and other connections between the emergent nineteenth-century field of statistics, on the one hand, and actuarial practice on the other, let alone how these practices might have orbited around accidents. Walford was an active member of the Statistical Society of London for many years before his untimely death in 1885,[67] while Alfred Legoyt (1815–85), whom Walford quotes as stating that 'accidental deaths nearly everywhere increase more rapidly than does the population',[68] was the head of the General Statistical Department of France and secretary of the Statistical Society of Paris. If, as seems likely, Legoyt's statement is an expression of fears for populations within the mechanical age, he was in harmony with, among others, the medical statistician William Farr who at mid-century expressed his concern over the 'progress of science ... creat[ing] new forces often fatal ... of which our forefathers had no knowledge'.[69] As many historians have shown, deep cultural anxieties were aroused by the encroachment of machines, whether on rails, streets, factories, battlefields, or in the home; many contemporaries came to regard violence as intrinsic to industrial technology.[70] At the very least, there was recognition that 'progress brings its own responsibilities', as was noted in 1881 by one of the advocates of ambulance services.[71] These and other such sources of fear and instability are crucial to an understanding of the moment of the accident. But precisely how the idea and practice of accident insurance might have animated and fed those anxieties must await further research.[72]

Far more obvious a source for the moment of the accident is the military, or, more exactly, the idealization and popularization of military concepts, values and practices as taken up from around the time of the American Civil War (1861–5) and especially after the Franco-Prussian War of 1870–1. Of course, in comprehending the moment of the accident we should not overlook the role of non-military antecedent circumstances as well as foreign example.[73] But to a large extent, the antecedent circumstances and the foreign models were themselves of a military kind. It was argued in 1884 that the only reason the English were behind in the civil ambulance movement was because of their insularity and freedom from the immediate 'realities of war' in Europe.[74] But by this date the English were in fact fairly committed to the movement largely as a result of military impetus. Without exception, all the principal advocates of ambulance services and first-aid classes had had military experience. For example, Benjamin Howard, the main agent behind the agitation in the early 1880s for an ambulance system for the 'quasi-battlefield of London',[75] was a New Yorker who had served in the Civil War and was particularly keen to promote the horse-drawn ambulance that he had designed for the Union Army.[76] Among Howard's active supporters was the Duke of Cambridge, the Commander-in-Chief of the British Army. In January 1882, a month before the Duke presided over a meeting at the Royal United Services Institute to raise funds for a 'London Ambulance Service' (of which he was to be President),[77] he declared that he looked upon the plans for an organized ambulance service for London 'from a military point of view as well as civil'.[78] In times of war, civilian organization and civil workers would constitute a vital reserve force.

Similar thoughts were entertained by the evangelists of the first-aid and ambulance movement in the Order of St John, all of whom also had military experience – a couple, even in the Prussian Army.[79] The Secretary-General of the Order, Sir Edmund Lechmere (1826–94), author of *Aid to the Injured* (1878), perhaps the least militarily minded, was nevertheless the captain of a company of rifle volunteers.[80] Francis Duncan (1836–88), the Secretary of the Order, first director of its ambulance department, and the author of *First Aid to the Injured* (1881), was a professional soldier in the Royal Artillery before becoming Conservative MP for Holborn.[81] Sir Vincent Kennett-Barrington (1844–1903), who divided his life between organizing humanitarian medical relief during the wars of the later nineteenth century, and promoting St John ambulance work at home and abroad, acquired his calling as a convoy agent for the British National Aid Society (i.e., British Red Cross) during the Franco-Prussian War. Between 1871 and 1878 Kennett-Barrington was also a lieutenant in the Middlesex militia.[82] Surgeon-Major Manley, who organized the ambulance service in Staffordshire (and manned it with ex-army orderlies), was then fresh from the battlefields of France where he had won the Victoria Cross.[83] Another Surgeon-Major, Peter Shepherd (1841–79), was the author of the first official textbook on first-aid, which in 1879, a year after its publication (and Shepherd's death in the Zulu War), was revised and reissued as *First Aid to the Injured*.[84] Sir Thomas Longmore, who appears in the records of the Order in 1870, was then Deputy Inspector-General in the Army Medical Service and the professor of military surgery at Netley. A veteran of the Crimean War and one of the architects of the Geneva Convention of 1864, Longmore was internationally well known for his *Treatise on the Transport of Sick and Wounded Troops* (1869), a work written in the shadow of the American Civil War, and the first to be devoted exclusively to the subject.[85]

Finally, mention must be made of John Furley (1836–1919), generally regarded, with Lechmere and Duncan, as one of the three founders of the St John Ambulance Association. Never happier than when playing soldiers, Furley had been involved with the volunteer militia in Kent since 1860.[86] During the Franco-Prussian War he organized the British voluntary ambulance services (as he would during the Russo-Turkish War of 1876), and acted as the director of the *ambulances volantes* of the French Army during the Commune war of 1871. It was Furley, with six other members of the Order of St John, who pressed for the organization of a British Red Cross in 1868 and secured the support of Colonel R.J. Loyd-Lindsay, the distinguished soldier, Tory MP, and pioneer of the volunteer movement. But Furley was unable to persuade Loyd-Lindsay to go further and commit the substantial reserves of the National Aid Society after the Franco-Prussian War to the creation of a standing peacetime organization to provide medical assistance in civilian emergencies.[87] Furley therefore led the succession from the NAS which resulted in the formation of the St John Ambulance Association (marking the end, incidentally, of other kinds of experiments at medical charity on the part of the Order of St John). It is thus hardly surprising that the Association should have consisted (much like the Salvation Army, founded only a year later) of 'corps', 'divisions' and 'brigades', designed to be 'uniform or interchangeable', with power ascending up a hierarchic chain of command to a central authority.[88] As Furley insisted, 'uniformity and discipline, which were formerly limited to military requirements, are of the first necessity to those who desire by means of organisation to minimize physical suffering'.[89] Like the Duke of Cambridge he also firmly believed that ambulance work in peacetime should be subservient to ambulance work in war.[90]

The military footing of civilian accident services is not merely a consequence of the place of the Order of St John in the ambulance movement by the late 1870s. It is in fact hard to see how the movement could have been conceived otherwise, given the thoroughly militarized vocabulary surrounding all aspects of the work. Even to use the word 'ambulance' around 1870 was to indulge in military parlance – specifically (and strangely to our ears) to refer to an assemblage of men, carriages, and medical and surgical stores and camp functions.[91] (Significantly, a section on 'Navy, Army, and Ambulance' became a regular feature of meetings of the British Medical Association towards the end of the century.) Indeed, there were some who objected to the use of the word 'ambulance' in connection with the work of the Order of St John as 'being too military'.[92]

Similarly, the expression 'first-aid' and its synonymous antecedents can scarcely be extricated from military deployments. 'First principles' was put forward in the 1850s in lectures to the Royal London Militia on 'the injuries incidental to warfare',[93] and one of the earliest uses of 'first-help' appears in the title of a work of 1864 by a professor at the Military Academy at Woolwich who had initially intended his book for the benefit of soldiers and sailors.[94] The practice of 'first dressings', which was to become integral to first-aid, was linked to 'first principles' and was also wholly military in its origins. In the 1870s the concept of first dressings had only recently been celebrated as a result of the introduction of antiseptic bandaging.[95] The modern military concept of a 'first field dressing' – an antiseptic bandage packaged for easy carriage and complete with instructions for use – was devised and first canvassed in 1869 by the eminent Prussian military surgeon, Friedrich von Esmarch (1823–1908)[96] – the same man who in 1875 delivered popular lectures on first-aid[97] and who was made an honorary member of the Order of St John for his various 'civilizing influences' on warfare.

Finally, the word 'accident' itself may have been more closely tied to military usage than has hitherto been appreciated. Much of our present-day association of 'accidents' with non-military matters, as opposed to our association of 'casualties' with the armed forces, dates only from around the middle of the nineteenth century – the same time that 'casualty insurance' was coming to be relabelled 'accident insurance'.[98] Before then, one could read in military medical textbooks about 'the diseases and accidents of soldiers and seamen'.[99]

As noteworthy as these etymologies is the wider construction of social reality after the Franco-Prussian War in terms of the 'civil' or 'civilian' space for dealing with accidents, i.e., in terms which only have meaning in reference to a military 'other'.[100] In works such as *The Ambulance in Civil Life* (1881), 'First Aid to the Wounded in Civil Life' (1884), and 'Ambulance Work in Civil Practice' (1888),[101] 'civilian' was not to be understood as non-military, but rather, the military secularized. These works took it for granted that the military offered the ideal model for the operation and organization of non-battlefield ambulance services. Implicit was a conception of cities as battlefields; indeed, increasingly, this was made explicit, as in the quotation from Benjamin Howard cited earlier. In a chapter on 'Civil Ambulance Work' in one of the handbooks of minor surgery issued in 1889, for example, it was stated that 'in recent years it has been recognized that circumstances much resembling those of war very frequently occur in civil life'.[102] The very scene of some accidents, it was claimed in another publication, was like a battlefield – but worse, since on the battlefield 'you find men prepared for what is happening' and 'regular systematic organization', whereas at the site of a major civil accident there was often little more than confusion.[103] Ergo, what was needed in the handling of and provision for civil accidents was military-style organization and control.

In a chapter on 'Civil Ambulance Arrangements' in *Ambulance Organization, Equipment, and Transport* (prepared by St John's activist, Surgeon-Major G.J.H. Evatt for the International Health Exhibition held in London in 1884), this idea of the battlefield organization of cities was more fully developed. Evatt anticipated the day when London and other British cities would be mapped into 'battle zones' with 'lines of communication' ('telephonic') running from the streets to the hospitals and police departments, where ambulance wagons would stand at the ready together with 'trained medical officials'.

> The existing hospitals, and the many other municipal hospitals needed, should be distributed with system over our great city. A chain of outposts in the shape of municipal dispensaries should bring medical relief within a quarter of a mile of every citizen. Here first aid should be ever ready, and here the outpatients now swarming and crowding at our great hospitals should be dealt with in detail and by districts. At certain hours in the morning, midday, and evening, the sick-transport wagons from the great central hospitals should call at these outlying dispensaries, and carry in comfort the cases chosen for admission to the district central hospital. But far more than this is

> needed, for a ring of great hospitals, combining in the same extensive grounds both convalescent and treating sections, should surround London at a distance far removed from the smoke and overcrowding of our great city. (25–6)

Very nearly, these were the arrangements which would become familiar during the First World War – the systematic movement of the injured from Regimental Aid Posts through to the Casualty Clearing Stations and on down to the base hospitals and convalescent camps.

The 'civilianization' of the accident can thus be seen essentially as an expression of a would-be militarization of urban space, or its public ordering and disciplining. Concurrent with this process was the transformation of the regard of accidents as more or less *private* (individualized) happenings to more or less *public* ones, affecting or concerning the whole of society. This change is all the more striking if we compare the early nineteenth-century literature on accidents with the later literature. The comparison, it emerges, is not between the civil and the military, but rather, between the private 'domestic' (often 'domestic-rural') and the public 'civilian-urban'.

What little writing there was specifically on accidents before the last third of the nineteenth century was almost all of the earlier variety – what Roy Porter in his chapter refers to as the literature of 'domestic *self*-help' (my emphasis). For the most part, as in the section on accidents in William Buchan's *Domestic Medicine*, the concerns were with the remedial action to be taken in cases of burns, dog bites, drownings, poisonings, falls and so on; here anecdotes mix freely with household antidotes. Framed in terms of the dangers of country and village life, this literature was frequently directed at the care of children. An early nineteenth-century example is Thomas Ayre Bromhead's *The Parent's Medical and Surgical Assistant: Intended for the Use of the Heads of Families, Parochial Clergymen and Others; Affording Familiar and Popular Directions for the Management of the Sudden Illnesses and Various Accidents That Require a Prompt and Judicious Treatment, and Will Not Admit of the Delay Necessary for Procuring Regular Advice*, published in London in 1821 and inscribed to 'the magistrates, parochial clergy, and country gentlemen, of Great Britain'. Bromhead, a Fellow of Christ's College, Cambridge, claimed to be responding to a medical colleague's call for clergymen to be educated in domestic medicine.[104] In this respect, as in his concern with accidental injury, the book conforms to a tradition stretching as far back as Stephen Bradwell's *Helps for Suddain Accidents*

Endangering Life (1633).[105] Typically, Bromhead wrote for those who might suffer 'a darling child, or a dear relative ... suddenly attacked with a fit, or injured by some accident'. Such literature was restricted to 'occurrences that may happen in a quiet household', for use in 'the domestic circle', as Karl Schaible, the above-mentioned professor at Woolwich, pointed out in his *First Help in Accidents* (1864).[106] Indeed, such works were often issued as wall charts to be nailed to 'the cottager's fireside' in 'promotion of domestic happiness'.[107] Still within this tradition was Alfred Smee's illustrated wall chart of 1848, *Accidents and Emergencies: A Guide For Their Treatment Before The Arrival of Medical Aid*, even though it also depicted a railway accident, and was widely distributed by the new accident insurance companies (see Appendix).

In contrast, Schaible's book had little to say about the bites and stings of venomous beasts, or the croup and convulsions of children. Drawing heavily on works of military surgery,[108] it emphasized the dressing of wounds, the handling of fractures, the effects of cold and heat, the dislodging of foreign bodies, and the 'hygienic rules for walking and for marches'. But *First Help in Accidents* was not wholly 'civilianized'; it can be seen as transitional, half-way between Bromhead's book and Shepherd's more or less civilian translation of military know-how in his *Aid to the Injured* (1878); half-way also between a medical text on minor surgery and a popular vade-mecum for the cottage gardener, valetudinarian, and traveller.[109] As the subtitle admits, it was in the nature of 'Being a Surgical Guide, In the Absence or Before the Arrival of Medical Assistance, for the Use of the Public, Especially for the Members of Both the Military and Naval Services, Volunteers and Travellers, etc.'. Unlike later full-blown 'first-aid' books, it did not wholly subsume the military under the presentation of 'civilian' requirements. Nevertheless, Schaible was conscious of transcending the pre-existing literature on accidents; unlike the readers of Bromhead or Buchan, Schaible's readers were deemed to have needs more akin to those of soldiers and sailors than rural parishioners.[110] Here was a literature motivated less by feelings for 'a darling child or relative' than by an ability to contend with the would-be hazards on the 'battlefield' of urban life. 'Inwardness' was displaced by 'outwardness', in a move that might be seen as parallel to (and perhaps constitutive of) the displacement of the 'internal' by the 'external' in the meaning of the words 'bodily accidents'. The notion of an internal accident (as in the title of Tissot's mid-eighteenth-century *Advice To The People in ... Acute Diseases, or Upon Any Inward or Outward Accident*) was used in medical discourse until the mid-nineteenth century.[111] Thereafter, with a few exceptions,[112] the word 'accident' tended to be reserved for injuries received from external sources.

The 'civilianization' of the accident in the late nineteenth century – the mapping of cities into rationalized battlezones, first-aid classes and drills, the organizing and uniforming of St John 'divisions' and the like – was not something simply driven by militarism, any more than the moment of the accident can be attributed solely to the advent of the railway.[113] Rather, the 'civilianization' process needs to be seen as a component of social and cultural contexts which were increasingly perceived as disordered. Henry James's depiction of London in 1876 as the 'largest chapter of human accident',[114] was but one expression of what Walkowitz refers to as 'the growing skepticism among men of letters about their capacity to read the city and to sustain a coherent vision of a structured public landscape'.[115] London, with a population soaring to 4.2 million in 1891, personified and clarified the condition of most large towns at the time. In such places the apparent sundering of long-standing and understood spatial boundaries between social classes legitimized and fed discourses on degeneration and decay, entropy and 'wastage', and generated the kinds of social gaze we associate with General Booth.[116] In such contexts, too, came calls for military-like unifying mechanisms and rationalized re-structurings, such as the networking of police and fire services, and the connecting up and co-ordinating across cities of underground water, gas and sewer systems[117] – i.e., large-scale rationalizations which for many late-Victorians were symbolized and epitomized in the railways and the Prussian Army.

Accident services were apiece with the call for rationalized public amenities; no less apparent than their military impetus is the fact that the plans for them were often discussed in terms of co-ordination with police services. Yet we might also regard accidents – insofar as they were seen as statistically predictable yet arbitrary events of violence – as symbols of the omnipresent potential dangers of the socially destabilized late-Victorian urban context. Street or railway accidents may have lacked the intensity of meaning that Jack the Ripper held for London prostitutes in the late 1880s, but something of the same sense of unpredictability, of lurking threat to personal safety was intrinsic to their discussion. The members of the Society for Preventing Street Accidents and Dangerous Driving may only have been a bunch of 'crotchety, fussy, busy bodies ... possessed with a monomania against rapid transit', as their arch-enemies, the Amalgamated Cab Drivers' Society, insisted.[118] But their rhetoric on 'the dangers of the street', the 'slaughter in the streets', conveys more than just a hankering after a safe and secure halcyon past. Simultaneously, it expresses fearfulness of an environment now composed not just of new risks (of larger and heavier-than-ever transport wagons thundering 'reckless and furious' through the narrow streets, unmindful of pedestrians), but also of dark and unpredictable forces (of unlit cabbies in night-time streets and fogs). The latter *bête noire* survived among the members of the Society even after it had been pointed out to them that many more pedestrians were run over during daylight hours than at night.[119] Of course, we can also read this rhetoric more explicitly in terms of class relations: who, after all, were the cabbies and the truckers who were seen to be literally free-wheeling across the social spaces?

My point is simply that preparation against accidents, through classes in first-aid, through the purchase of ambulance wagons, or through establishing effective communication networks between police stations and hospitals, needs to be read in terms wider than the 'practical', or the 'inevitable' or 'natural' response to perceptions of the increased incidence of accidents. The 'practical' is in any case virtually impossible to separate from the cultural and the ideological. Whilst the Fenian bombings in London in the 1880s might have served powerfully to justify the organization of accident services (though I have no evidence for this), they could equally serve to legitimize the militarized cultural construction of the urban landscape as a battlefield in need of rational social management.

Evidence for linking the moment of the accident more closely to the bourgeois cultural anxieties and insecurities of the late nineteenth century can also be derived from the lives of the individuals involved with first-aid and accident services. Sir James Cantlie, for instance, author of *Accidental Injuries: Their Relief and Immediate Treatment* (1884)[120] and the originator, in 1883, of the Army's volunteer ambulance corps (what would later become the Royal Army Medical Corps Territorial Force), was also the author of *Degeneration Amongst Londoners*.[121] In this he depicted an environment so lacking in vital 'ozoned air' as to be a source of 'urbomortis', or at least ennui and physical deterioration, and of stifled individuality and enthusiasm – in short, a London that was bad for health in both physical and ideological senses. 'There is', he grumbled, 'too much thought of the community and not enough of the individual.'[122] Subsequently, in *Physical Efficiency*, which was dedicated to a former Deputy Surgeon-General of the Army Medical Service, Cantlie reviewed 'the deleterious effects of town life' upon the population of Britain as a whole and offered similar 'suggestions for their arrest'.[123] The 'civilianization' of accidents was thus tied to what Cantlie and his social peers understood by the 'civilizing' process – the combating and reversing of the forces of degeneration through the disciplining of the body and the effective management of its physical and social environment, a view that Cantlie further broadcast through his founding of the *Journal of Tropical Medicine* in 1899 and through his imperial medicine in Hong Kong. In stark contrast to the accident as a symbol of the socially arbitrary, transgressive, unbounded, unstable and perilous, were the hierarchically organized and ordered, uniformed and 'de-individualized' but 'vitalized' volunteers whom Cantlie encouraged to fight in the war against 'accidental injury'.[124]

Similar anxieties, expressed pathologically, are also to be found in some of the contemporary texts on accidents. Minas Manook Basil's *The Commoner Diseases and Accidents to Life and Limb* (1887), for example, provides insight into a perception of society desperately in need of coming 'under intelligent control' – indeed, in need of being managed, ideally, through the aping of 'prisons and asylums'.[125] By deliberately seeking neither 'to *define* [an accident], nor to *describe*, nor to *limit*, nor to *delimit*, nor play any other logical or illogical tricks with the word', Basil was able to deploy the word 'in a very broad and very indefinite sense'.[126] He classified as 'medical accidents' not only conventional knocks and falls, but every manifestation of illness occasioned by an infective agent, as well as by those attributed to such new agents as kerosene and coal gas. Pursuing a secular point of view, he argued that

> a broken limb, poisoning by the reckless use of opium or carbolic acid or chloroform, no one would think of calling 'Providential dispensation' ... [therefore], why should poisoning by impure water, impure milk, poisonous drainage gas, &c, be called anything else but accidents due to want of the proper knowledge to avoid them, or to carelessness in availing ourselves of the means of their prevention in cases where we do possess such knowledge?[127]

By this reckoning a great many 'accidents' were not only arbitrary in their occurrence but, because of their invisible agency, ever emanant as perils. Furthermore, because of the invisibility and potential ubiquity of these agents of 'accidents', no boundary could be maintained between the 'private' and 'public'. What Nancy Tomes has called the domestic 'private side' of public health was, in Basil's reckoning, wholly part of the public realm.[128] Consequently, unlike industrial accidents, Basil's domestic accidents (the stuff of public health) did indeed threaten the splendour of the Victorian city. Yet, in ways slightly at odds with historians' views about late nineteenth-century public health propaganda, i.e., as disciplining the behaviour of individuals (especially women) within domestic environments,[129] Basil suggested that domestic *self*-help was no longer sufficient precaution against 'accidents'. His 'accidents' are 'civilianized' or at least 'de-privatized' in that they have become more amenable to 'the concerted action of society'.[130] Thus Basil called for collective vigilance to guard against such potentially dangerous private acts as kissing, touching unwashed hands, eating unsafe foods, drinking unboiled water, inhaling bad breath, occupying closed rooms, and contacting dirt of any kind – functions which hitherto in hygienic sanitarian discourse (like accidents in the conventional sense) had demanded individual responsibility. Although Basil's motive in casting such acts into the language of 'accidents' may only have been to heighten the impact of what was fast becoming a conventional sanitarian message about the threat of germs, there can be no doubt that he rendered the most trivial 'accidents' the subject of a class-specific public gaze. In the light of this gaze, both the 'domestic' and the 'accidental' were transformed and propelled into a perilous public space.

Basil's 'indefinite' application of the word 'accident' to all manner of threatening agencies was unusual. Most contemporary health popularizers kept their pathologizations of domestic environments separate from their messages on accident provision and prevention. Dr Andrew Wilson, for example, a prolific health popularizer, wrote *Common Accidents and How to Treat Them* (1886), before publishing his *A Healthy Home and How to Attain It* (1898) and *Infectious Diseases and How to Prevent Them* (1899).[131] Nevertheless, as the common authorship of these works suggests, there was an increasing proximity between popular works on accidents and illness.[132] This rapprochement may have been hastened by St John first-aid classes, insofar as these were extensively canvassed by housewives interested in the domestic application of such knowledge (often for purposes of home nursing).[133] Indeed by 1898 the St John Ambulance Association was publishing on 'Home Hygiene'.[134] Slightly later, this domestication was furthered through the promotion of household first-aid kits – which should be seen less as a down-market revival of the eighteenth century and earlier 'family medicine chest' of elite households, than as the extension of the first field dressing packets for soldiers advocated by Esmarch and others in the 1860s and implemented during the First World War.[135] To some extent, then, we can speak of a re-domestication of the accident stemming directly from its civilianization as embodied in the work of the St John Ambulance Association. (Perhaps, in more ways than one, then, we need to read the contemporaries' claims for the Association having become 'a household word' by the early 1880s.)[136] At any rate, by the mid-1880s, there was nothing untoward in publishing on 'First Aid To the Wounded' in a journal devoted to sanitary engineering.[137] By then the domestic accident and 'private' health had in effect been reconstituted within the same public space. Possibly in the greater utilization of the word 'emergency' towards the end of the century – as in J.B. Lawrence's *What To Do In Cases of Accidents and Emergencies ... Designed for Family and General Use* (1888)[138] – is signalled the synthesis of these socially constructed 'environments of risk' in the literature of domestic health promotion. But that is another story; here, it is sufficient to note that the domestic accident was no longer what it had been: a matter of private misfortune, largely of individual or local concern. It was now also part of a public domain, and of a cultural discourse directed towards social and ideological ends.

Accidents don't 'just happen', and neither did the interest in them. The multi-faceted growth of interest in accident prevention, treatment, and avoidance in the late nineteenth century is attributable to myriad forces, not least military ones. But the 'public' interest was also a part of deeper socio-cultural anxieties and fears. Whatever the statistical, medical and industrial 'realities' of accidents, the 'moment' of the accident was socio-culturally constructed within its urban setting.

The 'moment', however, was momentary. By the turn of the century its force was spent, both in the narrow sense of interest in the practical business around first-aid and accident provision, and in the wider sense of changes in the society and culture in which these activities occurred. For one thing, first-aid work became more specialized, professionalized and routinized amongst both the voluntary agencies and the volunteers. The journal *First Aid* was launched in 1892, and increasingly first-aid textbooks were split and rearranged for the adoption of particular users, such as policemen, firemen, shipmasters, railroad workers and women.[139] Secondly, concern with accidents, ambulances and rescue work became increasingly that of politicians and bureaucrats. The Consolidating (Factories) Act of 1901, which referred to first-aid in the course of empowering the Secretary of State to make regulations for dangerous trades, the Mines Rescue and Aid Act (1910), and the Home Office's Departmental Committee on the Ambulance Service in the Metropolis (1909) are but some of the many signs of what, for the most part, were delayed governmental responses to lay initiatives. After the war the initiatives largely came from government, with organizations such as the British Industrial Safety

First Association (1918–23), the Safety First Association (1923–41) and the Royal Society for the Prevention of Accidents (1924–) playing quasi-official roles.[140] But the cost was a dampening of the earlier voluntarist enthusiasm. Certainly, the fervour for ambulance services diminished once the municipal authorities began seriously to take charge of provision and co-ordination. Except for London, where the problems were more intractable and not fully resolved until after the First World War, most urban centres had introduced some form of organized ambulance service by 1900.[141] It may be that, as a result of the introduction of such services, there was a diminution of many people's anxieties over the cost of paying general practitioners to care for them in the one-in-ten chance of their sustaining an accidental injury. A 'free', telephonically accessible and reliable service which would transport an injured person to a hospital emergency department could obviate the need for personal accident insurance.[142]

Finally, although post-World War I fiction lent a degree of heroism and romance to ambulance drivers,[143] long before this the popular enthusiam for ambulance classes and practice suffered erosion. From within, among the rank and file in the St John Ambulance Brigades, there was dissent and disillusionment when it became clear that the leadership expected brigadeers to volunteer as stretcher-bearers for the war in South Africa.[144] From without, the medical profession organized themselves in a more militant and united manner against 'the reckless way in which we have taken to giving free instruction in what is called first aid in surgery ... to persons quite outside the profession'.[145]

Yet the late nineteenth-century concern over accidents and accident provision was far from being historically insignificant. The accident which was then forged is still with us. Most of the 'key words' touched upon in this chapter – 'accidents', 'ambulance', 'casualties', 'emergencies', 'first-aid' – have maintained the meanings they acquired during the period under discussion.[146] The resonance of militarism is clear in the retained notion of 'civilian accidents', 'civilian disasters', and 'civil defence'. Such terms remind us that, however much 'the accident' continues to be equated with the arbitrary, the extraordinary, the random, and the unplanned, public interest in accidents need not be so. History may have its accidents, but the late nineteenth-century interest in accidents cannot be numbered among them. That accidents had their 'moment' may surprise many; it might not have been predicted, but it can be explained.

Acknowledgements

I am grateful to Jonathan Morgan, archivist and curator of the Museum of the Order of St John of Jerusalem, for his helpfulness in the research for this chapter. For incisive comments on an earlier draft, I am indebted to John Hutchinson, Bill Luckin, John Pickstone, and Michael Worboys. For funding, my thanks to the Wellcome Trust.

Notes

1. See, for example, John Hodgson, *The Funeral Sermon of the Felling Colliery Sufferers* (Newcastle: E. Walker, 1813); James Brooks, *A Sermon Occasioned by a Melancholy Accident Which Occurred at Hyde, April 1st, 1829, By The Falling in of a Room, in Which Several Hundred Persons were Assembled, Twenty-nine of Whom Lost Their Lives* (Ashton: printed, 1829); Thomas Knox Talon, *The Tay Bridge Disaster. Was It Accident or Judgement? A Sermon* (Edinburgh: D. Douglas, 1880); *Awful Accident on the Ice in Regent's Park, And Loss of 40 Lives [a ballad]* (London: Henry Disley, 1867); *The Railway Accident: A Tale* (London: printed, 1855); Dick Browne, *Tom Downing, Miner. A Tale of a Staffordshire Colliery Disaster* (Stoke-on-Trent: Vyse & Hill, 1896); and Frederick Albert, *The Welsh Miners. A Song on the Recent Colliery Disaster in South Wales* (London: printed, 1877).
2. Newton Bosworth, *The Accidents of Human Life; With Hints For Their Prevention, Or The Removal Of Their Consequences* (London: Allen and Co., 1813), v. Few authors in this genre felt the need to distinguish 'accidents' from 'bodily accidents'; it was taken for granted that an 'accident' meant a sudden or violent bodily injury.
3. Quoted in Cornelius Walford, *The Insurance Cyclopaedia,* Vol. 1 (London: C. and E. Layton, 1871), 4.
4. A list of such 'Remarkable Causes of Violent Deaths' is provided in Cornelius Walford, 'On The Number Of Deaths From Accident, Negligence, Violence, and Misadventure in the United Kingdom and Some Other Countries', *Journal of the Statistical Society,* xliv (1881), 502–4. A glance at *Palmer's Index to 'The Times'* for any period in the nineteenth century wholly confirms Walford's remark that 'the list of examples is capable of great expansion'.
5. John Rule, *The Experience of Labour in Eighteenth-Century Industry* (London: Croom Helm, 1981), 91; Peter Bartrip and S.B. Burnam, *The Wounded Soldiers of Industry: Industrial Compensation Policy, 1833–1897* (Oxford: Clarendon Press, 1983), 68ff.; R.A. Lewis, 'Edwin Chadwick and the Railway Labourers', *Economic History Review,* n.s., iii (1950–51), 107–18; Terry Coleman, *Railway Navvies: A History of the Men Who Made the Railways* (Harmondsworth: Penguin, 1968); Lionel Rolt, *Red for Danger: A History of Railway Accidents and Railway Safety* (4th edn; Newton Abbot: David and Charles, 1982); Robert Colls, *The Pitmen of the Northern Coalfield:*

Work, Culture and Protest, 1790–1850 (Manchester: Manchester University Press, 1987), 40–1; P.E.H. Hair, 'Measuring the Blood on the Coal: The Use and Abuse of Medical Statistics', *Medical Historian*, no. 2 (1989), 3–10; John Benson, *British Coal Miners in the Nineteenth Century: A Social History* (Dublin: Gill & Macmillan, 1980), 43. For a list of colliery accidents in Britain, see Helen and Baron Duckham, *Great Pit Disasters: Great Britain, 1700 to the Present Day* (Newton Abbot: David & Charles, 1973).

6. These are rough calculations tallied from the columns of print on 'accidents' in *Palmer's Index to 'The Times'*. Not all such accidents involved humans and, of course, the meaning of 'accident' cannot be assumed to be consistent over this period.
7. 'Street Accidents', *Lancet*, 12 March, 1870, 387, which maintained that these figures were probably less than half the real numbers. See also the *Lancet* for 20 Aug. and 3 Sept., 1870, 269–70 and 345.
8. Nothing is known of the origins of the Society. It made a deputation to the Lord Mayor of London in October 1879. See the reports on the meetings of the Society in *The Times* of 14 Oct., 1879, and 6, 13, 15, 20, 28, and 31 Jan., 1880.
9. 'Street Accidents', *The Times*, 9 Jan., 1880, 8 col.a.
10. *The City Press*, 16 Feb., 1881, 3; 'Railway Accidents and Ambulance', *The Times*, 7 Sept., 1889; Board of Trade, Railway Department, *Railway Accidents ... During the Nine Months Ending 30th September, 1893* (London: HMSO, 1893). The Board of Trade had required railway companies to report accidents from 1848 but enforcement was lax.
11. See 'Playing at Surgery', *The Saturday Review*, 22 March, 1879 (in press cuttings, St John Ambulance Association Archives); and James Whitson, 'The Ambulance Movement in Scotland', *Edinburgh Medical Journal*, 30 (1884/5), 193–9.
12. On the latter groups in particular, see G.M. Ayers, 'Ambulance Services', in her *England's First State Hospitals, 1867–1930* (London: Wellcome Institute, 1971); Departmental Committee on the London Ambulance Service, *Report* and *Minutes of Evidence*, 2 vols (London: HMSO, 1909); and Desmond T. Tugwood, 'Coventry Ambulance Service: Its Origins and Development, 1872–1974', MA thesis, University of Warwick, 1984.
13. *Medical Press and Circular*, 11 March, 1885, 222. The journal *First Aid*, 16 (1910), 145–6 also likened the movement to the Boy Scouts.
14. 'Playing at Surgery', (ref.11). An analysis of the certificates issued in 1879 by the various St John Ambulance Association centres reveals that in fashionable areas of London, such as Belgravia and Mayfair, women vastly outnumber men (at these two particular centres 3,686 women completed a course of instruction, but only 874 men). However, the same source reveals that the sex ratio was nearly opposite elsewhere. St John Ambulance Association, *Annual Report*,

June 1880, 21–2. The *Annual Report for 1885* noted that of 10,123 certificates issued since the last report, 5,342 were conferred on male classes, 3,417 on female classes, and 1,364 on nursing classes. Cited in *BMJ*, 14 Nov., 1885, 926.

15. See, for example, the prefatory remarks in Minas Manook Basil, *The Commoner Diseases and Accidents to Life and Limb, Firstly, Their Prevention; Secondly, Their Immediate Treatment* (London: J. & A. Churchill, 1887).
16. See Donald Murdoch, *Remarks on the Origin of the First Aid Movement* (Ilfracombe: printed at the *Chronicle* Office, 1889).
17. See Ronnie Cole-Mackintosh, *A Century of Service to Mankind: A History of the St John Ambulance Brigade* (London: Century Bentham, 1986), ix; Nigel Corbet Fletcher, *The St John Ambulance Association, Its History and Its Part In The Ambulance Movement* (London: St John Ambulance Association, 1931), 197; *idem, Annals of the Ambulance Department, Being the History of the St John Ambulance Association and Brigade* (2nd edn, London: St John Ambulance Association, 1949); *idem, Ambulance Competition Tests etc.* (London: J. Bale, 1923); John Furley, *The Origin and Development of the St John Ambulance Association* (London: St John Ambulance Association, 1898 and various later editions); and Joan Clifford, *For the Service of Mankind: Furley, Lechmere and Duncan, St John Ambulance Founders* (London: Robert Hale, 1971). Whether such activity, and the wearing of para-military uniforms, represents subscription to militaristic values among sections of the working class is a matter of debate. See Patricia Morton, 'Another Victorian Paradox: Anti-militarism in a Jingoistic Society', *Historical Reflections*, viii (1981), 169–89; and Richard Price, *An Imperial War and the British Working Class* (London: Routledge, 1972).
18. The word first appears on 24 June, 1879 on page 7 of Francis Duncan's printed 'Report of the Ambulance Department of the Order of St John'. On page 53 of the report is a lecture syllabus entitled 'First Aid to the Injured': Archives of the St John Ambulance Association. The title banner to the *Annual Report* of the Association in June 1880 was 'First Aid to the Injured', the previous *Annual Report* having had merely 'Aid to the Injured'. Francis Duncan went public with 'first aid' when he delivered a paper explaining the aims of the Association to a meeting of the Social Science Congress in Dublin on 4 Oct., 1881: *First Aid to the Injured. The St John Ambulance Association; Its Aim And Objects* (printed as a pamphlet, London: St John Ambulance Association, 1881). Within a year, Peter Shepherd's handbook, *Aids For Cases of Injuries or Sudden Illness* (London: Order of St John, 1878), had been republished as *First Aid to the Injured*: see below.
19. A regulation by the College of Surgeons in the early 1860s requiring candidates for the diploma 'to show a practical acquaintance with the application of surgical apparatus' helps to explain the publication of works such as Thomas Annandale, *Surgical Appliances and Minor*

Operative Surgery (Edinburgh: Maclachlan & Stewart, 1866); William Fairlie Clarke, *Bandages and Splints* (being a supplement to the author's *Manual of The Practice of Surgery*), (London: H. Renshaw, 1868) – from whence the above quotation; and, possibly, Christopher Heath, *A Manual of Minor Surgery and Bandaging For the Use of House Surgeons, Dressers and Junior Practitioners* (London: J. Churchill, 1861). Hitherto most of the basic texts were either French or American, as for example Matthias Mayor's *Popular Surgery: Being Plain Directions Offered to the Public at Large But Particularly to Heads of Families, Captains of Ships, Emigrants, and Persons Engaged in Mines, Manufactories, and Public Works, for Affording Relief In All Cases of Accident, Dangerous Disease, Poisoning, etc. in the Absence of a Regular Practitioner*, trs. Thomas Cutler (London: Longman, Rees, Orme, 1836); Henry H. Smith, *Minor Surgery; or Hints on the Every-day Duties of the Surgeon* (Philadelphia: E. Barrington and G. Haswell, 1843); and John H. Packard, MD, *A Manual of Minor Surgery* (Philadelphia: J.B. Lippincott, 1863). An exception was John Flint South's *Household Surgery: or Hints on Emergencies* (London: John Murray, 1847) which reached a 4th edition ('17,000th') in 1859.

20. Established as a cottage hospital in 1863, it had been intended for the treatment of injured local iron and steel workers, but soon was attracting patients from as far away as Liverpool, Glasgow and London. In 1878, Queen Victoria's daughter, the Princess Imperial of Prussia, wrote for its rules in order to establish a similar institution for industrial casualties in Berlin. See Jo Manton, *Sister Dora: Life of Dorothy Pattison* (London: Methuen, 1971), 251, 341, 221. In 1890 the distinguished surgeon Lawson Tait declared it a shining example of what a cottage hospital could accomplish in the treatment of serious accidents: 'Address in Surgery', *BMJ*, 2 Aug., 1890, 271.
21. An example is the Poplar Hospital established in 1855 mainly for the employees of the East India Company Docks. By 1890 it was officially titled the 'Poplar Hospital for Accidents' and advertised itself as 'open all hours for the treatment of accidental injury or emergency'.
22. *City of Dreadful Delight: Narratives of Sexual Danger in Late-Victorian London* (London: Virago, 1992).
23. Walford, 'On The Number Of Deaths From Accident' (ref. 4), 515.
24. *Ibid.*, commentary by N.A. Humphreys and reply by Walford, 524–5 and 527.
25. Walford, 'Factory Accidents' in his *Insurance Cyclopaedia*, Vol. 3 (1874), 148.
26. Benson, *op.cit.* (ref. 5), 43.
27. See Peter Bartrip and P.T. Fenn, 'The Measurement of Safety: Factory Accident Statistics in Victorian and Edwardian Britain', *Historical Research*, lxiii (1990), 58–72. On the social construction of accidents, see Karl Figlio, 'How Does Illness Mediate Social Relations? Workmen's Compensation and Medico-legal Practices, 1890–1940', in P. Wright

and A. Treacher (eds), *The Problem of Medical Knowledge: Examining the Social Construction of Medicine* (Edinburgh: Edinburgh University Press, 1982), 174–224; and *idem*, 'What is an Accident?', in Paul Weindling (ed.), *The Social History of Occupational Health* (London: Croom Helm,1985), 180–206.

28. See, for example, Royal College of Surgeons of England, Commission on the Provision of Surgical Services, *Report of the Working Party on the Management of Patients with Major Injuries* (November 1988). In the USA, trauma is the number one cause of death in individuals aged between 1 and 44, and motor vehicles are the leading cause of death among those aged 1 to 34: Susan Baker *et al.*, *The Injury Fact Book* (Lexington, MA: D.C. Health, 1984), cited in Susan Baker, 'Injuries in America: A National Disaster', in Russell C. Maulitz (ed.), *Unnatural Causes: The Three Leading Killer Diseases in America* (New Brunswick, N.J.: Rutgers University Press, 1988), 135.
29. As provided in outpatient records from the *Annual Reports* of the London Hospital from 1842. The largest proportion of these 'accidents' were described as 'wounds'; next were 'fractures', then 'contusions'.
30. The word 'casualty' in the mid-nineteenth century had no fixed definition common to all hospitals. It could refer both to the most trivial cases as well as to the most urgent. See the *Lancet* commenting on St Bartholomew's Casualty Department in 1865, quoted in Nuffield Provincial Hospitals' Trust, *Casualty Services and their Setting: A Study in Medical Care* (Oxford: Oxford University Press, 1960), 25. Cf. J. G. Wood, 'Inner Life of a Hospital', *Cornhill Magazine*, v (1862), 462–77 at 463, according to whom 'casualties' were those cases with the slightest problems requiring the least assistance, whereas the graver cases were classified as 'outpatients'.
31. Ancoats Hospital, *Annual Report for 1892.* And see Roger Cooter and John Pickstone, 'From Dispensary to Hospital: Medicine, Community and Workplace in Ancoats, 1828–1948', *Manchester Region History Review*, vii (1993), 73–84.
32. A fact lamented by John Roberton in his paper 'On the Need of Additional As Well as Improved Hospital Accommodation For Surgical Patients in Manufacturing and Mining Districts, But Especially in Manchester', *Transactions of the Manchester Statistical Society*, 1860 (reprinted pamphlet), 1–2, and by Cornelius Walford in his 1881 paper to the London Statistical Society ('On the Number of Deaths From Accidents' (ref. 4), 444–5).
33. Wolfgang Schivelbusch, *Railway Journey: The Industrialization of Time and Space in the 19th Century* (Leamington Spa: Berg, 1986), 131. But the word 'accident' in 'first-aid' texts, from at least as far back as Stephen Bradwell's *Helps for Suddain Accidents Endangering Life* (London: T. Purfoot, 1633) was consistently about unpredictable injury not coincidence. In this sense, too, is Dr Johnson's 'Here malice, rapine, accident, conspire,/ And now a rabble rages, now a

fire ...', cited in Anne Dally, *Women Under the Knife* (New York: Routledge, 1991), 63. On shifts in the medical meaning of an accident, see below.

34. J.H. Baker, *An Introduction to English Legal History*, 2nd edition (London: Butterworths, 1979), 322.
35. Walford, *Insurance Cyclopaedia*, Vol. 1, 5, quoting figures for 1856, when 1,107 persons were killed by horses and horse conveyances. Walford adds that except in England, where 'burns and scalds', and in the USA where 'crushing and bruising' occupy the first place among accidents, 'submersion' is the cause of the greatest number of deaths. For anecdotal confirmation for London, see the breakdown of 'cases of accidents and emergencies' brought to Charing Cross Hospital to the year 1869, in Frank Hart, *The Roots of Service: History of Charing Cross Hospital 1818–1974* (Margate: Eyre & Spottiswoode, 1975), 36–7.
36. See Registrar-General, *Reports of Births, Marriages and Deaths.* In 1879 over 3,000 inquests were held on persons drowned in the inland waters of England. See *The City Press*, 16 Feb., 1881, 3.
37. Schivelbusch, *op.cit.* (ref. 33); Rosalind Williams, *Notes on the Underground: An Essay on Technology, Society, and the Imagination* (Cambridge, MA: MIT Press, 1990); and Walford, *Insurance Cyclopaedia*, Vol. 1, 7. On the theological implications, see James R. Moore, 'Theodicy and Society: The Crisis of the Intelligentsia', in Richard Helmstadter and B. Lightman (eds), *Victorian Faith in Crisis* (London: Macmillan, 1990), 153–86.
38. See Williams, *op.cit.* (ref. 37), 63. In 1858 the Board of Trade maintained that the 'large proportion' of accidents occurring to men employed on the railways was a result of their 'recklessness'. Cited in *Hand-book for Emergencies: Containing Hints and Cautions to Those Engaged in Dangerous Occupations, and to Sufferers by the Common Casualties of Life* (London/New York: Cassell, Petter and Galpin, 1861), 48. Of the 819 persons who died as a result of railways injuries in 1870, only 24 were killed by collisions; 670 were either crushed or run over, the majority, presumably, in the course of employment: *31st Annual Report of the Registrar-General* (London: HMSO, 1871).
39. Cited in Moore, *op.cit.* (ref. 37), 158.
40. From the reports of the Registrar-General it appears that, decennially from 1870 to 1900, only in 1880 did deaths from railway injuries (c. 1,200) outpace those from mines (c.950).
41. Calculated at 5-yearly intervals. Not all 'railway accidents' were serious; included in the category were often trivial mishaps to VIPs.
42. P.J. Waller, *Town, City and Nation: England, 1850–1914* (Oxford: Oxford University Press, 1983), 460.
43. *The Influence of Railway Travelling on Public Health. From the 'Lancet'* (London: Robert Hardwicke, 1862). See also William Camps, *Railway Accidents or Collisions; Their Effects, Immediate and Remote*

Upon the Brain and Spinal Cord and Other Portions of the Nervous System (London: H.K. Lewis, 1866; 2nd edn, 1867); Thomas Wharton Jones, *Failure of Sight from Railway and Other Injuries of the Spine and Head, Its Nature and Treatment* (London: J. Walton, 1869); Sir John Eric Erichsen, *On Railway and Other Injuries of the Nervous System* (London: Watton & Maberly, 1866); Allan Maclean Hamilton, *Railway and Other Accidents with Relation of Injury of the Nervous System. A Book for Court Use* (London: Bailliere, 1904); Thomas Bond, 'Railway Injuries', in Christopher Heath's *Dictionary of Practical Surgery*, 3rd edn (London: Smith, Elder, 1889), Vol. 2, 294–306; and Richard Davy, 'On the Surgical Aspect Of Our Present Mode Of Railway Travelling' (1879), in his *Surgical Lectures* (London: Smith Elder & Co., 1880), 68–73.

44. H.W. Porter, 'On the Influence of Railway Travelling on Public Health', *Assurance Magazine*, xi (Oct. 1863), 152–71 at 154.
45. See letters of Waynman Dixon to Sir Herbert Perrott, 19 August and 16 Sept., 1889, and 13 June, 1890 (Archives of the St John Ambulance Association, file 301–500); 'The Railway Regulation Bill and Ambulance and "First Aid" Work', *The Times*, 24 Aug., 1889; and *Report of Northern 'Crusade'* (London: Order of St John, 1889). The Mines Regulation Act of 1887 required that an ambulance or stretcher, splints and bandages be kept at every mine. However, enforcement was lax. Further pressure from various sources in the 1900s resulted in the Mines Rescue and Aid Act (1910).
46. See W.C. Mallalieu, 'Joseph Chamberlain and Workmen's Compensation', *Journal of Economic History*, x (1950), 45–57; Gilbert Stone, *A History of Labour* (London: Harrap & Co., 1921), 367–84; and Peter Bartrip and S.B. Burman, *The Wounded Soldiers of Industry: Industrial Compensation Policy 1833–1897* (Oxford: Oxford University Press, 1983). Following Anson Rabinbach ('The Body Without Fatigue: A Nineteenth-century Utopia', in Seymour Drescher *et al.* (eds), *Political Symbolism in Modern Europe* (New Brunswick, N.J.: Transaction Books, 1982), 42–62, especially 50) and Eric Hobsbawm ('Custom, Wages and Work-load in Nineteenth-century Industry', in his *Labouring Men: Studies in the History of Labour* (London: Weidenfeld & Nicolson, 1968), 344–70, especially 345), I argue elsewhere that interest in industrial injuries among industrialists and the State follows upon the higher valuation of labour – especially skilled labour – in the 1870s. See Roger Cooter, 'Die medizinische "Entdeckung" von Unfällen und die Industrialisierung medizinischer Sozialbeziehungen in Großbritannien um die Jahrhundertwende', in Dietrich Milles (ed.), *Gesundheitsrisiken, Industriegesellschaft und soziale Sicherungen in der Geschichte* (Bremerhaven: Wirtschaftsverlag NW, 1993), 85–100.
47. John Furley, 'On the Carriage and Removal of The Sick and Injured', *International Health Exhibition* (London: St John Ambulance Association, 1884), 3.

48. This role for the Association had been charted early in its history – sensationally, through the rescue work it performed during the sinking of the pleasure steamer the *Princess Alice* on the Thames on 3 September, 1878, when over 600 lives were lost. On the disaster, see Malcolm Stark, *The Wreck of the Princess Alice* (London: Haughton & Co., 1878).
49. Letter from C.H. Allfrey to Edmund Lechmere, 31 Jan., 1882: St John Ambulance Association Archives. See also 'Ambulance in Civil Practice', *Lancet*, 13 May, 1882, 794; John Furley, *On the Use of Ambulance Litters and Horse Carriages for the Removal of Sick and Injured Persons, Especially in Reference to the Metropolis* (London: Harrison & Sons, 1882); 'Pro Utilitate Hominum', *Medical Press and Circular*, 30 Jan., 1884; and Sir Edward Sieveking, John Furley *et al.*, *Invalid Transport Corps: Report of Meeting Held at St John's Gate, Clerkenwell, 30 March 1887* (London: J.R. Lockwood, 1887).
50. John Furley, *op.cit.* (ref. 47), 16.
51. Roberton, *op.cit.* (ref. 32), 1.
52. Williams, *op.cit.* (ref. 37), 62–3.
53. Edward Law Hussey, *Accidents to Volunteers. A Lecture Delivered to the City of Oxford Companies of the Oxfordshire Rifle Volunteers* (Oxford: E.W. Morris, 2nd edn 1866), 24n.
54. Roger Cooter, *Surgery and Society in Peace and War: Orthopaedics and the Organization of Modern Medicine, 1880–1948* (London: Macmillan, 1993).
55. Exceptional among the medical profession were Hugh Owen Thomas and his nephew Robert Jones who ran an accident hospital and private clinic for the treatment of fractures and orthopaedic conditions in Liverpool from the 1860s. See Cooter, *op.cit.* (ref. 54).
56. Only after members of the profession began to complain about the lack of rewards and recognition for their services as lecturers for the Association, did headquarters realize the need for some placating measures. See 'St John Ambulance Association and the Doctors', *Lancet*, 24 June, 1882, 1054; 'The St John Ambulance Association and the Medical Profession', *BMJ*, 4 and 18 Aug., 1888, 268, 391; and letters (dating from the 1880s) to John Furley and Herbert Perrot of the St John Ambulance Association, St John Ambulance Association Archives.
57. One of the first of which was that by the BMA activist, William Paul Swain, *Surgical Emergencies, Together with the Emergencies Attendant on Parturition and the Treatment of Poisoning. A Manual for the Use of General Practitioners* (London: Churchill, 1874; 5th edn 1896). Swain was surgeon to the Royal Albert Hospital, Devonport, an important place for St John Ambulance activity.
58. *BMJ*, 28 June, 1884, 1286. By 1800 this was a standard trope in popular works on the treatment of accidents. See, for example, Thomas Ayre Bromhead, *The Parent's Medical and Surgical Assistant*

(London: printed and sold by William Phillips, 1821), ix–x; and South, *op.cit.* (ref. 19), viii, who argued that such knowledge would not only deter people from quacks and render them 'less open to the tricks of cunning knaves, whether enjoying the honour of a diploma or not', but also make people 'more capable of estimating the value of honourable and upright practitioners'. The attack on quackery in such works was often allied with abuse of 'irrational' popular lore on the treatment of sudden accidents, such as the urgent need for bleeding. For evidence that St John instruction *contributed* to lay bonesetting and the like, see Roger Cooter, 'Bones of Contention? Orthodox Medicine and the Mystery of the Bone-setter's Craft', in W.F. Bynum and Roy Porter (eds), *Medical Fringe and Medical Orthodoxy, 1750–1850* (London: Croom Helm, 1987), 158–73.

59. 'Death in the Street', *Lancet*, 17 Dec., 1870, 866. The article refers to, but does not specify, 'the Act which prescribes these fees [and] ... the fund to which they are chargeable'.
60. Francis Caird and C.W. Cathcart, *A Surgical Handbook for the Use of Students, Practitioners, House-surgeons and Dressers* (London: C. Griffin, 1889), 157–8.
61. Hope's pamphlet was reprinted in 1871 with revisions and additions from *The Cottager and Artisan.* It was translated into Malagasy and other languages by the Foreign Bible Society.
62. Walford, *Insurance Cyclopaedia*, Vol. 1, 8.
63. Walford, *Insurance Cyclopaedia*, Vol. 1, 8. Many reasons might be assigned for the lack of working-class interest in accident insurance, beyond their alleged fatalism: existing provision in Friendly Societies could be one reason, unstable employment patterns another, and healthy distrust of self-serving insurance companies yet another.
64. Walford, *Insurance Cyclopaedia*, Vol. 1, 6. In colliery districts permanent relief funds were set up to insure miners and their dependants against the financial loss caused by colliery accidents. The first such fund was established in 1861; by 1881, when there were seven covering every major coalfield in England and Wales, a quarter of all coalworkers were thus insured. Benson, *op.cit.* (ref. 5), 187–8.
65. See Appendix: entries on Smee (1848) and Turner (1875).
66. Exceptional is the work of the sociologist Viviana Zelizer, who discusses changing attitudes to children in relation to the taking out of insurance on their lives in the late nineteenth century: Zelizer, *Pricing the Priceless Child: The Changing Social Value of Children* (New York: Basic Books, 1985). See also Zelizer, 'Human Values and the Market: The Case of Life Insurance and Death in 19th-century America', *American Journal of Sociology*, lxxxiv (1978), 591–610; and *idem*, *Morals and Markets: The Development of Life Insurance in the United States* (New York: Columbia University Press, 1979). Valuable theoretical insights can be gained from Francois Ewald, 'Insurance and Risk', in Graham Burchell, Colin Jones and P. Miller (eds), *The Foucault Effect: Studies in Governmentality*

(London: Harvester/Wheatsheaf, 1991), 197–210; Lorraine J. Daston, 'The Domestication of Risk: Mathematical Probability and Insurance 1650–1830', in Lorenz Krüger, L. Daston and M. Heidelberger (eds), *The Probabilistic Revolution*, Vol. 1: *Ideas in History* (Cambridge, MA: MIT Press, 1987), 237–60.

67. Untimely, because he had only reached the letter 'H' at the beginning of the sixth volume of his *Insurance Cyclopaedia*. On Walford, see the *Dictionary of National Biography*.
68. Walford, *Insurance Cyclopaedia*, Vol. 1, 5.
69. Farr, 1856, quoted in Walford, *Insurance Cyclopaedia*, Vol. 1, 5. Unfortunately, Legoyt, referred to, is not discussed in Theodore M. Porter, *Trust in Numbers* (Princeton: Princeton University Press, 1995), 79. Among Legoyt's works is *La France Statistique, au La France Intellectualle, Morale, Financière, Industrielle, Politique, Judiciaire, Militaire, Physique, Territoriale et Agricole* (Paris: Curmer, 1843).
70. Williams, *op.cit.* (ref. 37); Daniel Pick, *War Machine: The Rationalisation of Slaughter in the Modern Age* (New Haven: Yale University Press, 1993).
71. Reginald Harrison, *The Ambulance in Civil Life: Being An Address Delivered at the Liverpool Medical Society, 6 October 1881* (1881; 4th edn London: John Bale, 1902), 24.
72. An obvious starting-point would be the *Journal of the Institute of Actuaries and Assurance Magazine* which ran from 1850 to 1914; in particular, Edwin J. Farren, 'The History of Assurance', *Assurance Mag.*, i (1850), 40–6. See also W.A. Dinsdale, *History of Accident Insurance in Great Britain* (London: Stone & Cox, 1954).
73. For example, in Paris in the 1860s Thomas Longmore experienced the *Secours aux Blessés* stations dotted about the city, which were intended for the assistance of the victims of accidents or sudden illness: Longmore, 'Observations on the Preliminary Care and attention necessary for accidental bodily injuries and mutilations occurring in mines and establishments where many workpeople are employed', read at the Annual General Assembly of the Order of St John of Jerusalem, held in London on St John Baptist's Day, 1874 (printed by the Order, 1874), 23. A fully organized ambulance system was not established in Paris until 1884, largely on the initiative of the Franco-Prussian War veteran, Dr Herman Nachtel. See *Daily Telegraph*, 26 Dec., 1884; *Lancet*, 13 Dec., 1884, 1059–60, and Herman Nachtel, *Fonctionnement de l'ambulance urbaine de New York destinée à porter les premiers sucours sur la voie publique, et utilité qu'il y a d'établir un service de ce genre à Paris* (Paris, 1881). On the incremental and the accidental, see David S. Landes, 'What Room For Accident in History? Explaining Big Changes By Small Events', *Economic History Review*, xlvii (1994), 637–56.
74. John Furley, *op.cit.* (ref. 47), 7–8.
75. Howard, 'A Hospital and Accident Ambulance Service for London', *BMJ*, 4 Feb., 1882, 152.

76. See Howard, 'The New York Ambulance System', *BMJ*, 16 July, 1881, 72–3; *BMJ*, 24 Dec., 1881, 1027, 21 Jan., 1882, 97; *Lancet*, 28 Jan., 1882, 155, 22 July, 1882, 147–8. Howard first came to notice in London in 1878 as the demonstrator of a new method for resuscitating the drowned; see *Illustrated London News*, 6 April, 1878.
77. *Lancet*, 4 Feb., 1882, 202. See also Peter A. Young, 'City Ambulance Associations', *Edinburgh Medical Journal*, xxx (1884–5), 297–300.
78. MS 'Medical Meeting at St John Gate, 16 January 1882' (St John Ambulance Association Archives, Item 352).
79. Among those who attended the meeting at St John Gate in January 1882 (*ibid.*) were Thomas Bond (FRCS) who had been a surgeon in the Prussian Military Service in 1866, and Henry W. Page (FRCS) who had acted as assistant surgeon to the Hessian Division of Germany Army in the Franco-Prussian War. Another medical participant, William Henry Platt, had acted as a surgeon in the Union Army in the American Civil War.
80. Clifford, *op. cit.* (ref. 17), 63. See also Evelyn Shirley, *Hanley and the House of Lechmere* (London: Pickering & Co., 1883). Lechmere was also the Deputy Lieutenant and High Sheriff of Worcester.
81. Henry Blogg, *Francis Duncan: Soldier and Citizen* (London: Kegan Paul, 1892).
82. *First Aid to the Battlefront: Life and Letters of Sir Vincent Kennett-Barrington (1844–1903)*, ed. Peter Morris (Stroud: Alan Sutton, 1992).
83. Clifford, *op.cit.* (ref. 17), 78.
84. See Appendix. On Shepherd, see John Pearn, 'The Earliest Days of First Aid', *BMJ*, 24–31 Dec., 1994, 1718–20.
85. Neil Cantlie, *A History of the Army Medical Department*, Vol. 2 (Edinburgh: C. Livingstone, 1974), 406–10; Longmore, *On the Geneva Convention of August the 22nd 1864 With Some Account of the National Committees Formed For Aiding in Ameliorating the Condition of the Sick and Wounded of Armies In Time of War. A Lecture Delivered at the Royal United Service Institution, on 16th March, 1866, and Printed in the Journal of the Institution, vol. 10, p.162* (London: printed as a pamphlet, 1867); and see R.J. Loyd-Lindsay, *On Aid to the Sick and Wounded in War, A Lecture Delivered at the Royal United Services Institute* (printed pamphlet, 1871), 18.
86. See his *In Peace and War: Autobiographical Sketches* (London: Smith, Elder, 1905); and Clifford, *op.cit.* (ref. 17), 15ff.
87. On the succession, see Sir Henry Brackenbury, 'Philanthropy in War', *Blackwoods Edinburgh Magazine*, cxxi (Feb. 1877), 150–74; John Furley, 'The Red Cross', *Nineteenth Century*, xviii (Dec. 1885), 879–92; and Archie Kirkman Loyd, *An Outline of the History of the British Red Cross Society, From Its Foundation in 1870 to the Outbreak of the War in 1914* (London: n.p., 1917), 18ff.
88. See Cole-Mackintosh, *op.cit.* (ref. 17), 17ff.; Furley, *Autobiographical*

Sketches; Furley's evidence before the Home Office, *Departmental Committee on the London Ambulance Service, vol. II: Minutes of Evidence* (London: HMSO, 1890), Cmd 4564, 53–9; and Clifford, *op.cit.* (ref. 17). On Furley's contributions to the ambulance movement, see his *On the Use of Ambulance Litters* (ref. 49).

89. Furley, 'On the Carriage and Removal of The Sick and Injured' (ref. 47), 5.
90. See 'Ambulance Work and *Materiel* in Peace and War' (report on Furley's speech to the Royal United Service Institution), *BMJ*, 18 June, 1892, 1313–14. Furley was among those in the St John Ambulance Association who organized the Home Hospitals Reserve Corps in 1909. See A.K. Loyd, *op.cit.* (ref. 87), 29.
91. Furley, *op.cit.* (ref. 47), 1–2. Before the Franco-Prussian War the word 'ambulance' was almost unknown in Britain, except in connection with the army medical services. See John S. Haller, Jr, *Farmcarts to Fords: The History of the Military Ambulance, 1790–1925* (Carbondale and Edwardsville: Southern Illinois University Press, 1992), 32; Katherine T. Barkley, *The Ambulance: The Story of Emergency Transportation of Sick and Wounded Through the Centuries* (New York: Exposition Press, 1978); and Norman McLean, 'The English Military Ambulance 1870: the first field ambulance', typescript, RAMC Archives, Item 716, Wellcome Institute for the History of Medicine.
92. Furley, speech reported in *Aid to the Injured. Order of St John of Jerusalem in England. Proceedings of a Public Meeting held on Wednesday Evening, February 6th, 1878, at the Pall Mall Restaurant, Regent Street, London* (Woolwich: A.W. and J.P. Jackson, 1878), 20. 'Surely', he went on, 'it may be used in connection with work of a pacific character, in the same manner as "hospital," which is only suggestive of war when qualified by the word "field" or "military".'
93. George Borlase Childs, *A Few Practical Observations on the Injuries Incidental to Warfare, The Substance of Three Lectures Addressed to the Officers and Privates of the Royal London Militia* (London: J. Churchill, 1854), 32–3.
94. Karl [Charles] Heinrich Schaible, *First Help in Accidents* (London: Robert Hardwicke, 1864).
95. See, for example, A.W. Mayo Robson, 'First Aid to the Wounded in Civil Life', *BMJ*, 3 May, 1884, 854.
96. Esmarch, *Der Erste Verband Auf Dem Schlachtfelds* (Kiel: Schwers, 1869), which was translated into English by Thomas Guy as *The First Dressing on the Battle-field* (Kiel: Schwers, 1870). I am grateful to Claire Herrick for alerting me to this subject. From the start of its operations the St John Ambulance Association equipped itself with 'bandages (after Esmarch)': see report in the *Kentish Independent*, 22 Sept., 1877 (contained in the volumes of press cutting in the Association archives). See also 'The Treatment of the Wounded in Battle', *Daily News*, 18 Feb., 1884.

97. *Die Erste Bei Verletzungen: Ein Populärer Vortrag* (Hanover: Carl Rümpler, 1875). The lectures were translated into English by Esmarch's sister-in-law, HRH Princess Christian, as *First Aid to the Injured; Five Ambulance Lectures* (London: Smith, Elder, 1882); a 7th edition appeared in 1907. An American edition of 1883 was published as *Early Aid in Injuries and Accidents* (Philadelphia: Henry C. Lee, 1883).
98. Everywhere except in America. See Walford, *Insurance Cyclopaedia* (ref. 3), Vol. 1, 6.
99. Sir George Ballingall, 'Biographical Record of Works and Papers on the Diseases and Accidents of Soldiers and Seamen', appended to his *Outlines of the Course of Lectures on Military Surgery* (Edinburgh: Adam Black, 1833). Why and for how long it has been the custom to refer to 'accidents by fire', yet 'casualties at sea' remains to be discovered.
100. This 'civilianizing' discourse in relation to socio-medical issues seems first to appear in the mid-1860s in discussions on extending the Contagious Diseases Act beyond garrison towns. See, for example, 'The Prevention of Syphilis Among the Civil Population', *Lancet*, 4 March, 1865, 235. It is also implicit to writings such as A. Varona, 'The wounded in Times of Peace', *New York Medical Times*, ix (1881–2), 65–7.
101. Harrison, *op.cit.* (ref. 71) – a 5th edition appeared in 1902; Robson, *op.cit.* (ref. 95), 854; Richard Davy, 'Ambulance Work in Civil Practice', *BMJ*, 15 Feb., 1888, 345–7.
102. Caird and Cathcart, *op.cit.* (ref. 60), 157.
103. Baron Mundy, 'On the Urgent Necessity for Making Surgical Provision for Railway Accidents', a lecture delivered at the Royal United Services Institution, 29 July, 1884 (London: printed, 1884), 5; and see Longmore's commentary on p.15.
104. In his preface (vi–vii) Bromhead acknowledges 'a Course of Lectures on Domestic Medicine in the University of Cambridge [by Sir Buswick Harwood, Downing Professor of Medicine], avowedly for the purpose of making their branch of knowledge an indispensable element in the education of clergymen'. Given that the practice of physic had long been bound up with the duties of the clergy, such advocacy might be read as reaction to changes in the professional spheres of doctors and clergymen. See W.J. Sheils (ed.), *The Church and Healing* (Oxford: Oxford University Press, 1982).
105. See Norman Gevitz, '"Helps for Suddain Accidents": Stephen Bradwell and the Origin of the First Aid Guide', *Bulletin of the History of Medicine*, lxvii (1993), 51–73.
106. Schaible, *op.cit.* (ref. 94), vi. Schaible (1824–99), MD, Ph.D., worked mostly as a teacher and liberal journalist in Britain. A participant in the Baden-Palatinate uprising of 1849, he fled to France before arriving in London in 1853. See Karl Marx and

Frederick Engels, *Collected Works*, Vol. 42 (London: Lawrence & Wishart, 1987), 706, and Rosemary Ashton, *Little Germany: Exile and Asylum in Victorian England* (Oxford: Oxford University Press, 1986), 38 *et passim*. He appears to have taught physical drill at Woolwich from about 1862. In Baden, Germany he had been a member of the Medical Officers for the Advancement of Public Medicine.

107. Publisher's advertisement for James Parkinson, *The Way to Health, Being a Selection of Maxims For the Preservation of Health From 'The Villagers Friend and Physician'* [1800] (London: H.D. Symonds, c.1804), price 4d, on the back page of the 1804 edition of Parkinson's *Villager's Friend* (London: H.D. Symonds, 1804).
108. In particular Schaible drew on the work of Dr Beck of Baden, who was also (with Longmore) one of the signatories of the Geneva Convention.
109. For examples of the latter categories, see Appendix: entries on Beecher (1841), Crosby (1881), *Hints and Helps* (1860), Hogg (1853), Kittoe (1837) and Mann (1861).
110. Interestingly, the last nineteenth-century edition of Buchan's *Domestic Medicine* listed in the National Union Catalogue was that of 1863 – the year before the publication of Schaible's book. *Domestic Medicine* seems to have been most popular between the 1770s and 1840s.
111. Samuel A.A.D. Tissot, *Advice To The People In General, With Regard To Their Health: But Particularly Calculated For Those, Who Are The Most Unlikely To Be Provided In Time With The Best Assistance, In Acute Diseases, Or Upon Any Inward Or Outward Accident*, translated from the French edition of 1761 by J. Kirkpatrick (London: T. Becket, 1767). A 7th edition appeared in 1801. On the continuance of this usage, see, for instance, Michael Ryan 'Introductory Lecture on the Theory and Practice of Midwifery', *Lancet*, ii (1827–8), 394–400, and Heath, *Manual of Minor Surgery* (ref. 19).
112. The medical profession still speaks of cardio-vascular 'accidents' when meaning an unexpected haemorrhage, and of neurological accidents in reference to strokes. Some unexpected complications in pregnancy are also thus labelled. My thanks to Dr Peter Mohr for this information.
113. In truth, as Schivelbusch points out (*op.cit.*, ref. 33), 'in the creation of the modern military there was a mechanization of the "human material" analogous to the mechanization in the more or less simultaneously emerging process of mass manufacture' (153); 'the technical and organizational development of the military is a paradigm for the simultaneous or immediately subsequent analogous development of the civilian productive forces' (158).
114. Cited in Walkowitz, *op.cit.* (ref. 22), 15.
115. *Ibid.*, 39. For other contemporary perceptions of disorder in London, cast especially in bodily metaphors of ill-health, see James Winter, *London's Teeming Streets, 1830–1914* (London: Routledge, 1993),

especially chapter 1, 'Imagining'. See also Dina M. Copelman, 'The Gendered Metropolis: Fin-de-Siècle London', *Radical History Review*, lx (1994), 38–56.

116. Walkowitz, *op.cit.* (ref. 22), 31. See also Daniel Pick, *Faces of Degeneration: A European Disorder, c.1848–c.1918* (Cambridge: Cambridge University Press, 1989); Anson Rabinbach, *The Human Motor: Energy, Fatigue and the Origins of Modernity* (Berkeley: University of California Press, 1992); Schivelbusch, *op.cit.* (ref. 33); Robert Wiebe, *The Search for Order, 1877–1920* (New York: Hill and Wang, 1967); Stephen Kern, *The Culture of Time and Space, 1880–1918* (Cambridge, MA: Harvard University Press, 1983); Mikulas Teich and Roy Porter (eds), *Fin de Siècle and its Legacy* (Cambridge: Cambridge University Press, 1990); Gareth Stedman Jones, *Outcast London: A Study in the Relationship Between Classes in Victorian Society* (Harmondsworth: Penguin, 1976), especially chapter 16: 'From "Demoralization" to "Degeneration": the Threat of Outcast London'; and Eric Hobsbawm, 'Mass-Producing Traditions: Europe, 1870–1914', in Hobsbawm and T. Ranger (eds), *The Invention of Tradition* (Cambridge: Cambridge University Press, 1983), 263–307.

117. See Joel A. Tarr and Gabriel Dupuy (eds), *Technology and the Rise of the Networked City in Europe and America* (Philadelphia: Temple University Press, 1988); Joel A. Tarr *et al.*, 'The City and the Telegraph: Urban Telecommunications in the Pre-telephone Era', *Journal of Urban History*, xiv (1987), 38–80; Thomas P. Hughes, *Networks of Power: Electrification in Western Society, 1880–1930* (Baltimore: Johns Hopkins University Press, 1983); Bill Luckin, *Pollution and Control: A Social History of The Thames in the Nineteenth Century* (Bristol/Boston: Hilger, 1986), and *idem*, *Questions of Power: Electricity and Environment in Inter-war Britain* (Manchester: Manchester University Press, 1990).

118. *The Times*, 15 Jan., 1880, 10, col.e. At least one member of the SPSADD, Viscount Templetown, was also on the Council of the Order of St John.

119. *The Times*, 20 Jan., 1880, 11, col.f.

120. ... *How to Prevent Accidents Becoming More Serious. With a Chapter on the Various Methods of Conveying the Sick and Wounded, Including the Stretcher Exercises in Use by the St John Ambulance Association*, printed and published for the Executive Council of the International Health Exhibition and for the Council of the Society of Arts by Wm. Clowes and Sons. It had run to a 12th edition by 1887. See also Nigel Corbet Fletcher, *A Compendium of Aids to First Aids ... With An Introduction by James Cantlie* (London: John Bale, 1913; 7th edn 1930).

121. (London: Field & Tuer, 1885) – originally a lecture delivered to the Army's Parkes Museum of Hygiene. On the volunteer medical staff corps, see James Cantlie, 'Ambulance Service (Volunteers)', *Medical*

Annual 1884–1885 (Bristol: John Wright, 1885), 333–4; and Jean Cantlie Stewart, *The Quality of Mercy: The Lives of Sir James and Lady Cantlie* (London: Allen & Unwin, 1983), chapter 3.

122. *Degeneration Amongst Londoners*, 47–8.
123. *Physical Efficiency: A Review of the Deleterious Effects of Town Life Upon The Population of Britain, With Suggestions For Their Arrest*, with a preface by Sir Lauder Brunton, MD, FRS, and foreword by Sir James Crichton-Brown, MD, FRS (London/New York: G.P. Putnam's Sons, 1906). Cantlie (1851–1926), a consultant surgeon at Charing Cross Hospital, was a pioneer in tropical medicine/public health in China.
124. Other senior medical men who were voluntarist enthusiasts include Edward Law Hussey (1816–99), surgeon to the Radcliffe Infirmary; Andrew Clark (1847–1913), surgeon to the Middlesex Hospital, a Knight of the Order of St John, a member of the first Volunteer Rifle Corps from 1867, Chairman of the Voluntary Aid Detachments Association, 1890–1908; and Samuel Osborn (1848–1936), chloroformist to St Thomas's Hospital, who was surgeon to the Royal Navy Volunteers before becoming chief surgeon to the St John Ambulance Brigades. On all three men, see Plarr's *Lives of the Fellows of the Royal College of Surgeons*; for their publications, see Appendix.
125. Basil, *op.cit.* (ref. 15), 82.
126. *Ibid.*, 3.
127. *Ibid.*, 5.
128. Tomes, 'The Private Side of Public Health: Sanitary Science, Domestic Hygiene, and the Germ Theory, 1870–1900', *Bulletin of the History of Medicine*, lxiv (1990), 509–39. See also Caroline Hannaway, 'From Private Hygiene to Public Health: A Transformation in Western Medicine in the Eighteenth and Nineteenth Centuries', in T. Ogawa (ed.), *Public Health* (Tokyo: Saikon Pub. Co., 1981), 108–28; and Naomi Rogers, *Dirt and Disease: Polio Before FDR* (New Brunswick: Rutgers University Press, 1990), 31ff.
129. Hence the strong resistance to the logic of germ theory, that infection was random rather than morally ordered. See Charles Rosenberg, 'Florence Nightingale on Contagion: The Hospital as Moral Universe', in Rosenberg (ed.), *Healing and History* (Folkestone, Kent: Dawson, 1979), 116–36.
130. Basil, *op.cit.* (ref. 15), 5.
131. He also wrote *Common Ailments and Their Cures* (London: Bellairs & Co., 1897); *Brain and Body: The Nervous System In Social Life* (London: J. Bowden, 1900); *Health for the People* (London: Sampson Low & Co., 1886); and *Homely Talks on First-aid* (Leeds: Zam-Buk Co., 1907).
132. Several works combined the treatment of accidents with the treatment of illness, though usually without the Basil-like appeal to sanitarian rhetoric. For examples, see Appendix: entries on Cowper (1885), W.J. Mackenzie (1890), and Morten (1896).

133. See, for example, Henry Crookshank, *The Theory and Practice of Sick Nursing: Being A Course of Five Lectures Delivered to a Ladies Advanced Class of the St John of Jerusalem Ambulance Association* (London: St John Ambulance Association, 1880); Appendix, entries on J.W. Martin (1890), J.M.H. Martin (1886), Osborn (1885), W.R. Smith (1898); and Nigel Corbet Fletcher, *A Compendium of Aids to Home-Nursing* (London: J. Bale, 1915). On this subject and on women and the first-aid movement generally, I am indebted to Anne Summers' Stopford Lecture, 'Battlefields and Bandages: Medicine, War and First Aid Charities, 1848–1914', Manchester, 10 June, 1992. See also Anne Summers, *Angels and Citizens: British Women as Military Nurses* (London: Routledge, 1988).
134. J.F.J. Sykes, *Home Hygiene* (London: St John Ambulance Association, 1898).
135. But not without considerable debate during the 1880s as to the wisdom of thus equipping soldiers for self-aid. See Thomas Longmore, 'On the Issue of First Field Dressing Packets to Soldiers in Time of War', *Trans. International Medical Congress*, 9th session, Washington, D.C., 1887, Vol. 2, 116–20; and Esmarch, *The Surgeon's Handbook on the Treatment of Wounded in War*, trs. H.H. Clutton (Hanover: C. Rümpler, 1878), 136. For the debate by the First World War, see J. Magill, 'First Field Dressing', *The Red Cross* (Feb. 1914), 61–2. See also James Evelyn Pilcher, 'Some New First-Aid Packets', *J.Amer.Mil.Surg.* (1906), 56–9. 'First Aid Cabinets', 'Hampers' and 'Haversacs' (large and small and costing between £1 and £4) are illustrated in publications of the St John Ambulance Association from the turn of the century. However, these were intended mostly for police surgeons, nurses and ambulance workers on railways etc. Smaller, cheaper kits do not appear until the 1910s, though even then 'domestic use' is not specified. For illustration of the earlier family medicine chest and its contents 'in Domestic and Private Practice', see Reece & Comp. (Chemists to Her Majesty), *A Description of Family Medicine Chests* (London: S. Highley, 1807).
136. Duncan, *op.cit.* (ref. 18), 6.
137. W.H. Clarke, 'First Aid to the Wounded', *The Health Journal and Record of Sanitary Engineering, A Monthly Review of Sanitary Science, and of Voluntary Effort for the Public Good*, serially, Oct. 1884–Sept. 1886.
138. See Appendix: entries on Butler (1889), Crosby (1881), Dulles (1880), Fleury (1879), Lawrence (1888), and for examples of earlier usage in domestic medicine, see *The Poor Man's Medical Guide in Emergency* (1855), and *Hints and Helps* (1860). See also Charlotte Vetter Gulick, *Emergencies*, in L.H. Gulick, *The Gulick Hygiene Series*, Vol. 2 (Boston: Ginn & Co., 1906).
139. For example in 1913 the general edition of Charles Lynch's *American Red Cross Abridged Text-book on First Aid* was issued in three separate parts: *Police and Firemen's Edition*, *Railroad Edition*, and a *Women's*

Edition. All were published in Philadelphia in 1913. See also W.H. Smith, *Medical and Surgical Help for Shipmasters, Including First Aid To The Injured* (London: Griffin's Nautical Series, 1900). Much ambulance lecturing was now addressed at 'advanced' levels. See, for example, Francis J. Warwick and A.C. Tunstall, *First Aid to the Injured and Sick: An Advanced Ambulance Handbook* (Bristol: John Wright & Co., 1901; 5th edn – 30,000 rev. 1908; 17th edn – 197,000 – 1939; and editions to 1952); and Nigel Corbet Fletcher, *Efficiency in First-Aid: A Manual of Aids For Senior Students etc.* (London: John Bale & Sons Co., 1916; 3rd edn 1934).

140. Not only was the concern with accidents now far more industrially orientated than during the late nineteenth century, but the rhetoric was cast more in terms of cost-cutting prevention. See, for example, the section on 'first aid' in the Holman Gregory Report on Workmen's Compensation (1920), quoted in Arnold Wilson and H. Levy, *Workmen's Compensation* (London: Oxford University Press, 1939), Vol. 2, 203.
141. 'The Street Ambulance Service in Great Britain', *Medical Record*, 20 Jan., 1900, 106.
142. I am grateful to Michael Worboys for this intriguing suggestion. One is again reminded of the need for research into life insurance and its medical relations.
143. See Mark C. Carnes's Introduction to Guy E. Bowerman, Jr, *The Compensations of War: The Diary of an Ambulance Driver During the Great War* (Austin: University of Texas Press, 1983), especially xv.
144. Summers, *op.cit.* (ref. 133).
145. Quoted in 'Ambulance and the Medical Profession', *First Aid*, 1 Oct., 1897, 224. In Stockport the medical profession boycotted teaching at the St John Ambulance Centre: *Lancet*, 15 July, 1899. See also the attempt to rebut the renewed accusation that first-aid instruction 'might do great mischief in making people fancy they knew far more than they did': Alfred Crespi, 'The St John Ambulance Association', *The Medical Magazine*, ii (1893–4), 44–58.
146. Thus conventionalized, they could become available for wider usage, as for example by Dr Margaret Marriner in *First Aid to Marriage* (London: Williams & Norgate, 1933).

Appendix

Popular Works on 'First Aid', 1800–1900 (English Language Only)

Accidents, what to do in the absence of the medical attendant (London: Junior Army and Navy Stores, [**1883**]).

Austin, John Alfred, *Ambulance sermons: being a series of popular essays on medical and allied subjects* (London: G. Redway, **1887**). 384pp.

————, *Manual of first aid; being a text-book for ambulance classes and a work of reference for domestic and general use* (London: Low, Marston, **1898**; edns 1902, 1904). 203pp.

Basil, Minas Manook (MB, CM Edin), *The commoner diseases and accidents to life and limb, firstly, their prevention; secondly, their immediate treatment* (London: J. & A. Churchill, **1887**). 104pp.

Beatson, Sir George Thomas (1848–1933), *Ambulance hand-book on the principles of first-aid to the injured* (Glasgow: St Andrews Ambulance Association, **1891**). 414pp.

Beecher, Catharine E. (1800–78), 'On Accidents and antidotes', in her *A treatise on domestic economy, for the use of young ladies at home and at school* (Boston: Marsh, Capen, Lyon and Webb, **1841**). Reprinted 1970, New York: Source Book Press, 245–50.

Begbie, James Warburton (MD; 1826–76), *Handy book of medical information and advice. By a physician* (London: Hogg, [**1860**]; 2nd edn 1872). 352pp. *Begbie was employed by the Scottish Widows' Fund Life Assurance Society to write their reports on causes of death as drawn from their statistics. His* Handy book *was less accessible than Buchan's* Domestic medicine, *the main focus being on diseases, which were arranged alphabetically.*

Benton, Samuel (medical writer), *Home nursing, and how to help in cases of accident* (London: David Bogue, **1880**). 133pp.

Bernhard, Oskar (surgeon; 1861–1939), *First aid to the injured. With special reference to accidents occurring in the mountains; a handbook for guides, climbers and travellers,* trs. from the German by M.G. Foster (London: Unwin, **1900**). 136pp.

Black, George (medical popularizer), *First aid; a book of ready reference in times of emergency. A manual of instruction for ambulance students, and a plain practical guide to the rendering of help in case of accident or sudden illness* (London: Ward, Lock & Co., **1887**; 2nd edn 1889). 215pp.

————, *Every-day ailments and accidents* (London: Ward, Lock & Co., **1892**). 426pp.

The book of accidents; designed for young children (New Haven: S. Babcock, **1831**; 1840 edn re-subtitled 'or, warnings to the heedless'). 23pp. *Cautionary tales.*

Bosworth, Newton (d.1848), *The accidents of human life; with hints for their prevention, or the removal of their consequences* (London: Allen and Co., **1813**; 2nd edn: T. Ward and Co., 1834). 209pp.

Brodie, John Ewan, *Manual of stretcher drill and exercises* (Glasgow: St Andrew Ambulance Association, **1894**). 67pp.

Bromhead, Thomas Ayre (MB; Christ's College, Cambridge), *The parent's medical and surgical assistant: intended for the use of the heads of families, parochial clergymen and others; affording familiar and popular directions for the management of the sudden illnesses and various accidents that require a prompt and judicious treatment, and will not admit of the delay necessary for procuring regular advice* (London: printed and sold by William Phillips, **1821**). 156pp.

Bruce, Robert (MRCS, DPH; MO for Holborn), *First aid to the injured* (London; Cassell & Co., **1885**; editions to 1928). 78pp. *A revision of Peter Shepherd's* Handbook *(1878). See also B. Morton.*

Buchan, William (1729–1805), 'Of Casualties', in his *Domestic medicine; or the family physician* (**1769**; with editions to 1863; 1804 edn Leominster: Adams and Wilder), 408–29. *Discusses the treatment of sudden accidents; he regarded his comments on this subject as 'happily anticipated' by 'the learned and humane Dr. Tissot'.*

Butler, Glentworth Reeve (MD; 1855–1926), *Emergency notes. What to do in accidents and sudden illness, until the doctor comes. ... With eighteen original illustrations* (New York: Funk & Wagnalls, **1889**). 102pp.

Cameron, Angus, *Practical hints on ambulance* (Manchester: J. Heywood, **1895**). 32pp.

Cantlie, James (1851–1926; FRCS), *Accidental injuries: their relief and immediate treatment. How to prevent accidents becoming more serious. With a chapter on the various methods of conveying the sick and wounded, including the stretcher exercises in use by the St John Ambulance Association* (printed and published for the Executive Council of the International Health Exhibition and for the Council of the Society of Arts by Wm. Clowes and Sons, **1884**). The 4th edition is entitled *First aid to the injured ... with a chapter on stretcher transport by John Furley [and] a chapter ... for females only* (London: St John Ambulance Association, 1901; 22nd edn 1908). 215pp.

Clark, Andrew (1847–1913; FRCS), *First aid to the injured, a course of five lectures* (2nd edn London: Polytechnic Young Men's Christian Institute, **1888**). 79pp.

Clarke, Sir Arthur (1778–1857; FRCS; physc. Bank of Ireland and Dublin Metrop. Police), *A code of instructions for the treatment of sufferers from railroad and steam-boat accidents ... until medical aid can be procured* (Dublin: printed for the author, 1849). 176pp. *'The work which may be considered as the* germ *of this* essay, *is a sheet published by Alfred Smee ... headed "Accidents and Emergencies, a Guide for their Treatment".'*

Cowper, (Countess) Katrine (1845–1913), *Help at hand; or what shall we do in accidents or illness?* (London: Gardner, Darton, **1885**). 36pp.

Crookshank, Harry (1856–1914), *Manual of home nursing and hygiene: including first aid to be rendered in cases of accidents and emergencies* (London: W. Whiteley, **1881**). 232pp.

Crosby, Albert Harrison (1825–86), Alpheus Benning Crosby (1832–77) and John T. Hodgen (1826–82), 'Accidents and Emergencies', in *[George B.] Wood's household practice of medicine, hygiene and surgery. A practical treatise for the use of families, travellers, seamen, miners, and others,* edited by Frederick A. Castle, MD, Vol. 1 (London: Sampson, *et al.*, **1881**), 585–768.

Darwin, George Henry, *Ambulance lectures* (Manchester: J. Heywood, **1892**). 95pp.

Doty, Alvak Hunt (1854–?), *A manual of instruction in the principles of prompt aid to the injured, designed for military and civil use* (New York: Appleton & Co., **1889**; further edns of 1894, 1898, 1902 and, London, 1912). 224pp.

Dowie, Minnie L., *Mrs. Minnie Dowie's cookery book and household management: comprising 900 cookery recipes and general hints for the home, first aid and nursing instructions* (London: Maclaren, n.d. [c.**1890**]). 280pp.

Drinkwater, Harry (MD; 1855–?), *First aid to the injured and ambulancer drill* (London: J.M. Dent, **1900**; 2nd edn 1907). 104pp.

Dulles, Charles Winslow (1850–1921; MD), *What to do first, in accidents or poisoning* (Philadelphia: Blakiston, **1880**; 2nd edn 1883). Editions after 1888 entitled: *Accidents and emergencies. A manual of the treatment of surgical and other injuries in the absence of a physician* (Philadelphia: Blakiston, 1888; 8th edn 1918).

Duncan, Francis (1836–88; first director of St John Ambulance department), *First Aid to the injured. The St John Ambulance Association; its aim and objects. To which are appended a selection from authenticated cases in which first aid to injured persons has been rendered by certificated pupils of the Association, pending the arrival of surgical assistance ... including reports from the surgeons of London hospitals and others.* Read at the Dublin meeting of the Social Science Congress, 4 Oct., **1881**. Reprinted as a pamphlet, London, 1881.

Emergency cards (London: Houlston & Sons, 1898). *Six cards for handy home use.*

Esmarch, Johannes Friedrich August von (1823–1908), *Die erste bei verletzungen: ein populärer vortrag* (Hanover: Carl Rümpler, **1875**). Translated into English by HRH Princess Christian in **1882** as *First aid to the injured; five ambulance lectures* (London: Rümpler, 1882; 'enlarged' editions to 1916). It was also translated into many other languages.

Evatt, Surgeon-Major George J.H. (1848–1921), *Ambulance organisation, equipment, and transport* (printed and published for the Executive Council of the International Health Exhibition and for the Council of the Society of Arts by Wm. Clowes and Sons, **1884**). 122pp.

First aid to the injured. The ambulance pupil. By a pupil of the St John Ambulance Association (London: Crosby, Lockwood & Co., **1887**; 2nd edn 1888). 64pp.

First aid. The independent journal for the ambulance and fire services. **1894**–1947. 2 pence per issue.

First help in accidents and in sickness. A guide in the absence, or before the arrival, of medical assistance (Boston: A. Moore, **1871**). 264pp.

Fleury, Charles Robert, *Modern household medicine. A guide to the mode of recognition and the ... treatment ... of diseases and emergencies incidental to daily life* (London: E. Gould & Son, **1879**; 2nd edn 'enlarged', 1884; 3rd edn 1893).

Foster, Philip (popular health writer), *What to do in accidents and sudden illness* (2nd edn Leeds: Fred R. Spark, **1883**). 76pp.

Furley, John (1836–1919), *On the use of ambulance litters and horse carriages for the removal of sick and injured persons, especially in reference to the metropolis* (London: Harrison & Sons, **1882**).

———, *The carriage and removal of the sick and injured* (printed and published for the Executive Council of the International Health Exhibition and for the Council of the Society of Arts by Wm. Clowes and Sons, **1884**).

Gell, Henry Willingham, *Aids to the injured and sick* (London: National Health Society, **1892**). 32pp.

Gibb, William (LRCS), *First aid to the injured. Ambulance lectures* (London: Griffith, Farran *et al.*, **1886**). 97pp.

Hamilton, John Brown (1847–98), *Hand-book for the ship's medicine chest* (Washington: Government Printing Office, 1881; further edns authored by George W. Stoner, 1900, 1904). 45pp. *Issued by US Public Health Service.*

Hamilton, Walter Moffat, *Common accidents and their treatment*, Manchester and Salford Sanitary Association Health Lecture (London: J. Heywood, **1893**). 23pp.

Hand, William M., *The house surgeon and physician; designed to assist heads of families, travellers, and sea-faring people in discerning, distinguishing, and curing diseases ... all in plain English* (Hartford: P.B. Gleason & Co, **1818**; 3rd edn 1849). 288pp. Price $1. *Deals with accidents under 'Surgery': 'I have endeavoured to describe what every man may do, (and they may do much;) in many cases, immediate and effectual assistance may be afforded, where people are now idle spectators; and frequently departing life may be staid, till a surgeon arrives to make all safe' (vi).*

Hand-book for emergencies: containing hints and cautions to those engaged in dangerous occupations, and to sufferers by the common casualties of life, 'Cassell's Elementary Hand-books' (London/New York: Cassell, Petter and Galpin, **1861**). 90pp. *Intended 'to inculcate certain habits of precaution, and prepare the reader to act in emergencies with a better intelligence than heretofore', this work is also uniquely informative on the statistics of railway and mining accidents etc.*

Headland, Frederick William (1830–75; FRCP), 'Accidents and Emergencies', in his *A medical handbook, comprehending such information on medical and sanitary subjects as is desirable in educated persons, with hints to clergymen and visitors of the poor* (London: Seeley *et al.*, **1861**). 348pp.

Henderson, George (Physician of Washington), *Preservation of health: simple remedies for ordinary ailments; care of wounded, sunstroke, freezing, cuts, bruises, burns, and all ordinary accidents* (Lecture 9 to the National Guard in Service) (Washington, D.C.: n.p., n.d. [**c. 1880**]), 219–33.

Hints and helps for every-day emergencies, in connection with social economy, legal difficulties, domestic economy, rural economy, household medicine, casualties and accidents, ipecunary embarassments, legal difficulties, etc., etc. (London: Ward, Lock & Sons, **1860**; 2nd edn 1880). 112pp. *Directed to the housewife, the traveller and the valetudinarian, among others.*

Hogg, Jabez (1817–99; MRCS), *The domestic medical and surgical guide, for the nursery, the cottage, and the bush; giving the best advice, in the absence of a physician or surgeon, in cases of accident or sudden illness; useful to families, emigrants, travellers, missionaries, village clergymen, and sea captains* (London: Ingram, Cooke, and Co., **1853**; 2nd edn 1853; 4th edn 1857). 156pp.

Home nurse (The). Comprising useful suggestions by an experienced physician on the care of the sick, dressing of wounds, and what to do in an emergency (London: Seabury & Johnson, **1894**). 32pp.

Hope, George H., *Till the doctor comes and how to help him* (London: Religious Tract Society, **1870**; 2nd edn 1871; New York: Putnam's, 1879, 1901). 160pp.

Howe, Joseph William (1843–1890; medical popularizer), *Emergencies and how to treat them. The etiology, pathology, and treatment of the accidents, diseases, and cases of poisoning which demand prompt action, etc.* (New York: Appleton, **1871**; at least six editions to 1901). 267pp.

Hussey, Edward Law (FRCS; 1816–99), *Accidents to volunteers. A lecture delivered to the City of Oxford companies of the Oxfordshire Rifle Volunteers* (Oxford: E.W. Morris, **1864**; 3rd edn Oxford: Horace Hart, 1889). 56pp.

Hutton, Surgeon-Major George Allan (1830–1907), *Facts and figures connected with first aid. With an addendum by Waynman Dixon* [and an appendix containing the syllabus of instruction and rules for local ambulance corps; adopted by the St John Ambulance Association] (London: St John Ambulance Association, **1884**). 12pp.

Hyett, William Henry (1795–1877; horticulturalist), *Prompt remedies for accidents and poisons, adapted to the use of the inexperienced, till medical assistance arrives* (2nd edn London: Trübner & Co., **1884**). Price 3s 6d *('For the benefit of the Gloucester Infirmary'.) Double-sided sheet (16" x 18") 'To be hung up for quick reference in country schools or vestries, workshops, offices of factories, mines, and docks, in railway stations, yachts, remote shooting quarters, Highland manses, and even private houses.'*

Instant remedies for accidents and emergencies of daily occurrence, 'A Book for Every Home' series (London: S.J. Brown, **1856**). 16pp. Price 4d. *Alphabetically arranged.*

Kittoe, William Hamilton (MD; author of *Boudoir companion*), *The pocket book of practical medicine; or, manual for emergencies* (2nd edn, 'enlarged and improved', London: R. Jackson, **1843**; 3rd edn London: Sherwood, Gilbert & Piper, 1844). 278pp. The first edition was entitled *The domestic medical pocket-book: or, family vade mecum* (Southampton: Fletcher, **1837**). 288pp. *A listing of common diseases; little on accidents, though fractures and minor surgical operations are discussed.*

The labour we delight in: a handbook for persons, explaining ... the treatment of wounds before the arrival of a doctor (London: Russell & Everett, **1885**). 24pp. *The Preface is signed 'R.'*

Lawless, Edmond James, *The bearer's companion. First aid to the injured, and management of the sick. An ambulance handbook and elementary manual of nursing for volunteer bearers and others* (Edinburgh/London: Y.J. Pentland, **1894**; 2nd edn, published by The Scientific Press and without 'The Bearer's Companion' in the title, 1898). 262pp.

Lawrence, Joseph B., *What to do in cases of accidents and emergencies, describing the symptoms in each case, and how to treat them on the moment ... designed for family and general use* (New York: J. Vail, **1888**). 139pp.

Lechmere, Sir Edmund A. H. (1826–94; MP; Sec. St John Order from 1867), *Aid to the injured. Order of St John of Jerusalem in England. Proceedings of a public meeting held on Wednesday evening, February 6, 1878, at the Pall Mall Restaurant, Regent Street, London* (Woolwich: printed by A.W. and J.P. Jackson, **1878**). 29pp. Sixpence.

Life Saving Society, *Illustrated hand-book for the rescue of the drowning* (London: LSS, **1897**, and 1901). 101pp.

Longmore, Thomas (1816–95), *Observations on the preliminary care and attention necessary for accidental bodily injuries and mutilations occurring in mines and establishments where many workpeople are employed*, read at the Annual General Assembly of the Order of St John of Jerusalem, held in London on St John Baptist's Day, 1874 (published by the Order, **1874**). 29pp.

Lowe, George May, *Accidents*, Practical Nursing Series no. 4 (London: Roxburghe Press, **1894**). 76pp.

Mackenzie, William James (MD), *Home medicine and surgery. A dictionary of diseases and accidents, and their treatment when the services of a doctor are not obtainable; with illustrative diagrams, showing how to apply surgical bandages, splints, etc.* (London: L. Upcott Gill, **1890**; another edn 1901). 170pp.

Mann, Robert James (1817–86; MRCS Edin.; government super. of education in Natal, S.A.), *Medicine for emergencies; for the use of settlers in colonies, sailors on shipboard, and students of every class* (London: Jarrold & Sons, **1861**). 463pp. *Aimed at 'persons of fair education and intelligence'. Does not propose to be 'a "Domestic medicine" in the familiar sense'. Pages 400–40 deal with 'casual injuries'.*

Marshall, Major John James de Zouche, *Stretcher drill illustrated* (London: Clower, **1898**; 2nd edn [... *compiled from the Manual of the Royal Army Medical Corps, 1904 Regulations for army medical services*], HMSO and J. & A. Churchill, 1904). 83pp.

Martin, John Michael Harding (1847–1906; FRCS), *Ambulance lectures; to which is added a nursing lecture in accordance with the regulations of the St John Ambulance Association for male and female classes* (London: J. & A. Churchill, **1886**; 4th edn 1895). 120pp.

Martin, John Wise (1846–1911), *Questions and answers on nursing, for St John's [sic] Ambulance Association and others* (London: Baillière *et al.*, **1890**; 6th edn, 23rd thousand, 1916).

——————— and John Martin (FRCSE, of Huddersfield and a St John Ambulance Assn examiner), *Ambulance work: questions and answers upon first aid to the injured* (London: Baillière, Tindall and Cox, **1886**; 2nd edn 1887; 18th edn 1915). 57pp.

Mayor, Matthias Louis (1775–1847), *Popular surgery: being plain directions offered to the public at large but particularly to heads of families, captains of ships, emigrants, and persons engaged in mines, manufactories, and public works, for affording relief in all cases of accident, dangerous disease, poisoning, etc. in the absence of a regular practitioner*, trs. Thomas Cutler (London: Longman, Rees, Orme, **1836**). 125pp.

Merrimack Humane Society, *The institution of the Merrimack Humane Society with the methods of treatment to be used with persons apparently dead from drowning and other accidents* (Newburyport, Mass.: W.H. Huse, printer, 1870). 31pp. *Printed by the Society for gratuitous distribution.*

Moore, Sir William James (1828–96; late surgeon-general with the government of Bombay; wrote on medicine in India; health resorts; family medicine), *The immediate and general treatment of accidents and injuries* (London: J. & A. Churchill, **1889**). 54pp.

Morgan, Llewellyn, *Ambulance card* (Liverpool: Winstanley & Watkins, **1893**).

Morten, Honnor (1861–?; writer on nursing), *How to treat accidents and illnesses. A handbook for the home* (London: Sampson Low & Co., **1896**). 147pp.

Morton, Bowditch (1857–1909; MD), *First aid to the injured* (New York: G.P. Putnam's Sons, **1882**). *A revised and supplemented edition of Shepherd's* Handbook *(1878), produced at the request of the First Aid to the Injured Association of New York. See also R. Bruce (1885).*

Murdoch, Donald (MRCS; wrote on fever), 'Projections to instruct police in simple surgery'. (*Listed among Murdoch's publications in the Medical Directory after 1881, where it is noted as 'first aid'.*)

Osborn, Samuel (1848–1936; FRCS), *Ambulance lectures: first aid to the injured* (London: H.K. Lewis, **1890**; 2nd edn 1891; 4th edn London: Lewis, 1899). 156pp. 2 shillings. Translated into French, as *Premiers secours à donner aux malades et aux blessés* (Paris, 1894), and into German, Italian, Spanish, Greek, Japanese, Chinese and Hindustani.

————, *Ambulance lectures on home nursing and hygiene* (London: H.K. Lewis, **1885**; 2nd edn 1891). 95pp.

Paris, Lieut-Col. Charles B., *St John Ambulance Association. Aid-ology or first aid to the injured* (Liverpool: E. Howell, **1887**). 106pp.

Parkinson, James (1755–1824; FRS), *The villager's friend and physician; or the familiar address on the preservation of health, and the removal of disease, on its first appearance; supposed to be delivered by a village apothecary: with cursory observations on the treatment of children on sobriety, industry, etc. Intended for the promotion of domestic happiness* (**1800**; 2nd edn London, printed by C. Whittingham, Deans Street, and sold by H.D. Symonds, Paternoster Row, 1804). 71pp. Price 1s. *Parkinson rarely ever uses the word 'accident'; instead, as in discussing the breaking of bones and how to handle such injuries, he refers to those 'rendered so by violence' or those who suffer 'after a blow by a fall'.*

————, *The way to health, being a selection of maxims for the preservation of health from the Villager's Friend and Physician* (n.p.: n.d., **c.1800**). Printed on a single sheet 'for the cottagers fireside'. Price 4d.

———, *Dangerous sports, a tale addressed to children warning them against the wanton, careless and mischievous exposure to those situations from which alarming injuries so often proceed* (2nd edn London: H.D. Symonds, **1808**). 198pp.

Partridge, Sydney, *Practical ambulance tablets* (London: J. & A. Churchill, **1890**; 2nd edn 1895). 59pp.

Pilcher, James Evelyn (1857–1911; medical author and organizer of Assn of Military Surgeons of USA, 1891), *First aid in illness and injury, comprised in a series of chapters on the human machine its structure, its implements of repair, and the accidents and emergencies to which it is liable* (New York: Scribner's Sons, **1892**; revised edns to 1915). 322pp.

Poor man's medical guide in emergency. By a Fellow of the Royal College of Surgeons, Ireland (Dublin: Fannin & Co., **1855**). 30pp. 'Price in cloth, Sixpence; Poor Man's Edition, Twopence'. *A deeply sympathetic dispensary surgeon provides alphabetically listed advice. Page 29: 'Do not trust to bonesetters (so-called) and other quacks. It is madness to do so.'*

Questions on first aid to the injured (Preston: Guardian Printer Works, **1896**). 15pp.

Raye, J. Ardavon (military surgeon), *Ambulance handbook for volunteers and others* (London: J. & A. Churchill, **1884**). 138pp.

Ready remedies in medical and surgical emergencies. By an Edinburgh Practitioner (London: Edmonston & Co., **1881**). 94pp. *'Not intended ... to interfere with some excellent publications already in high favour, such as a "Book of Medical Information and Advice" by the late lamented Dr. Warburton Begbie'.*

Richmond, D., *Accidents of childhood, or cautionary stories for heedless children. With twenty illustrations by J.D. Watson, engraved by the Brothers Dalziel* (London: Routledge, **1861**). 175pp.

Riddell, John Scott (1864–1929; Asst-Surg. Aberdeen R.I. and Examiner to St Andrew's Ambulance Association), *A manual of ambulance* (London: Griffin, **1894**; 6th edn 'much enlarged and especially prepared for the use of voluntary aid detachments', 1913 and 1916). 214pp.

Rivers, Henry Wheaton, *Accidents: popular directions for their immediate treatment with observations on poisons and their antidotes* (Boston: T.H. Webb, **1848** [1st edn: printed for the author; Providence, R.I.]).

Roberts, Richard Lawton (MRCS; St John lecturer), *Illustrated lectures on ambulance work* (London: H.K. Lewis, **1885**; 5th edn 1895). 179pp.

Robertson, Joseph M'Gregor (1858–1925), *The household physician: a family guide to the preservation of health and to the domestic treatment of ailments and disease, with chapters on food and drugs and first aid in accidents and injuries* (London/New York: Blackie, **c.1890**; 2nd edn, rev. and enl., published by Gresham Publishing Co., 1899). 2 vols.

Robertson, William (1865–1941; MD, DPH), *Practical first aid* (Perth: Scottish News Agency, **1899**; 3rd edn Paisley, 1902).

S.C.S., *Ambulance hints* (Glasgow: Bryce & Son, **1889**). 31pp.

St John Ambulance Association, *Advantages of ambulance instruction* (London: St John, **1895**). 56pp.

Sargent, Dudley Allen (1849–1924; writer on physical education and body building), *In case of accident* (Boston: D. Lothrop, **1884**; 2nd edn 1893). 125pp.

Schaible, Karl [Charles] Heinrich (1824–99), *First help in accidents: being a surgical guide, in the absence or before the arrival of medical assistance, for the use of the public, especially for the members of both the military and naval services, volunteers and travellers, etc.* (London: Robert Hardwicke, **1864**). 228pp. Price 2s 6d.

Shepherd, Surgeon-Major Peter (1841–79), *Handbook. Aids for cases of injuries or sudden illness* (London: Order of St John, **1878**). *For revised editions (*as First aid to the injured*), see B. Morton (1882) and R. Bruce (1885).*

Smee, Alfred (1818–77; FRS; Surgeon to the Bank of England; also wrote on the eye; nutrition; potatoes; and mind), *Accidents and emergencies: a guide for their treatment before the arrival of medical aid* (London: J. Churchill, **1848**). Price 6d. Tenth edition, London, n.d.; French trs., Paris, 1872; German trs., Berlin, 1895; American editions (sometimes entitled *The house surgeon, or the doctor at home, containing instructions for the prompt treatment of accidents and emergencies before the arrival of medical aid*), with appendix by Dr R.T. Trall, published in N.Y. by Fowler, 1850, 1851, 1856, 1876, 1888. *A wall chart approximately 3' x 2' with 60 complaints and conditions set out pictorially in alphabetical order, from 'bleeding' to 'supposed death', including usefully 'bites of mad dogs' (break all but one tang off a fork and then heat it and place it all around the bite). According to Cornelius Walford (*Insurance Cyclopaedia, *Vol. 1, 6) Smee's chart was prepared for the Accident Insurance Company and was widely distributed to agents and policy holders.*

Smith, William Henry (1846–?), *Self treatment or everyone his own physician* (Chicago: Chicago Medical Co., **1887**). 44pp.

Smith, W.H., *Medical and surgical help for shipmasters, including first aid to the injured* (London: Griffin's Nautical Series, **1900**). 349pp.

Smith, Sir William Robert (1850–1932), *Text-book of first aid work and home nursing for the use of ambulance classes* (London: Allman & Son, **1898**). 150pp.

Society (The) for Instruction in First Aid to the Injured, *Its object, plan of work, and system of instruction* (New York, 1883). *See Morton (1882).*

South, John Flint (1797–1882), *Household surgery: or hints on emergencies* (London: Cox, **1847**). 340pp. Second edition, 1850; 4th edn (17,000th 'with an additional chapter on Poisons by Dr. Gladstone'), 1859. American editions (Philadelphia) from 1850.

Sutherland, John Francis (1854–1911), *The ambulance pupil's vade-mecum* (Glasgow: J. Menzies & Co., **1894**; 46th edn rev. by H.G. Sutherland [E. & S. Livingstone] 1957). 32pp.

Thompson, Charles John Samuel (1862–1943), *'The best thing to do'. First aid in simple ailments and accidents* (London: Record Press, **1892**; 2nd edn 1893 and 1900). 53pp.

Tissot, Samuel A.A.D. (1728–97), *Advice to the people in general, with regard to their health: but particularly calculated for those, who are the most unlikely to be provided in time with the best assistance, in acute diseases, or upon any inward or outward accident,* translated from the French edition of 1761 by J. Kirkpatrick (London: T. Becket, **1767**). A 7th edition appeared in **1801**. *According to Buchan in his section on accidents in* Domestic medicine, *Tissot had said it all.*

Turner, Alexander Paul (1840–92), *Plain directions for accidents, emergencies, and poisons. By a Fellow of the College of Physicians of Philadelphia* (New York: Powers, Macgowan and Slipper, **1875**). 125pp. *Originally published anonymously as* Accidents, emergencies and poisons *(Philadelphia: Hammond, 1874) and distributed through the Howard Hospital and Infirmary for Incurables, Philadelphia. Reissued in 1875 by the Mutual Life Insurance Society of New York and distributed to its policy holders.*

Weatherly, Lionel A. (1852–?), *Ambulance lectures; or, what to do in cases of accident or sudden illness* (London: Griffith & Farran, 1880; other edn 1882). 65pp.

Webb, Henry, *Conversation-lessons on prompt aid to the injured* (Bury: W. S. Barlow, **1887**; 2nd edn 1888). 129pp.

White, James William (1850–1916), *First aid to the injured. An abstract of lecture delivered* (Philadelphia: n.p., **1883**). 25pp.

Williams, Alfred (Sec. MS & L Railway Company's Ambulance Corps, Gorton, and a teacher of ambulance classes, Manchester), *Accidents and emergencies. Adapted for use in day and evening schools, etc.* (Manchester: Higher Openshaw, **1896**). 31pp. Price 2d.

Wilson, Andrew (1852–1912; FRCSE, medical popularizer), *Common accidents and how to treat them* (London: Chatto & Windus, **1886**). 122pp.

———, *What to do in emergencies* (London: C. Arthur Peason, **1897**; 2nd edn 1900). 180pp.

7

Civilian Ambulances and Lifesaving Societies: The European Experience, 1870–1914

John F. Hutchinson

What accounts for that 'great wave of ambulance enthusiasm'[1] that swept across continental Europe in the four decades following the Franco-Prussian war? From Bordeaux to Budapest and from Milan to Kiel, the plight of accident victims was rapidly and definitively transformed. In 1870, those struck down by sudden injury or illness were dependent on family and friends, compassionate passers-by, or the police for whatever assistance might be rendered in an emergency; by the turn of the century, accident victims in most European cities could typically expect organized assistance from persons trained in first-aid techniques who would quickly arrive at the site, probably in a horse-drawn ambulance staffed and equipped by the local volunteer lifesaving society.

To be sure, this transformation was by no means an exclusively European phenomenon. In the major American cities, most hospitals began to organize their own horse ambulance services; Bellevue Hospital in New York City had led the way in 1869, and within twenty years hospital ambulances could be found in all the important northeastern cities, as well as in Chicago, St Louis, and New Orleans. In England, the St John Ambulance Association was founded in 1877, and the northern industrial centres of Liverpool and Manchester soon established municipal ambulance services under the direction of the police. Although Europeans were initially strongly influenced by what had happened in England and America, this chapter will argue that on the Continent both the establishment of urban ambulances and the growth of the lifesaving movement took on distinctive features, and that what happened in Europe was much more than a pale reflection of developments elsewhere.

Until the present decade, the origins of civilian ambulances attracted relatively little scholarly attention. John S. Haller, Jr, who recently published a volume on the history of the military ambulance, ascribes the beginnings of urban ambulance services in the United States and England to 'an outgrowth of military experiences in both Europe and America'. Haller's principal interest was in the development of ambulance technology,[2] and he naturally emphasized the influence of those military surgeons who profited from Civil War experience to design and market ambulance vehicles in the post-war decades. Haller's straightforward approach is arguably too simple: it fails to explain why some major cities – notably London and Paris – resisted for decades the blandishments of American military surgeons turned ambulance salesmen; nor does it explain why some European military surgeons – notably Friedrich Esmarch – responded to civilian accidents not by selling ambulance vehicles to hospitals, but rather by organizing a Samaritan League of trained civilian volunteers, and by establishing accident or first-aid stations in major cities throughout Germany. Nor does Haller explore those specific changes in the organization of nineteenth-century cities, for example the growth of police communication networks, that were so much a part of the successful development of urban ambulance services.

The use of mobile first-aid units in the American Civil War and the three Wars of German Unification (1864–71) demonstrated that an organized and effective response to sudden injury was possible on the battlefield. To convince people that a rapid response was possible in an urban setting, however, more was involved than simply adapting military ambulance vehicles for use in city streets. Existing networks of police and fire-fighters already subdivided cities into smaller units (precincts, districts) that were connected by telegraph and telephone to a central exchange; the same lines that were used to report fires or robberies could also be used to summon a mobile first-aid unit. Without the availability of these police communication networks, it is questionable whether the creation of civilian ambulance services would have been regarded as feasible.

In his contribution to this volume, Roger Cooter explicitly rejects the idea that the ambulance movement was merely 'the "practical", or the "inevitable" or "natural" response to perceptions of the increased incidence of accidents'. Instead, he links 'the moment of the accident' to 'the bourgeois cultural anxieties and insecurities of the late nineteenth century'; to, especially, a middle class that feared social disorder and destabilization. He suggests that we regard accidents 'as symbols of the omnipresent potential dangers of the socially destabilised late-Victorian urban context' (see pages 123–4). This interpretation is suggestive, perhaps even provocative; however, little of Cooter's evidence pertains directly to those individuals who established the St John Ambulance Association, or who organized and operated the urban ambulance services in Britain. Whether it provides a convincing explanation of their motives remains an open question.

For Cooter, the importance of ideology is paramount. In turning from the English to the European experience, however, one is quickly struck by the limitations of explanations based on ideology. This is not to suggest that politics and ideology played no significant role on the Continent; indeed, in most European countries those individuals who promoted the lifesaving movement and the development of urban ambulances were generally right-of-centre, if not solidly right-wing in their political views. They shared a deep aversion to revolutionary ideologies such as socialism and communism. At the same time, they took pride in the fact that their movement was a voluntary one, a spontaneous upwelling of concern for the unfortunate, which arose independently of the action or wishes of any government, and which, they believed, crossed the boundaries of social class and economic inequality. The rending conflicts of 1848 and 1871 were to be replaced by a more harmonious society, of which this new concern for accident victims was to be a concrete manifestation. Yet, as will be shown below, appeals based on ideology sometimes fell on deaf ears, while more practical approaches often yielded impressive results. Thus, although the spectre of the Paris Commune can rightly be seen as one element in explaining that great wave of ambulance enthusiasm, yet it is only one; for a more comprehensive explanation, the net must be cast more widely.

Following Thomas Haskell, I believe it is necessary to explain why, at certain times and in certain places, sufficient support builds within a society to push the humanitarian sensibility 'over the threshold' and into practical activity.[3] In the case of accidental injuries, which did not suddenly begin to happen in the mid-nineteenth century, how does one explain the apparently growing conviction that accidents now demanded an organized, no longer a haphazard, response? Did it not stem from the belief that life in an increasingly urban and industrial society was obviously dangerous, and likely to become more so? Certainly the explanations given by contemporaries stressed danger, above all the danger of living in a world of growing cities and of ubiquitous machines. Typical is the following, written in 1890 by Dr Émile Mauriac of Bordeaux, himself a strong advocate of urban ambulance services:

> Among all civilised peoples, the number of accidents on roads, in factories and workshops increases daily as a consequence of the incessant growth of urban concentrations, the rapidity and multiplicity of means of transport, the expansion of huge public works, and especially the almost universal substitution of machinery for the hands of men in factories and workshops.[4]

This growing awareness of the dangerousness of modern life was to have profound consequences.

Misadventures involving injury had been occurring for centuries, but the response to them was almost always contingent, haphazard, and ineffective, or even positively harmful. It was the great innovations of the nineteenth century – the railway, the omnibus, the tram and the bicycle; the more powerful, and potentially more dangerous machinery in factories, mills, and foundries; the theatres, opera houses, and other large public buildings where fire and suffocation were ever-present dangers – that prompted contemporaries to perceive a need to respond to these threats in some organized fashion. The very idea of a planned response implies a growing awareness that accidents were themselves predictable events – not in the sense that the precise time of their occurrence or the identity of the victim(s) could be known in advance, but rather in the sense that some places, processes, or occupations were plainly more dangerous than others. It followed, therefore, that the probable occurrence of accidents was taken as a basis for planning an appropriate response, regardless of the fact that the circumstances of any particular accident could scarcely be known in advance.

What were the general characteristics of this organized response? It was strongest, naturally enough, in cities, because it was there that the congestion was so obvious.[5] Although it was in some sense a reaction against the consequences of innovation, it would nevertheless depend for its effectiveness on the use of two more innovations: the telegraph and the telephone. It may not have been sparked, although it was certainly shaped, by the growing understanding and acceptance of the germ theory of disease, upon which were based the use of antiseptic dressings and the practice of antiseptic surgery. Moreover, however much the focus of the ambulance movement was on accidents in civil life, Europeans never lost sight of the potential usefulness in war of persons already trained in first-aid techniques and familiar with ambulance procedure. Indeed, the roots of the movement to organize assistance to civilian accident victims lie in what might be called a timely conjunction between the perceived increase in the physical danger of urban life, and the need to find a useful peacetime role for the societies that had recently been formed for the purpose of aiding sick and wounded soldiers.

During the 1860s, societies to aid wounded soldiers – they were not yet called 'Red Cross' societies – were established in most European countries.[6] During the Franco-Prussian War, they had been active not only in the belligerent states but also in neutral countries. Once the war was over, however, these newly-formed societies – most were only five or six years old in 1871 – were faced with adjusting to what might be called the problem of peace. What they might do to ensure their survival in peacetime was first discussed at an international conference held in Berlin in 1869. At that time, there was considerable disagreement among the various delegations. The Prussians had argued that national societies and local committees should undertake the training of nurses to care for the sick poor, a work which would both popularize the societies and create a pool of trained females who would be useful in future conflicts. The Hessians, by contrast, argued for a more limited role: the promotion of hygienic improvements in barracks, hospitals, prisons, and schools; combined with the propagation of knowledge about the principles and practices of hygiene. The French delegates, on the other hand, questioned whether such grandiose plans were in fact practical, and also expressed the fear that even a limited involvement in disaster relief might consume all the available funds and energy of the societies; at most, they were prepared to contemplate a far more limited role, that of assisting accident victims in civil life. The Russians were even more outspoken, warning against the danger of turning societies formed to aid the wounded into 'committees to do everything': with considerable force, they argued that the societies had no right to do anything with donors' contributions except to employ them for relieving sick and wounded soldiers: to do otherwise, said one of the Russian delegates, would be both bad philanthropy and bad political economy.[7]

The debate in Berlin in 1869 largely foreshadowed the responses of the various societies to the period of peace which began in Europe (except for the Balkans) in 1871. Under Prussian influence, the societies in the German states did as planned: they got on with relieving the victims of the last war and preparing their human and material resources for future wars. Elsewhere, however, the idea of providing assistance to civilian accident victims found its supporters. In England, the President of the National Aid Society, Colonel Robert Lloyd-Lindsay, found himself under a good deal of pressure from the partisans of an active peacetime programme of preparation and training. The latter included Thomas Longmore, who had represented the British government at Geneva in 1864 and Berlin in 1869, and three members of the recently-revived Order of St John of Jerusalem: John Furley, Captain Henry Brackenbury, and Captain John Burgess. Furley and Burgess had also attended the Berlin Conference, and were clearly impressed by the arguments made by those who advocated providing assistance to accident victims. In 1872, they recommended that the National Aid Society begin training lifesaving teams which could provide assistance to victims of road, railway and industrial accidents, and which could also be employed as stretcher-bearers by the army in wartime.

Lloyd-Lindsay, a Crimean veteran and recipient of the Victoria Cross, was adamantly opposed to this proposal. Like the Russians in 1869, he and his supporters took the position that using for other purposes monies which had been donated for the relief of the sick and wounded in war was a violation of the trust of the donors. They also argued that assembling storehouses of ambulance equipment and *matériel* was a foolhardy enterprise, because both might well become obsolete before they were required. This claim was tied to another: that because Britain was unlikely to be involved in a major war with another European power, there was no need for such grand preparations. By 1873, John Furley realized that he would be unable to carry the day against the National Aid Society's Executive Committee, so he resigned from that body in order to form

> another society which should more fully realise the object of my aspirations in respect to the organisation of work for the relief of suffering in time of peace, and which should also be fitted to accomplish the same purpose for our army and navy in time of war ....[8]

In 1877, Furley became one of the principal organizers of the St John Ambulance Association, which was soon to exercise considerable influence upon the development of the lifesaving movement on the Continent.[9]

Meanwhile, the French Society for Assistance to Wounded Soldiers was also being urged to take on the task of organizing assistance to accident victims, especially those injured in industrial accidents. In 1872, Drs Ricord and Demarquay, who had been attached to the *Ambulance de la Presse* during the war, urged the

Society to establish a large hospital for the teaching of surgery and the care of the wounded; soon they went further, arguing that the Society should also create several smaller hospitals for the victims of industrial accidents. Making heavy use of analogies with the military, they claimed that the industrial worker should be recognized as 'a soldier of industry who struggles daily against the forces of nature with means that are no less dangerous than the destructive forces routinely employed by armies'.[10] While affirming that they had no intention of weakening the Society's commitment to the needs of wounded soldiers, they were nevertheless bold enough to ask

> why the wounded from the industrial army, who admittedly do not defend our native land, but who enrich it by their labour, who struggle against the elements, who create wonders that bring honour and glory to our country in peacetime, why should these labourers – these other combatants, as it were – not also become the object of your attention in peacetime? [11]

If the Society were to accord the same status to *les mutilés du travail* as it did to *les mutilés de la guerre*, the doctors continued, its beneficent services to the country would be doubled at a stroke.

What lay behind this new-found concern for injured workers? In the pages which followed, Ricord and Demarquay made it plain that they regarded the Paris Commune – 'this monstrous attempt against the family and the moral order'[12] – as a dreadful reminder that too little had yet been done to improve the living and working conditions of industrial workers and their families. With considerable skill, they painted an evocative picture of the present fate of the injured worker: rejected by his employer, unable to spend time with his friends, a burden to his family, unable even to beg because begging was illegal, he would eventually and inevitably become an insurgent against the social order. (From their language, they apparently conceived of both workers and insurgents as male.) Although they conceded that modern industry had created fresh miseries and misfortunes, and that these new forms of suffering deserved assistance, they were resolutely opposed to state intervention on behalf of the victims: society, they firmly asserted, 'must not burden the state with responsibilities that it cannot accept'.[13] On the other hand, they continued, it would be most unwise to leave these matters to the workers themselves, because workers' associations were obviously bent on destroying the social order, the Christian religion, the family, and the institution of property. Instead, it was – as they saw it – the duty of the Society for Assistance to Wounded Soldiers to broaden its horizons and take up *la question sociale* in a practical and tangible way.

Where would the money come from to pay for the care of injured workers? From the great and the rich, apparently; they recommended that the Society approach big companies and wealthy industrialists, who might well prefer assisting the injured to paying damages to widows and orphans whose claims might be pressed by greedy lawyers. Moreover, there were long-term gains for both industry and society in assisting workers to recover from their injuries: without proper care and nourishment, wounds would not heal properly, and then the injured would become unemployable, bringing misery upon themselves and their families, and adding to the numbers of the destitute. If an assistance scheme were to be started successfully in Paris, they speculated, the entire country would soon respond with praise, money would come pouring in, and the Society would be able to depend on the support of a wider circle of benefactors. With a final flourish, they predicted that these endeavours would teach the workers that 'the true socialists are not those who want a society without the family, without property, without God, but those who are animated by a living faith, by a faith that impels them to create fruitful associations that promote well-being ...'. [14]

Despite its frank appeal to ideology, this grand scheme went nowhere. The leaders of the Society for Assistance to Wounded Soldiers simply ignored the proposals of Ricord and Demarquay, and instead spent the rest of the decade attempting to salvage the Society's reputation from the attacks of those who found fault with its performance during the war. By far the most acerbic and trenchant of these critics was Professor Léon Le Fort of the Paris Faculty of Medicine, who delighted in exposing what he regarded as the incompetence of the Society's aristocratic leadership.[15] For the World Exposition held in Paris in 1878, the Society tried to demonstrate its vitality by organizing an extensive display of ambulance wagons and other devices useful in caring for the wounded, but Le Fort used the occasion of a conference on army medical services – held in conjunction with the Exposition – to inflict further damage on the Society's reputation before an international audience, insisting repeatedly on the need to subordinate the quixotic enthusiasm of devotees of battlefield charity to the sobering authority of military medical officers.[16]

Meanwhile, Le Fort's colleague, Dr Auguste Duchaussoy, who had also directed an *ambulance volante* in 1870, advanced the argument that the Society ought to learn from the Germans (following the example of the Baden Ladies' Association and the Patriotic Union of German Women) and establish a school for the training of nurses and ambulance personnel. When he received no encouragement from the Society's leaders, he turned instead to the Paris Society for Practical Medicine – he was its President in 1876 – and with its support established such a school – *l'École de gardes-malades et d'ambulancières* – in 1878. On the strength of the school's initial success, Duchaussoy went on to found his own patriotic charitable society – *l'Association des Dames Françaises* – in 1879. The association attracted a large following, but Duchaussoy's autocratic style and political conservatism soon provoked a confrontation with feminists and democrats who seceded *en bloc* in 1881 to found their own organization, the *Union des Femmes de France.* This body, under largely but not exclusively female leadership, established its own training programmes for nurses. These events produced a legacy of personal animosity and mutual recrimination that lasted into the early years of the twentieth century. The French government officially recognized all three associations as 'organizations of public utility' that were permitted to assist the army medical services. Consequently, Red Cross work in France was divided among three societies, one of which was for decades congenitally inactive, while the other two, both of them proclaiming the need for action, refused to co-operate with one another. These facts help to explain why no French counterpart to the St John Ambulance Association was formed during the 1870s; and also why, when the lifesaving movement finally sprouted in France in the 1890s, it did so outside the framework of the French Red Cross.

Across the Rhine, on the other hand, enthusiasm for the idea of civilian lifesaving was greater than anywhere else in Europe. The moving spirit behind the lifesaving movement in Germany was Friedrich Esmarch, Professor of Surgery at the University of Kiel. Like Thomas Longmore in England and Baron Mundy in Austria, Esmarch had a lifelong interest in the treatment of wounds and injuries, and in the techniques of first-aid and ambulance transport. He was also a good friend and correspondent of John Furley, whom he had first met during the Schleswig war of 1864, and whom he had seen again at the Berlin Conference in 1869. A decade later, Esmarch visited England, and Furley proudly showed him the ambulance corps that were being trained by the St John Ambulance Association. Greatly impressed, Esmarch returned home determined to promote a similar development in Germany. With Furley's assistance, he unveiled his plan for the formation of a 'lifesaving league' at a conference which he organized in Kiel in 1881, and a year later the German Samaritan Association (*Deutscher Samariter Verein*) was officially established. The stated goal of the Association was the establishment of 'Samaritan schools', through which knowledge of first-aid would be spread as widely as possible; all those in positions of authority in business and industry, in government, in the armed forces, and in civil society were called upon to lend their support to the growth of the Samaritan movement.

And support it they most certainly did: within a year, Samaritan societies and schools had been established in some 69 towns and cities throughout Germany, including all of the most important urban centres.[17] The Samaritan cause was taken up by the German Federation of Associations of Factory Foremen, which organized first-aid training courses for its members in Dusseldorf, Magdeburg, Kassel and several other places. In Saxony and Hesse, members of the already popular gymnastic societies not only attended courses but also set up first-aid posts. Cologne was one of several cities where the driving force was the local veterans' association, and in some places the local branch of the German Red Cross Society undertook to organize first-aid training. The directors of the most important technical schools – of agriculture, mining, brewing, etc. – encouraged their students to form Samaritan societies. By the end of the decade, in virtually every German city of any size, policemen and fire-fighters were attending first-aid courses organized by the local Samaritan society. Throughout Germany, respectable society rushed not only to support the Samaritan cause, but to be seen doing so. At court, where Empress Augusta's strong support for the Red Cross set the tone for patriotic philanthropy, the imperial princesses and their ladies-in-waiting attended a course in first-aid that was specially organized for them by the Berlin Samaritan Society. In Saxony, where the philanthropic King John actively promoted the lifesaving idea, the response was so overwhelming that the Leipzig society quadrupled its membership in one year. First-aid had become fashionable.

What did German physicians think of all this? When Esmarch was trying to organize the Samaritan Association, some physicians predictably expressed the fear that the condition of accident victims might be made worse by well-meaning but incompetent assistance. However, Esmarch made a point of ensuring that the Association's statutes defined first-aid as 'assistance given prior to the arrival of a physician', and himself wrote a handbook of first-aid procedures that became the movement's catechism. According to one commentator, what convinced sceptical physicians was the realization that the more numerous Samaritans became, the less business there was for quacks and charlatans.[18] One may question this claim, but there is no doubt that many German physicians were ready to participate in first-aid classes for the Samaritans.

By the mid-1890s, Berlin had the most elaborate arrangements for dealing with accidents of any city in Germany.[19] First-aid courses for fire-fighters and for the police had already been in operation for a decade, and every police station and fire company had sufficient trained men and appropriate equipment to function as both a stationary and a mobile first-aid post. Railway employees and postal workers had also been trained in first-aid techniques. In addition, the city boasted ten 'accident stations' (*Unfallstationnen*), each of which had its own 'pavilion' for the duty physicians and medical equipment, its own stable, and a shed in which the horse-drawn ambulance vehicles were kept, with harness at the ready.[20] The accident stations had been established by the Berlin Samaritan Society; they were maintained with funds contributed to the society by the city's commercial and industrial enterprises and associations (the latter including associations of workers as well as employers). Each station was staffed twenty-four hours a day by three qualified physicians who took day and night duty in rotation. The three principal stations – seven others were classed as auxiliary – had emergency medical clinics attached, so that in many cases it was possible to deal with the injury or illness at the accident station, although where necessary the victim could be transported to one of the city's hospitals. More than a dozen large hospitals in the Greater Berlin area provided emergency treatment in what were called 'ambulance stations', but victims had to be taken or find their own way to the hospitals, none of which possessed their own ambulance vehicles. All of the Samaritan Society's accident stations were connected first by telegraph with the police stations, and later with the hospitals as well, via a central telephone switchboard installed at the Town Hall. Published statistics for the years 1895 through 1897 reveal that the accident stations recorded a total of 31,983 cases of injury or sudden illness, of which almost all (29,386) were attended to at one of the stations or attached clinics.[21] More than half of these cases took place in 1896, when Berlin hosted an international commercial exposition.

In the course of the next decade, this enthusiasm for establishing accident stations was taken up by two more voluntary associations: the Berlin Society for Sanitary Stations, and the Berlin Red Cross Society for Accident Stations. By 1905, these two bodies were operating another 34 'sanitary' or 'Red Cross' first-aid stations scattered around the city and its suburbs. Although more modestly equipped than the larger stations run by the Samaritan Society, these smaller facilities were accessible day and night to those in need, particularly the poor, who were treated for free. Those better off were charged fees for their treatment, and the proceeds were used to offset a portion of the operating expenses; other sources of revenue came from individual donations, subsidies from local authorities, house-to-house collections, and charity fêtes. Expenses were substantial because every one of these 34 first-aid stations had a qualified physician and an assistant – probably a medical student – on duty at all times; at some of them, a nurse was also on duty.[22]

In order to co-ordinate their work, the three voluntary associations agreed to work together as the Berlin First Aid Society, appointing Professor George Meyer as medical director. However, in April 1907, these arrangements were superseded by the municipal government, which took over the personnel and equipment of the Samaritan Society, and established a new Berlin Ambulance Department under the direction of Professor Meyer. This municipal intervention resulted in some reorganization of the main accident stations, but it apparently left the smaller first-aid stations in the hands of the voluntary associations that had created them.

Although the St John Ambulance Association had served as Esmarch's original model, the accident stations and emergency medical clinics run by the Berlin Samaritans put them well beyond the achievements of their English counterparts. True, the St John Ambulance Brigade had been formed in 1887, but its members – though numerous, well-trained and disciplined – were deployed largely on special occasions when great crowds were assembled, or in response to particular disasters, especially in the coal-mining areas. Although the Association had established a small permanent first-aid post at St Paul's Cathedral in the City of London, neither the Association nor the Brigade operated civilian ambulances that were always on duty, nor had they begun to plan the creation of accident stations or emergency clinics in urban areas. Clearly, the Germans had outstripped their English mentors; yet the formidable achievements of the Berliners were certainly equalled, if not overshadowed, by those of the lifesaving societies in the two great cities of Austria-Hungary.

The Austrians had not participated in Esmarch's conference, but almost simultaneously the inhabitants of Vienna were prodded into action by a civil disaster of spectacular proportions: 449 persons lost their lives when the Ring Theatre burned down in December 1881.[23] The fire served as the catalyst for an appeal, launched by philanthropic members of the aristocracy, for funds to establish a volunteer lifesaving society (*Wiener freiwillige Rettungs-Gesellschaft*). Baron Mundy of the Austrian Red Cross became its first secretary-general and, in effect, its physician-administrator. Under his direction, the active members of the Society – almost 1000 of them, between the ages of 18 and 40 – attached themselves to one of three sections. The first section was a 300-man volunteer fire brigade, with its own apparatus and equipment, that formed an auxiliary to the municipal fire department. The second section specialized in flood relief: it was composed of almost 300 members, most of whom belonged to boating or gymnastic societies, and by the early 1890s it possessed two lifeboats and several cooking and supply wagons. The third section, organized to respond to accidental injuries, was composed of 200 physicians, assisted by another 200 medical students. The work of the active members was supported by the contributions of a roughly equal number of other (inactive) paying members and benefactors, and by small subsidies from the Austrian government, the city of Vienna, and the Savings Bank.

During the first decade of its existence, the Vienna Voluntary Lifesaving Society operated three permanent first-aid posts in various parts of the city. Unlike the Berliners, the Viennese staffed these posts with medical students trained in first-aid rather than with physicians, and communication between the posts and the police was by telephone rather than telegraph. Besides the first-aid posts, the Society placed stretchers for public use at nearly two dozen stops along the municipal tramway; these were fastened to a nearby wall, together with a notice which politely requested users to bring them back when finished and rebuckle the belts, the notice itself a revealing commentary on the level of propriety expected of the general public a century ago. According to its own statistics, during the first seven years of its existence the Society responded to nearly ten thousand accidents, more than half of which required the services of physicians as well as medical students; the volunteer fire brigade turned out more than 1800 times; the lifeboat crew 350 times; and the tramway stretchers were employed more than 1100 times.[24] By 1890, the Society had come to an agreement with the military authorities concerning its role in the event of war: while its fire brigade would take charge of security at military barracks, hospitals and storage depots throughout the city, its first-aid teams would take charge of the disembarkation of wounded soldiers in the city's railway stations and at the landing stations along the Danube river.[25]

At the end of its first decade, the Vienna Society decided to concentrate its first-aid operations in one central location, on a site offered by the government. The new building, which cost 30,000 florins (about half of the Society's annual revenue), was imposing as well as functional. Its central block of two storeys provided an office for the physicians, a duty room for the medical students, space for the treatment of the sick and injured, a bath and WC, a library, secretarial offices, and sleeping accommodation for the medical students, nurses, servants and drivers. One wing held the refectory, and another the garage and a five-horse stable.

The Vienna Society's decision to centralize its work may have been taken to profit from economies of scale, but ethnic rivalry may also have played a part, because it was in the Kingdom of Hungary that the European lifesaving movement had reached its apogee. A volunteer lifesaving society had been founded in Budapest in 1887, and after only three years of operation it moved into a newly-constructed building, 'a grand edifice in the Renaissance style, which conforms to all the requirements of modern hygiene'.[26] The new building, which replaced an earlier first-aid station in the old town, was deliberately located close to the industrial districts, but also near enough to the bridges to provide easy access to other parts of the city. While the earlier station (which comprised six rooms, three ambulance wagons and an omnibus) had been serviceable, the new building, which boasted central heating throughout, was nothing short of lavish. Among its noteworthy features were a fully-equipped medical clinic, including an operating table and disinfecting equipment; an elaborate telephone switchboard, connecting it with the city's police stations and hospitals; offices for the two physicians who, in alternating 24-hour shifts, served as medical director; a dormitory for the twelve senior medical students who, working in teams of four, made up its regular staff; a guardroom for those on duty and a library/recreation room for those off duty; a meeting and seminar room, where classes in first-aid were held; and, on the top floor, a five-room apartment for the administrative director. In addition to the main building, there was also a huge two-storey outbuilding, its lower floor occupied by sheds holding twenty vehicles and by two separate stables (one for the duty horses and another for those in reserve); above the stables were dormitories for the drivers and (male) nurses, while over the garage was a loft where fodder and additional stretchers were stored.

In the impressive fleet of ambulance transport operated by the Budapest Society were some remarkable vehicles: a horse-drawn omnibus for multiple-victim accidents; a propeller-driven lifeboat that patrolled the urban portion of the Danube; a windowless carriage specially designed for transporting the insane, with a skylight/grill in the top for light, a rubber-padded interior, and a hidden alarm which permitted the guard inside to communicate with the driver outside; and finally, two landaus (the favourite vehicles of the aristocracy), which were used exclusively for transporting sick or injured members of the upper class, 'their exteriors looking exactly like those of ordinary carriages, so as not to arouse the curiosity of passers-by'.[27] Given that one of the vehicles used by the Society for transporting victims of industrial accidents had slatted sides and resembled a railway cattle-car, it seems that lifesaving in Budapest had reached an almost Marxian level of class consciousness. Certainly the work done by the Society met with a high degree of public approval: half of its annual operating expense (20,000 florins in 1890) was defrayed by a subsidy from the city, while the remainder was covered by donations and legacies from benefactors.

But what of the French? Despite their earlier lack of interest in the Ricord/Demarquay plan, the French could not remain entirely aloof from this wave of enthusiasm for ambulances and lifesaving, and before the end of the century ambulances had appeared in the streets of Paris. For inspiration, the Parisians had looked neither to the English practice of training a volunteer first-aid corps, nor to the central European model of increasingly elaborate 'accident stations' and emergency medical centres; instead, they borrowed from the United States – specifically from New York City – the practice of basing ambulance vehicles at hospitals, and sending a hospital surgeon to the scene of the accident. If the victim required more care than could be given at the site, the same vehicle could be used to transport him/her back to the hospital, where the surgeon could speedily arrange for admission.

The leader of the campaign for urban ambulance services in Paris was Dr Henri Nachtel, who had been much impressed during a visit to New York in 1880 by the ambulances operated by Bellevue Hospital, and by the House of Relief Society (dating from 1869 and 1876 respectively). As soon as he returned, Nachtel rushed into print with a series of pamphlets which praised the New York arrangements and called for the establishment of similar services in Paris.[28] His proposal was discussed and approved by the Academy of Medicine, the Council on Hygiene and Salubrity of the Department of the Seine, and the Municipal Council of Paris. 'But,' as Dr Mauriac of Bordeaux commented, 'in France it's a long way from the expression of a wish to its realisation'[29] and the plan soon became bogged down in interminable discussions between the Prefect of Police and the Director of Public Assistance. In 1887, the exasperated Dr Nachtel decided to form a private society, known as *L'Oeuvre des Ambulances Urbaines*, to support a more limited version of his plan in one area, centred on the St Louis Hospital in the northeast quadrant of the city. Within a fixed perimeter, 28 public call-boxes were erected, so that anyone witnessing an accident could immediately summon help from the ambulance station at the Hospital. The scheme was so popular that in 1890 plans were forthcoming to create a second station at the Beaujon Hospital, but the Paris Municipal Council refused a requested subsidy, and for the moment, the scheme stalled.

At this point Bordeaux rather than Paris became the centre of attention. Here Dr Mauriac, Inspector of Salubrity of the Department of the Gironde, was the driving force behind the creation of an urban ambulance service. An active participant in the work of international congresses of public assistance, Mauriac had visited Germany and Austria-Hungary while compiling a report on first-aid to accident victims, which he presented to the 1889 Congress. Captivated by what he had seen in Berlin, Leipzig, Vienna and Budapest, Mauriac was convinced that French cities needed first-aid posts run by trained staff who would be instructed in first-aid, as would the general public, by physicians and pharmacists who would donate their services to an ambulance or lifesaving society. In matters of public assistance, Mauriac was a strong advocate of private initiative:

> In France we have an unfortunate tendency to ask the State and the Municipalities to do everything. It is important to react against this tendency towards a veritable State socialism which results in the incessant increase in the number of civil servants, the growth of administrative red tape, loans, and new taxes; all of which paralyse individual effort, promote selfish feelings, and in the end lead people to abandon any interest in philanthropic work, while persuading themselves that the State and the Municipalities are obligated to deal with all the miseries, needs, and demands of the community.[30]

The Bordeaux Urban Ambulance Society, set up in 1890 as a result of Mauriac's initiative, modelled itself on the central European societies: it aimed to establish first-aid posts around the city, to offer first-aid courses to the public, and to offer its services to the authorities in the event of war.[31] A dozen years later, it was operating three ambulance stations (two of them on the waterfront) and 25 first-aid posts in the district police stations, all of these connected by telephone with the city's hospitals and with the office of the director of ambulance services at the Society's headquarters. At one of its ambulance stations, the Society also operated a dispensary for the sick poor. Nevertheless, Dr Mauriac admitted in a report written in 1903, financial support for the Society had been declining recently, and its involvement in industrial accidents had been sharply reduced by the passage of a law (in 1900) requiring injured workers to obtain certificates that were available only from physicians employed by accident insurance companies. Because of falling revenues, Mauriac lamented, the Society could not afford to put rubber tyres on its horse-drawn ambulance vehicles. In these straitened circumstances, the erstwhile ideologist of voluntarism soon modified his views on state subsidies: 'Without doubt [he wrote in 1903] private initiative is best, the ideal way to proceed; but when private initiative becomes insufficient, it is the duty of the State, of the department, or the commune to come to its aid'.[32]

The absence of strong voluntary societies continued to plague the lifesaving movement in France. In Paris, the city government changed its mind in 1894 and took over Dr Nachtel's ambulance scheme, promising to extend its scope by creating new ambulance posts on both the left and the right banks of the Seine; nevertheless, the Parisian ambulance service continued to be based at hospitals rather than accident stations. French advocates of Samaritan societies continued to call for a broader approach: Émile Cacheux, President of the French Hygiene Society and one of the organizers of the international lifesaving congress, proposed a 'model society' that, like the Vienna Society, was organized to assist victims of submersion, fire, and accident. He emphasized that each group could play a special role in wartime: the submersion experts dealing with floods, the fire experts protecting the supplies of the military health service, and the accident experts serving in Red Cross auxiliary hospitals. The central European model also attracted Professor Félix Terrier of the Faculty of Medicine, who argued that what Paris and other French cities needed were ambulance posts or accident stations, specialized emergency facilities staffed by organized groups of senior medical students; these could be funded partially by aid societies and partially by subventions from accident insurance companies whose payouts would be substantially reduced if good first-aid treatment were available to the injured.[33] In his lectures Terrier put considerable emphasis on the close connection between emergency surgery and military surgery, telling his students that if they worked at civilian ambulance stations, 'you would render great service to the injured ... and you will prepare yourselves for the moment when France will need you to care for her wounded'.[34] Nevertheless, despite the urgings of Cacheux, Terrier and other like-minded physicians, the *Société de secouristes français* (founded 1892) never became an organization comparable in size and influence to the lifesaving societies in other European states.

What distinguishes the European experience with ambulances and lifesaving from developments in England and the United States? Two features stand out immediately: first, the enormously important role played by the voluntary lifesaving movement; and secondly, the clear preference of European cities – Paris excepted – for free-standing accident stations, institutions that were quite separate from municipal and charity hospitals.

The absence of a voluntary lifesaving movement in the United States is striking. Earlier in the century, Alexis de Tocqueville had proclaimed the principle of voluntary association to be a remarkably strong feature of American life, and on that basis one might have expected a voluntary lifesaving movement to flourish in this environment. However, the truth is that nothing comparable to the St John Ambulance Association – let alone the more ambitious European Samaritan societies – ever appeared in the United States. It is true that under Clara Barton's leadership, the American Red Cross Society involved itself in civilian disaster relief, but disasters are of a different order of magnitude than accidents, and accident victims did not form part of the constituency of the American Red Cross. Teaching and practising civilian first-aid never became the popular, even fashionable, cause in America that it did in England or Germany. Instead, it became the accepted practice in American cities to transport accident victims directly to hospitals in vehicles owned and operated by the hospitals themselves. Support from municipal governments and from the police ensured that the practice quickly became firmly entrenched, and there was thus no reason to conceive of a possible role for organized volunteers or for institutional alternatives to big city hospitals. In any case, postbellum Americans believed that their nation's great armed struggle was already behind them; hence they could imagine no future military role for persons trained in first-aid and ambulance techniques.

In England, as on the Continent, the humanitarianism of those who promoted ambulances and lifesaving was undoubtedly coloured by their enthusiasm for the potential wartime usefulness of trained ambulance workers. Yet this blending of patriotism and humanitarianism did not produce comparable results: although the vitality of the voluntary lifesaving movement in England is indisputable, its aspirations and achievements were of a different order of magnitude from those of the Samaritan societies in Germany and Austria-Hungary. Why this should have been so is a difficult question to answer. Although the St John Ambulance Association may have provided the initial inspiration for the *Deutscher Samariter Verein*, the latter quickly made itself a force to be reckoned with in civil society, while the former was apparently content to teach first-aid to those in hazardous occupations and to provide highly visible trained ambulance brigades for parades and state occasions. Furley and other leading St John figures made no effort to involve the Association or the Brigade in the ambulance services that were organized in Liverpool and Manchester, nor did they campaign for the establishment in London of decentralized, easily accessible accident stations. If Cooter is correct in emphasizing the fear of disorder as their principal motivation, one has to ask why it did not impel them to seek a more active and extensive social role.

More definitive conclusions will have to await further research, but at least some important questions can be identified. In explaining the extraordinary success of the ambulance movement in Central Europe, one could ask how far state and municipal authorities welcomed the appearance of Samaritan societies and accident stations largely because they relieved the police of the burden of caring for, and providing transport for, the sick and injured, thereby allowing them to concentrate on the maintenance of public order, and the pursuit of criminals. If it emerges that this was indeed an important consideration, then one would need to explain why a similar sense of relief was not felt in Paris, or indeed anywhere in England. Why did it take so long for the popularity of lifesaving to spread to France? Does Germanophobia explain why the Parisians preferred to follow New York and Boston rather than Berlin and Vienna? Finally, to what extent was the movement fuelled by concerns far less elevated than patriotism or humanitarianism? Cooter rightly draws attention to the need for further study of the idea and practice of accident insurance.[35]

How many of the promoters of ambulances and lifesaving, it may be asked, had connections with accident insurance companies, the latter having a direct financial interest in the fate of accident victims? Dr Mauriac of Bordeaux, for example, was for many years in the employ of the Zurich Insurance Company, which furnished him with most of the statistical evidence that he used to make the case for better urban first-aid services. Was it perhaps to be expected that the lifesaving movement would arise in a Europe where both armaments and profits increasingly occupied the thoughts of those in authority?

Notes

1. Joan Clifford, *For the Service of Mankind. Furley, Lechmere and Duncan, St John Ambulance Founders* (London: Robert Hale, 1971), 85.
2. John S. Haller, Jr, 'The Beginnings of Urban Ambulance Services in the United States and England', *Journal of Emergency Medicine*, 8 (1990), 743. See also his *Farmcarts to Fords: A History of the Military Ambulance, 1790–1925* (Carbondale: Southern Illinois University Press, 1992).
3. Thomas Haskell, 'Capitalism and the Humanitarian Sensibility', *American Historical Review*, 90 (1985), 339–61, 547–66.
4. E. Mauriac, *L'organisation des secours publics en cas d'accidents en Allemagne et en Autriche-Hongrie* (Bordeaux: Feret & Fils, 1890), 5–6.
5. On the congested city see James M. Winter, *London's Teeming Streets, 1830–1914* (London: Routledge, 1993).
6. For a more detailed account, see John F. Hutchinson, *Champions of Charity: War and the Rise of the Red Cross* (Boulder and Oxford: Westview Press, 1996); *idem*, 'Rethinking the Origins of the Red Cross', *Bulletin of the History of Medicine*, 63 (1989), 557–78.
7. Hutchinson, *Champions of Charity*, 97–101. In fact, the position taken by the Russian delegates in Berlin was soon abandoned by the Russian Red Cross Society, which then undertook extensive peacetime work that went far beyond disaster relief.
8. Sir John Furley, *In Peace and War. Autobiographical Sketches* (London: Smith, Elder, 1905), 384.
9. On the origins and activities of the St John Ambulance Association, see Cooter, 'Moment of the Accident', in this volume; also Anne Summers, *Angels and Citizens: British Women as Military Nurses, 1854–1914* (London: Routledge and Kegan Paul, 1988), 166–71.
10. *Deuxième rapport fait à la Commission des Études de la Société de Secours aux Blessés sur la necessité de créer des ambulances modèles pour les blessés d'industrie par Mm. les Drs. Ricord et Demarquay* (Paris, n.d. [1873?]), 2.
11. *Deuxième rapport*, 4.
12. *Deuxième rapport*, 7.

13. *Deuxième rapport*, 6.
14. *Deuxième rapport*, 10.
15. See, for example, Léon Le Fort, *La Chirurgie Militaire et les Sociétés de Secours en France et à l'Etranger* (Paris: Germer Ballière, 1872).
16. His unrelenting assaults may be followed in *Congrès international sur le service médical des armées en campagne, tenu à Paris les 12, 13 et 14 août 1878* (Paris: Imprimerie Nationale, 1879).
17. What follows here summarizes the more detailed discussion in Mauriac, *L'organisation des secours publics*, 11–21, and J. Grunberg, *De l'organisation des secours aux blessés dans les grands villes (Les ambulances urbaines de l'Hôpital Saint-Louis)* (Paris: Société d'éditions scientifiques, 1897), 139–44.
18. Émile Cacheux, *Le Sauvetage en France et à l'étranger* (Paris: Paul Baudry, 1896), 173–4.
19. For a detailed treatment of the situation in Germany, see George Meyer, *Das Rettungs- und Krankenbeförderungswesen im Deutschen Reiche* (Jena: Gustav Fischer, 1906).
20. Grunberg, *De l'organisation des secours*, 142–3.
21. Grunberg, *De l'organisation des secours*, 144.
22. This information about Berlin was supplied by Professor George Meyer to the London Ambulance Committee, and appeared in *Report of the Ambulance Committee* (London: HMSO, 1909), 1: 113–14.
23. This summary is based on the descriptions in *Report of the Ambulance Committee*, 125–31; Cacheux, *Le Sauvetage en France et à l'étranger*, 185–91; and Mauriac, *L'organisation des secours publics*, 22–9.
24. Mauriac, *L'organisation des secours publics*, 26–7.
25. Cacheux, *Le Sauvetage en France et à l'étranger*, 190.
26. Grunberg, *De l'organisation des secours*, 133.
27. Grunberg, *De l'organisation des secours*, 135.
28. Henri Nachtel, *Fonctionnement de l'ambulance urbaine de New-York, destinée à porter les premiers secours sur la voie publique, et utilité qu'il y a d'établir un service de ce genre à Paris* (Paris: G. Masson, 1881); *idem, L'organisation à Paris d'ambulances urbaines analogue à celle des grandes villes d'Amérique* (Paris, 1881).
29. [E. Mauriac] *La Société des Ambulances Urbaines de Bordeaux. Son organisation et son fonctionnement* (Bordeaux: Imprimerie C. Gounouilhou, 1890), 7.
30. [E. Mauriac] *La Société des Ambulances Urbaines*, 8.
31. *Statuts de la Société des Ambulances Urbaines de Bordeaux, adoptés 28 mars 1890.*
32. E. Mauriac, *Les Ambulances Urbaines de Bordeaux de 1890 à 1903* (Bordeaux: Feret et Fils, 1903), 12–13.
33. Terrier's opening address to his students, entitled 'Les soins à donner aux blessés dans les grandes villes', is reprinted in Grunberg, *De l'organisation des secours*, 24–38.
34. Grunberg, *De l'organisation des secours*, 38.
35. Cooter, 'Moment of the Accident', 115–16.

8

What are Occupational Diseases? Risk and Risk Management in Industrial Medicine in Germany, c.1880–1920

Dietrich Milles

Production of Risks and Production of Security

The discussion of risk is a modern trend in German sociology.[1] There are still the 'pleasures and pains' of war, natural catastrophes and famine to attract the onlooker; but society is now becoming a 'risk to itself',[2] and even human beings are regarded as 'risk factors'.[3] Of course, there are various explanations for this growing perception of risk, ranging from social change, economic crises[4] and individualization,[5] to global and ecological crises.[6] I want to argue, however, that there are specific links between present-day concerns with risk and the industrial society that began to take shape towards the end of the nineteenth century. Economic, social, technological and market processes all demanded the application of strictly calculable factors; at the same time the complexity of 'risk' and the significance of chronic processes were growing. Yet, the sociopolitical construction of risk was still founded on a general belief in technological safety and welfare which was only threatened by the random occurrence of singular, acute 'accidents' – literally, in German, those events which were not supposed to happen (*unfall*, i.e., 'non-case').

It has become a part of everyday life for our society and its subjects to suffer and overcome crises.[7] Today, only the extent of such phenomena is found to be irritating. This appears to be connected with the advance of liberal social intercourse, which has been described by Karl Polanyi as the 'Great Transformation',[8] and 'has created a fundamental sense of insecurity in society as a whole'.[9] The fact that all the necessities for a modern 'civilized' existence are produced in the material world and by human 'rational' design[10] does not simply form the foundation for, and legitimize, civil liberties, but also gives rise to reciprocal claims to security between individuals, the community and the state. The 'securement of security' (*Sicherung der Sicherheit*)[11] was the objective behind the foundation of the welfare state. In a society which was alleged 'artificially' to create and thus ensure all the conditions for social existence, action was necessary to regulate those hazards which manifestly proclaimed the opposite. The security of the risk-producing and compensating community has become a central value in our society.[12] However, two questions central to the concept of security – to what extent security should be ensured, and what people could reasonably be expected to tolerate – were then evaluated and reduced to the insurance formula: probability of 'hazard x' multiplied by extent of the expectable damage. This formula, which combined the illusion of controlling nature by compensation strategies, is today being questioned in the light of the growing complexities of hazards, widening areas of risk and increasingly incalculable damage.[13]

One particular aspect of the modern conception of risk – the development of accident insurance from its introduction in 1884 to the enactment of the German Occupational Disease Ordinance (*Berufskrankheit-enverordung*) in 1925 – will be presented here. The central issue is the context within which perceptions of risk developed in industrial society. This is seen, for example, in the differentiation between accidents and diseases. The inclusion of work-related diseases in accident insurance as laid down in 1925 in the Occupational Disease Ordinance, which contained a list of recognized diseases, will serve to illustrate more clearly the perception of risk in German industrial society.

Emphasis will be laid on specific developments in Germany which, particularly in comparison to England, were influenced by a stronger socially integrative state policy. In discussions of different types of welfare state (following Goesta Esping-Andersen)[14] it has been argued that in Germany compulsory state insurance can reasonably be attributed to the combined influences of a conservative labour policy and a weak parliament.

Over and above the relationship between paid work and welfare, reference can here be made only to the interesting relationship between paid work and unpaid work and welfare, and, with it, the gender-specific control mechanisms of the welfare state.[15] It is important to note, however, that in Germany, under the influence of the social doctrine of Catholicism, a socialization of industrial risk took place which was differentiated and organized through corporations (e.g. trade associations), which shaped the German social insurance system. This was different from England, where more emphasis was laid on voluntary insurance contributions, and where the role of the state was on the whole regulatory. Reference can only be made here to some of the more striking differences in the development of the English social insurance system, one of which is the surprisingly stable foundations of the German insurance system.[16]

The Construction of Risk in the Development of German Industrial Society

The hazards to life and health which accompanied industrial development from the end of the seventeenth century onwards were first recognized by their frequency in specific occupational groups and regions, as for example mercurial poisoning among mirror workers in Fürth. The causal connections with the generally difficult living conditions of the workers as well as certain working materials, working postures and working environments, were blatant. Whether these causal connections were valid, or whether the exact causes and the laws governing them could be determined, was not questioned. Likewise, no difference was made between the hazards which afflict us 'externally' and the risks which are a consequence of human actions and decisions.[17] Until the mid-nineteenth century hazards and risks were therefore perceived as conditions peculiar to certain occupations. At that time, the term 'occupational diseases' covered, on the one hand, social evils of a general nature and, on the other, concrete problems relating to 'artificial' work processes.[18]

Simultaneously there emerged a further category of health risks. Modern society did not offer everyone or every family the opportunity to secure a decent livelihood by means of property ownership, or the acquisition of property by the fruit of one's own labour. *Poverty* became the main obstacle to integrative social reform and manifested itself in the form of immoral and unclean, i.e. 'unhealthy', lifestyles.[19] Poverty became the focal point of the conception of risk in a society which justified itself on the basis of its ideals of equality but which was in effect socially and economically unequal.

In this respect Salomon Neumann, one of Germany's first notable medical officers of health, drew the logical conclusion when in 1847 he defined health risk as a problem of property ownership, particularly for those who had no property other than their own bodies with which to secure a livelihood and had no access to medical care.[20] He claimed that the only means of securing a livelihood was therefore by the guarantee of a right to work. This 'social question' became the dominant social problem in Germany throughout the nineteenth century.[21]

Ironically, while poverty was initially a threat, it also had a sociopolitical stabilizing and regulatory function[22] by facilitating a description of the situation and a terminological classification on the basis of goods and 'lacks'.[23] However, major accidents accompanying industrialization threw this construction of risk (including health risks) into disorder.[24] These accidents were symbolic of the risks inherent in industrial production and signalled the limitations of human control over nature. From the point of view of optimists, though, these accidents were nothing more than processes which were technically imperfect or maladjusted: disruptions that could be corrected.

It was only with the recognition of accident risks in industrial society in the first half of the nineteenth century that the health hazards in general which accompanied industrial production – 'industrial pathogenicity' – were again acknowledged as a salient problem. Among affected workers and in public debates, the links were recognized between work-related diseases, poverty and hardship on the one hand,[25] and spectacular accidents and fatalities on the other. Socio-politically, occupational diseases attained menacing proportions, illustrating the irresponsible egotism of industrialists as well as the just demands of the workers' movements. After the Paris Commune of 1871, during the wave of strikes in the Great Depression, the issue became potentially explosive.

From the dominant scientific and technological point of view, work-related health hazards were problematic because of their long latency period, and because the relation between cause and effect was difficult to determine or prove. From the 1870s onwards, there was a tendency within industrial society to rule out their existence as far as possible, or at least to maintain that they could be kept under control. This tendency tied in with the logic of controlling nature, which was purported to be following its own laws, maintaining an apparently objective approach, and not requiring any justification for the consequences. The complex and pervasive health hazards and injuries which nevertheless prevailed were then attributed to the workers themselves, who were examined for deviations, peculiarities or susceptibilities according to their age and constitution. A prominent example of this category of risk was workers' diseases as defined in the German Occupational Disease Ordinance. These conditions[26] were unpleasant and a burden for the persons affected, but at the same time they were difficult to account for; they were abnormal and puzzling. Even natural processes such as ageing might be perceived and treated as 'unnatural' conditions. The holistic approach to disease corresponded less and less with the diseases which were diagnosed, for which the victims were increasingly reproached and generally called upon to adopt a 'better', more healthy behaviour.[27] It was replaced by the concept of disease as a defect in need of repair.[28] Great pains were taken to diagnose direct organic connections between cause and effect in the diseased body and to treat them accordingly.

The perception of risk was structured by institutions which initially came into existence to deal with economic and social concerns. These were mainly private insurance companies on the one hand, and trade union friendly societies, on the other.[29] Later, however, agencies were founded to mediate between affected civilians or workers and the state. The principles of the 'Société Industrielle' in Mulhouse (occupied by Germany from 1871)[30] formed the root of the German social insurance system as it first developed around accident insurance in the late 1870s and early 1880s. Participating employers applied patriarchal principles not just within their factories but also within united trade associations for the purposes of controlling and regulating technological standards and especially accident prevention, as a means of 'pacification'. This construction fitted in well with the development of Bonapartiste Prussian Germany. The central concern of these intermediate agencies was the prevention of accidents by technological means, and compensation for accidents and industrial pathogenicity. Thus, although the Accident Insurance Act was the first and fundamental social insurance legislation to be discussed, it was only passed by the Reichstag in 1884 after the establishment of general statutory health insurance a year earlier.[31]

From its foundation until the early 1880s there was no coherent risk structure within the German social insurance scheme. Initially, this meant that those suffering from work-related diseases were either granted general compensation through statutory health insurance according to the poverty model, or they had to substantiate their compensation claim with proof that their condition, its development and all its ramifications were caused by a sudden event, that is, an 'accident'.

Industrial Pathogenicity as an Inherent Component of Industrial Society

From the pre-1848 revolutionary period at the latest, the functional differentiation of modern society[32] was closely related to that of industry.[33] Even within the workers' movements there were many who viewed economics from a technological perspective; they assumed that industrial development and general public well-being, as well as social security, went hand-in-hand.[34]

Social responsibility for the negative consequences of industrial-technical development was therefore only acknowledged in extraordinary and acute circumstances. The 'accident paradigm' – the fundamental concept of an accident as a sudden occurrence of external origin causing health damage to the human body – was thus effective for all injuries to people who themselves had no decisive influence over cause. Within the legal framework, liability law was intended to compensate for such injuries and at the same time impose a form of behavioural control on the responsible party. The Liability Act of 1871 (*Haftpflichtgesetz*), however, placed the onus on the injured worker to prove the relationship between work-related causes and the injury. In view of the workers' dependency on their employers and on their jobs, this was difficult to accomplish.[35] Liability for intentional and negligent acts as defined by civil law still lay with the employers, but the scope of behavioural control was restricted. Industrial development was of greater sociopolitical significance than possible impairments to the health of individual workers. Injured workers therefore had to prove, firstly, that an accident – and *not* a disease – had actually occurred and, secondly, that the responsibility for the accident lay with the employer. The definition of an accident as 'a sudden occurrence of extrinsic origin' ruled out a whole range of risks and injuries which were systematically ascribed to the personal responsibility of individual workers.

The normative legal justification for the welfare state implied the protection of employers from state intervention and the protection of workers from the disadvantages of industrial progress. Throughout the nineteenth century this justification was of considerable significance to the growing acceptance of industrial capitalism as the inherently 'natural' form of production within German society: there was a degree of legitimacy in health hazards and injuries since they lay 'in the nature of industry'. On 6 July, 1888, for instance, the Third Civil Senate of the Imperial Insurance Court (*Reichsversicherungs-Amt*) ruled that the term 'accident' be defined in a narrow sense as a 'temporally determinable occurrence'. However, they argued that the occupational disease in question,

> could not be attributed to the gradual onset of the effects of a particular occurrence, but was an intoxication which had developed over a number of years as a result of constantly handling white lead, it was a chronic disease caused by continual exposure [to white lead]. This is directly connected with the occupation of the Plaintiff, and must be regarded as an occupational disease, the nature of which is unalterable even if, as the Plaintiff asserts, the Defendant

> failed to meet the regulations and make the necessary provisions to avert the danger. Diseases arising gradually out of the effects of industrial production are however not accidents, but the common and foreseeable drawbacks of an inherently unhealthy industry which must be taken into account by everyone participating in that industry. The Accident Insurance Act does not provide for insurance against such diseases or invalidity resulting from them.

Industrial pathogenicity was thus no longer an 'artificial', i.e. abnormal, additional and produced risk, but had become a 'natural' unalterable risk. This understanding of work-related diseases as 'natural risks' contributed to what has been defined by Ulrich Beck as 'the mistake of the century in the administration of hazards' within the field of work-related diseases.[36]

It should also be pointed out that Kant's theory of reason provided an effective philosophical foundation for the sociopolitical context within which these developments took place.[37] According to this theory, causality is an *a priori* form of thought, and the laws of nature comply with human knowledge. In the course of the nineteenth century, 'reason' was usurped by mechanical science by simply inverting Kant's argument.[38] Hermann Helmholtz, for example, one of Germany's most eminent natural scientists, acknowledged in the 1870s the necessity of general philosophical reflection, but at the same time argued that clarity and certainty grew with empirical facts, becoming manifest in the formulation of natural laws.[39] Helmholtz thus paved the way for the general conviction among industrialists that although *homo faber* may not be in a position to comprehend all the vital forces of the world, to control nature one simply had to dissect it, carve it up into measurable sizes and reconstruct its simple regularities. Consequently a simple, linear principle of causality prevailed which, although disproved by reality, could be asserted by active and rational humans.[40] In this respect it was possible for the scientific point of view, in interaction with the scientific control of nature, to predominate, while natural philosophy and ethics were suppressed.[41]

In this way a new relationship was established between endeavours to overcome human physiological limitations by technological means [42] and the belief in progress which was predicated on increased productivity. This progressivism was justified naturalistically by the 'laws' of social Darwinism.[43] The principle of vital forces was set forth in the course of discussions on *das wahre Kraftmaß* ('the real measure of power'), which gave rise to the belief that greater efficiency could be achieved through technological progress. Its similarity to the principles of economy lay in a mutual concern for weights, measures and figures, rational philosophy and lifestyle and an optimistic approach to the Enlightenment.[44]

These philosophical, ideological and practical precepts had a marked influence on work-related risks. Some were categorized as natural, acceptable risks, like lightning, the effects of which could be alleviated, while the rest were deemed to be a problem relating to the technological development of industry. The implication here was that the progressive control of nature brought new hazards with it which would be overcome during the next phase of technological development.

Insurance – an Institutional Framework for Technological Progress

Politically, the institutional control of risks imposed on industrial society by itself was executed at two levels: insurance, and through the principle of meritocracy. Insurance evolved with modern society's desire for security, the calculability of hazards and injuries and the protection of civil property. Simultaneously it eased the manageability of industrial pathogenicity. It made it possible to treat the problem of risk as a problem of risk management, which was essentially a question of normalization. Risks which occurred despite human control over nature were perceived as hazards, and in extreme cases as catastrophes, and were dealt with as claims problems rather than those of prevention.

In terms of claims settlement, risk implied that there were uncontrollable hazards: a great many possibly controllable hazards should be treated as such because of financial and similar constraints. It also implied that all social problems were related to property ownership or earnings and could be solved by employment, and that all specific causes should be objectified and all specific effects placed under the responsibility of society (*vergesellschaftet*). The consequence was a certain degree of protection against the blows of fate, but mainly in the form of employment-related compensation.

Strictly speaking, the consequence of this was a right to work (as Salomon Neumann had argued), because only through work could the obligation to secure a livelihood for everybody be upheld.[45] This was a sociopolitical problem which the modern state was not so keen to solve, and it was also a claim which legally could not be met because the dynamics of the market economy were already in force. This is where sociopolitical control took over by substituting the right to work with the state provision of a small subsistence allowance, which at the same time served as a social control mechanism and imposed the obligation to increase productivity. This in turn was based on the idea of technological and industrial progress and the illusion of industrially produced security and public well-being.

The meritocratic control of risk can be explained as follows. The coupling of risk management with growing social efficiency – welfare provision and social control – was in principle linked to the association of power and capital, as epitomized by the rivalry of the German empire with England, and expressed in the relation between economic expansionism and militaristic nationalism. The underlying ideology was expressed by the term 'human economy' which, founded on the doctrine of social Darwinism, described the structural combination of technological and industrial development with social policy and economic expansion with national well-being.[46] This term was first coined by Rudolf Goldscheid in 1911 and was soon embedded in theories on evolution and the world market.[47]

The doctrine of human economy attributed a reciprocal dynamic force to technological progress and population growth. During and after the First World War this theory permeated and dominated public opinion so thoroughly that it was even reinforced by events which pointed to the contrary, such as the defeat of Germany, mass unemployment or serious accidents as a result of accelerated production. Biologically and medically, it was argued that the optimum performance of workers and social well-being could be combined if maximum human capacity and efficiency were established scientifically and applied, together with technological improvements, to obtain better productivity. Most important were the monitoring of soldiers' or workers' actual capabilities and their deployment in the right place. This fixation on a better future attained by human productivity reduced emphasis on the problem of risk perception and management. Henceforth, certain risks for individual workers were deemed acceptable for the sake of the nation and society as a whole; taken even further, this reasoning meant that the selection of efficient workers also created a better biological basis for the competition for a world market and for world power.

The growing significance of meritocracy helped to overcome a problem relating to risk management which developed towards the end of the nineteenth century. At this time the German social constitution, centring on the interaction between accident and health insurance, had just been established when a new, unforeseeable risk-related problem arose. The increased use of chemicals and the intensification of work processes gave rise to hazards to the health and life of workers which did not take the form of accidents but were nevertheless inseparably linked to work processes. The health injuries which arose were chronic diseases attributable to a multitude of factors, but were not infectious or traumatic. This type of disease risk no longer fitted in with the German construction of social insurance, as it could be categorized neither as an accident nor as a disease.

The establishment of social security gave rise to many discussions in the late nineteenth century about entitlement to security and benefits, and it was during these discussions that the distribution and accumulation of hazards to health and life among certain social strata and classes, which did not fit into the accident paradigm, became a subject of considerable debate. Such diseases were defined as 'workers' diseases' – a prominent example being tuberculosis. Most industrial diseases, also, were not recognized as 'accidents' and neither for the purposes of health insurance were they 'diseases'.

Socially committed doctors and politicians sought to prove that some industrial diseases (especially intoxication) had all the characteristics of accidents and should be recognized as such for the purposes of accident insurance. One reason for this was that the benefits of accident insurance were substantially better than those for sickness insurance. Simultaneously such authorities wanted to call direct attention to the cause of the problem. But it remained an open question whether industrial doctors would develop a widened conception of risk and bring it into discussions on the sociopolitical management of industrial pathogenicity, or whether the institutional risk management of the social insurance system would force industrial doctors to redefine risk. It was a question of whether these disease processes would gain significance in their own right, or whether the central concern would be simply to marginalize, de-emphasize and 'de-thematize' the connections between accident risks and poverty risks. Politically, this was a highly explosive line to take.

Towards the end of the century, work-related diseases took on a different, more comprehensive sociopolitical quality. They contradicted the illusions of technological progress and the shift towards national efficiency. In fact, the realization grew that industrial pathogenicity and the scope of sociopolitical control should be reconsidered. It is, therefore, not surprising that the most important discussions on the 'social question' in Germany at the turn of the century revolved around alcohol and the chemical industry, so-called *Giftküchen und Giftkocher* ('devil's kitchens' and 'poison mixers'). In many speeches in the Reichstag and at meetings,[48] in agitated scientific debates,[49] and in official circles this new constellation of risks and possible ways of dealing with it was debated. An increasing and explicit need for a sociopolitical course of action and regulation was reflected in the endeavours of the International Association for Statutory Worker Protection (*Internationale Vereinigung für gesetzlichen Arbeiterschutz*) which finally published a list of toxic substances and diseases that proved to be an important prerequisite for the enactment of the German Occupational Disease Ordinance in 1925.[50]

The construction of the risks known from 1925 onwards as 'occupational diseases' did not, however, resolve the discrepancies within the different branches of German social insurance. Indeed, the construction of occupational disease risk still involves a systematic flaw. A new category of risk had been woven into the structure where it could not be treated as a process in its own right; it was – and still is – very difficult to claim compensation or to prove the existence of a possible cause and its relation to risk. In this interplay between accident and sickness insurance, occupational diseases are less problematic the less frequently they occur.

Conceptually, the construction of risk by segregating accident insurance and health insurance is inherently confusing. According to the construction of occupational diseases, which is still valid today, work-related diseases are on the one hand comprehended as accidents. A narrowly defined terminology and the complicated procedures involved – a worker still has to prove the existence of the disease and that it is work-related – have a severely restrictive effect on the management of problems relating to causes and to possible preventive measures. Simultaneously, such states are perceived as diseases: with the exception of a few recognized occupational diseases, they are dealt with within the framework of statutory health insurance which does not single out specific causes or look into working conditions and labour relations.

Industrial pathogenicity has thus become a critical term as distinct from 'occupational disease' and its underlying concept of risk. It describes a type of risk not laid down in the procedures and definitions established in the early 1880s within the framework of social insurance for the management of accidents, incapacity to work or even occupational diseases. Instead, it reactivates the call for sociopolitical control which had been implicit in the demand for the recognition of work-related diseases at the turn of the century.

Notes

1. This paper draws on research currently carried out in Sub-Project D1, 'Construction of Biographical Risks in Occupational Disease Proceedings 1889–1929', as part of the Special Collaborative Programme No. 186, 'Status Passages and Risks in Life Course' (Deutsche Forschungsgemeinschaft) at the University of Bremen. For translating the paper and her support I would like to thank Vicki May.
2. See Ulrich Beck, *Risikogesellschaft, Auf dem Weg in eine andere Moderne* (Frankfurt/M.: Suhrkamp, 1986); *idem* (ed.), *Politik in der Risikogesellschaft* (Frankfurt/M.: Suhrkamp, 1991). See also Gotthard Bechmann, *Risiko und Gesellschaft: Grundlagen und Ergebnisse interdisziplinärer Risikoforschung* (Opladen: Westdeutscher Verlag, 1993).
3. See Max M. Wambach (ed.), *Der Mensch als Risiko* (Frankfurt/M.: Suhrkamp, 1983).
4. For a general approach, see Adalbert Evers and Helga Novotny, *Über den Umgang mit Unsicherheit: Die Entdeckung der Gestaltbarkeit von Gesellschaft* (Frankfurt/M.: Suhrkamp, 1987), 18; Burkart Lutz, *Der kurze Traum immerwährender Prosperität: Eine Neuinterpretation der industriell-kapitalistischen Entwicklung im Europa des 20. Jahrhunderts* (Frankfurt/M.: Campus, 1984); Reinhard Spree, *Lange Wellen wirtschaftlicher Entwicklung in der Neuzeit: Historische Befunde, Erklärungen und Untersuchungsmethoden*, Historical Social Research Suppl. 4, 1991. See, also, Roland Bogun, Martin Osterland and Günter Warsewa, *'Was ist überhaupt noch sicher auf der Welt?' Arbeit und Umwelt im Risikobewußtsein von Industriearbeitern* (Berlin: Edition Sigma, 1990).
5. See Hans-Joachim Hoffmann-Nowotny, 'Gesamtgesellschaftliche Determinanten des Individualisierungsprozesses', *Zeitschrift für Sozialreform*, xi (1988), 659–70; Wolfgang Zapf *et al.*, *Individualisierung und Sicherheit: Untersuchungen zur Lebensqualität in der Bundesrepublik Deutschland* (Munich: Beck, 1987).
6. See Klaus Michael Meyer-Abich, *Wege zum Frieden mit der Natur: Praktische Naturphilosophie für die Umweltpolitik* (Munich/Vienna: Hanser, 1984), 52 et passim. For historical research, see Franz-Joseph Brüggemeier and Thomas Rommelspacher (eds), *Besiegte Natur: Geschichte der Umwelt im 19. und 20. Jahrhundert* (Munich: C. H. Beck, 1987); Hamburger Stiftung für Sozialgeschichte (ed.), *Arbeitsschutz und Umweltgeschichte* (Cologne: Volksblatt, 1990).
7. The fact that risk perceptions are always subjective and ambiguous was pointed out by A. Rapoport, 'Risiko und Sicherheit in der heutigen Gesellschaft. Die subjektiven Aspekte des Risikobegriffs', *Leviathan* (1988), 123–36. On the historical genesis see Klaus Wahl, *Die Modernisierungsfalle: Gesellschaft, Selbstbewußtsein und Gewalt* (Frankfurt/M.: Suhrkamp, 1989).
8. Karl Polanyi, *The Great Transformation* (New York: Farrar & Rinehart, 1944).

9. Christoph Sachße and H. Tristram Engelhardt (eds), *Sicherheit und Freiheit: Zur Ethik des Wohlfahrtsstaates* (Frankfurt/M.: Suhrkamp, 1990), 9.
10. This is thoroughly analysed in Max Weber, *Die protestantische Ethik. Eine Aufsatzsammlung* (5th edn Gütersloh, 1979). For one of the many contributions to more recent discussions, see Artur Bogner, *Zivilisation und Rationalisierung. Die Zivilisationstheorien Max Webers, Norbert Elias' und der Frankfurter Schule im Vergleich* (Opladen: Westdt. Verlag, 1989).
11. Franz-Xaver Kaufmann, *Sicherheit als Soziologisches und Sozialpolitisches Problem. Untersuchungen zu einer Wertidee hochdifferenzierter Gesellschaften* (Stuttgart: F. Enke, 1970). See also Ulrich K. Preuß, 'Verfassungstheoretische Überlegungen zur normativen Begründung des Wohlfahrtsstaates', in Sachße and Engelhardt, *op.cit.* (ref. 9), 106–32; Stephan Leibfried, 'Sozialstaat Europa? Integrations-perspektiven Europäischer Armutsregimes', *Nachrichtendienst des Deutschen Vereins für Öffentliche und Private Fürsorge*, ix (1990), 295–305; and Peter M. Baldwin, *The Politics of Social Solidarity: Class Bases of the European Welfare State* (Cambridge: Cambridge University Press, 1990).
12. This is analysed thoroughly in Kaufmann, *op.cit.* (ref. 11).
13. 'With the increase of knowledge we exponentially increase our ignorance': Thomas Blanke, 'Der Fortschritt der Wissenschaft und der Untergang des abendländischen Weltbildes', *Vorgänge*, lxxxvii (1987), 3 et passim; and Anim v. Gleich, *Der wissenschaftliche Umgang mit der Natur. Über die Vielfalt harter und sanfter Naturwissenschaften* (Frankfurt/M., New York: Campus, 1989).
14. Goesta Esping-Andersen, *The Three Worlds of Welfare Capitalism* (London: Polity Press, 1990).
15. See Jane Lewis, *Women and Social Action in Victorian and Edwardian England* (Aldershot: Edward Elgar, 1991); Jane Lewis and Ilona Ostner, *Gender and the Revolution of European Social Policies* (Papers of the Centre for Social Policy Research, no. 7, 1992).
16. See Wolfgang J. Mommsen and Wolfgang Mock (eds), *The Emergence of the Welfare State in Britain and Germany 1850–1950* (London: Croom Helm, 1981); and Peter A. Köhler, and Hans F. Zacher (eds), *Ein Jahrhundert Sozialversicherung in der Bundesrepublik Deutschland, Frankreich, Großbritannien, Österreich und der Schweiz* (Berlin: Duncker & Humblot, 1981); Jens Alber, *Vom Armenhaus zum Wohlfahrtsstaat. Analysen zur Entwicklung der Sozialversicherung in Westeuropa* (Frankfurt/M.: Campus, 1982); Gerhard A. Ritter, *Social Welfare in Germany and Britain* (Leamington Spa: Berg, 1983); Deborah Stone, *The Disabled State* (Philadelphia, 1984); E. P. Hennock, *British Social Reform and German Precedents. The Case of Social Insurance 1880–1914* (Oxford: Clarendon Press, 1987); Franz-Xaver Kaufmann and P. Wolters (eds), *Papers of the First European School of Historical and*

Comparative Sociological Research on Social Policy, IBS-Materialien Nr.32 (Bielefeld, 1991); and especially Vicki May and Katherine Bird, 'Berufskrankheiten in England unf Deutschland: Historische Entwicklungen und Forschungsfragen', in Dietrich Milles (ed.), *Gesundheitsrisiken, Industriegeseilschaft und soziale Sicherungen in der Geschichte* (Bremerhaven: Wirtschaftsverlag, 1993), 389–417.

17. On this epistemological problem, see Reinhard Löw, 'Evolution und Erkenntnis. Tragweite und Grenzen der evolutionären Erkenntnistheorie in philosophischer Absicht', in Jost Herbig and Rainer Hohlfeld (eds), *Die zweite Schöpfung. Geist und Ungeist in der Biologie des 20. Jahrhunderts* (Munich/Vienna: Hanser, 1990), 231 ff.; on the differentiation between 'hazard' and 'risk', see Niklas Luhmann, 'Sicherheit und Risiko aus der Sicht der Sozialwissenschaften', in Rheinisch-Westfälische Akademie der Wissenschaften (eds), *Vorträge* (Opladen, 1987), 63–6; for a thorough survey of current discussions, see Thomas Blanke, 'Zur Aktualität des Risikobegriffs. Über die Konstruktion der Welt und die Wissenschaft von ihr', *Leviathan* (1990), 134–43.
18. See the standard works by Ramazzini, Halfort, Thackrah, Patisier, and Villerme referred to in the historical overview of Karl-Heinz Karbe, *Die Entwicklung der Arbeitsmedizin in Deutschland 1780 bis 1850 im Spiegel der zeitgenössischen medizinischen Literatur* (Dissertation, Leipzig, 1978), and discussed in Franz Koelsch, *Beiträge zur Geschichte der Arbeitsmedizin* (Munich, n.d.); Rainer Müller and Dietrich Milles (eds), *Beiträge zur Geschichte der Arbeiterkrankheiten und der Arbeitsmedizin in Deutschland* (Bremerhaven: Wirtschaftsverlag, 1984) and Paul Weindling (ed.), *The Social History of Occupational Health* (London: Croom Helm, 1985).
19. See S. Leibfried and F. Tennstedt (eds), *Politik der Armut und die Spaltung des Sozialstaates* (Frankfurt/M.: Suhrkamp, 1985).
20. See Karl-Heinz Karbe (ed.), *Salomon Neumann 1819–1908. Wegbereiter sozialmedizinischen Denkens und Handelns. Ausgewählte Texte* (Leipzig: J.A. Barth, 1984).
21. Volker Hentschel, *Geschichte der deutschen Sozialpolitik 1880–1980* (Frankfurt/M.: Suhrkamp, 1983), who emphasizes that social policy was not intended to provide security *and* social equality, but '[to act] as a substitute for social equality and [as] an instrument against proletarian aspirations' (10). See also Leibfried and Tennstedt, *op.cit.* (ref. 19).
22. See Stefan Breuer, 'Sozialdisziplinierung. Probleme und Problemverlagerungen eines Konzepts bei Max Weber, Gerhard Oestreich und Michel Foucault', in Christoph Sachβe and Florian Tennstedt (eds), *Soziale Sicherheit und soziale Disziplinierung* (Frankfurt/M.: Suhrkamp, 1986), 45–69.
23. See Franz-Xaver Kaufmann's systematic survey in 'Elemente einer soziologischen Theorie sozialpolitischer Intervention', in Kaufmann (ed.), *Staatliche Sozialpolitik und Familie* (Munich/Vienna: Oldenbourg, 1982), 49–86.

24. For the viewpoint of trade associations, see Ernst Wickenhagen, *Geschichte der gewerblichen Unfallversicherung. Wesen und Wirken der gewerblichen Berufsgenossenschaften* (Munich/Vienna: Oldenbourg, 1980).
25. See, for example, the regular articles in the social democratic newspapers on the 'Neue Socialdemokrat' and on the 'victims of labour'.
26. On the conceptualization, see Karl Erich Rothschuh, *Was ist Krankheit?* (Darmstadt: Wiss. Buchgesellschaft, 1975); a survey of the important theories is given by Uta Gerhardt, *Ideas about Illness. An Intellectual and Political History of Medical Sociology* (London: Macmillan, 1989).
27. For the history of the perception and treatment of such problems in the field of medicine, see Gerd Göckenjan, *Kurieren und Staat machen. Gesundheit und Medizin in der bürgerlichen Welt* (Frankfurt/M.: Suhrkamp, 1985), 139 et passim.
28. For an early critique, see Viktor v. Weizsäcker, *Soziale Krankheit und soziale Gesundung* (Göttingen: Vandenhoek & Ruprecht, 1955).
29. See Leibfried and Tennstedt, *op.cit.* (ref. 19), 305 et passim.
30. See Sandrine Kott, 'Attitudes ouvrières face à la médicalisation. L'usage des assurances sociales dans l'Alsace allemande', *Prevenir*, xviii (1989), 109–28; *idem*, 'Gesundheitsvorsorge in der Fabrik zwischen elsässischem Patriarchalismus und staatlicher Sozialpolitik', in Milles (ed.), *op.cit.* (ref. 16), 69–84.
31. *Tennstedt, Florian und Winter, Heidi:* "Der Staat hat wenig Liebe – activ wie passiv". Die Anfänge des Sozialstaats im Deutschen Reich von 1871. In *Zeitschrift für Soziale Reform*, 39 (1993), 362–92. *dies.:* "Jeder Tag hat seine eigenen Sorgen, und es ist nicht weise, die Sorgen der Zukunft freiwillig auf die Gegenwart zu Übernehmen." Die Anfänge des Sozialstaats im Deutschen Reich von 1871. In: *Zeitschrift für Soziale Reform*, 41 (1995), 671–706.
32. For a fundamental and carefully argued international comparison, see Heide Gerstenberger, *Die subjektlose Gewalt. Theorie der Entstehung bürgerlicher Staatsgewalt* (Münster: Westfäl Dampfboot, 1990); on modern society see Richard Münch, *Die Struktur der Moderne. Grundmuster und differentielle Gestaltung des institutionellen Aufbaus der modernen Gesellschaften* (Frankfurt/M.: Suhrkamp, 1984).
33. As Eckart Pankoke has concluded, 'The changing evaluation of risks and chances, thresholds and limits, division and distribution of social work reflect the historical points of departure, expansion and reconstruction of modern industrial society.' In E. Pankoke, *Die Arbeitsfrage. Arbeitsmoral, Beschäftigungskrisen und Wohlfahrtspolitik im Industriezeitalter* (Frankfurt/M.: Suhrkamp, 1990), 7; see also Leibfried and Tennstedt, *op.cit.* (ref. 19), 90 et passim.
34. See Ingeborg Nahnsen, 'Bemerkungen zum Begriff und zur Geschichte des Arbeitsschutzes', in Martin Osterland (ed.), *Arbeitssituation, Lebenslage, Konfliktpotential* (Frankfurt/M.: Europ. Verlagsanstalt, 1975), 145–84; and E. Pankoke, *op.cit.* (ref. 33), 27 et passim.

35. For a general comparison, see Ulrich K. Preuβ, *Zur Internalisierung des subjektiven Rechts* (Frankfurt/M.: Suhrkamp, 1979); and Angelika Pensky, *Schutz der Arbeiter vor Gefahren für Leben und Gesundheit. Ein Beitrag zur Geschichte des Gesundheitsschutzes für Arbeiter in Deutschland* (Bremerhaven: Wirtschaftsverlag, 1987), 70 et passim.
36. Beck, *Risikogesellschaft*, (ref. 2), 9.
37. See Reinhard Löw, *Philosophie des Lebendigen. Der Begriff des Organischen bei Kant, sein Grund und seine Aktualität* (Frankfurt/M.: Suhrkamp, 1980). Löw refers to the general mechanization and mathematization of the world concept in the sixteenth and seventeenth centuries, traces the supersession of the teleological foundation by one of causal mechanism in Kant's works, and gives evidence of the unilateral appropriation of mechanical lines of reasoning by Neo-Kantians. This philosophical tradition seems to differ quite markedly from that of English philosophers, if one assesses the significance of David Humes or the current critiques of Bertrand Russell.
38. This is explained in detail in Anson Rabinbach, *The Human Motor. Energy, Fatigue, and the Origins of Modernity* (New York: Berg, 1990).
39. Helmholtz defined 'experiments as the real basis of science' and declared 'the terminological formulation of natural laws' as the 'ultimate purpose' of natural research, in his *Die Thatsachen in der Wahrnehmung* (Berlin, 1879). See also Helmholtz, *Das Denken in der Medizin* (Berlin, 1877).
40. The German judiciary, for example, did not try to define the principle of causality which was demanded of medical experts, perhaps because in matters of accident insurance practical jurisdiction was not based on the assumption of causalities, but on probabilities. See Heinz Barta, *Kausalität im Sozialrecht. Entstehung und Funktion der sogenannten Theorie der wesentlichen Bedingung. Analyse der grundlegenden Judikatur des Reichsversicherungsamtes in Unfallversicherungssachen (1884–1914)* (Part 1, Berlin/Munich: Ducker & Humblot, 1983), 520 et passim.
41. Reference is made, for instance, to the position of Hermann Lotze, who was 'still ... convinced ... that I am on the right track when I look at the way things should be to find the reason for the way things are' (Lotze, *System der Philosophie.* Part 2, 604). On the current relevance of ethical reasoning see Robert Spaemann and Reinhard Löw, *Die Frage wozu? Geschichte und Wiederentdekung des teleologischen Denkens* (Munich/Zurich: Piper, 1981).

Most historians of technology, in the wake of Conrad Matschoβ, had a correspondingly deterministic understanding of technological progress. 'They perceived it as a purposeful, one-dimensional process of improving size, complexity and efficiency, the optimisation of functions and the minimalisation of space requirement, losses and costs which went hand in hand with "natural necessity" and "inherent laws". History, however, is then reduced to the mere pre-history of the absolute present-day "state of technology" and alternative possibilities are ruled out from the start.' Hans Dieter Hellige, 'Die gesellschaftlichen und historischen Grundlagen der Technikgestaltung als Gegenstand der Ingenieurausbildung', *Technikgeschichte*, iv (1984), 280.

42. See Rabinbach, *op.cit.* (ref. 38) for a thorough analysis.
43. Paul Weindling, *Health, Race and German Politics Between National Unification and Nazism 1870–1945* (Cambridge: Cambridge University Press, 1989); Jost Herbig and Rainer Hohlfeld (eds), *Die zweite Schöpfung. Geist und Ungeist in der Biologie des 20. Jahrhunderts* (Munich/Vienna: Hanser, 1990), 17–31.
44. Gerd Zweckbronner, 'Das Prinzip der lebendigen Kräfte, ein Bindeglied zwischen rationeller Mechanik und praktischem Maschinenbau im Zeitalter des Industrialismus', *Technikgeschichte*, i (1981), 106.
45. Karbe, *op.cit.* (ref. 20), and Pankoke, *op.cit.* (ref. 33), 84.
46. The close relationship between economic and eugenic strategies was most blatantly expressed in the Friedrich Krupp prize competition. Wilhelm Schallmeyer won 30,000 Marks in 1903 for a paper on 'heredity and selection in the life course of nations', which referred to biological vitality and national efficiency. The clever politician 'must recognise that the future of his nation depends on the skilful administration of its generative property'. See also Weindling, *op.cit.* (ref. 43), 112.
47. 'Of all those things which will of natural necessity succeed in the course of development, the economic improvement of production processes is one of the most important.' The consequence of this is 'the permanent necessity for technological improvements', but also the need for 'relatively highly qualified human resources', which in turn could be obtained by human economy. Human economy is thus the application of social Darwinism to a society which was dedicated to industrial progress. Rudolf Goldscheid, *Höherentwicklung und Menschenökonomie. Grundlegung der Sozialbiologie* (Leipzig: W. Klinkhardt, 1911), 522 et passim.
48. Dietrich Milles, '"Künstliche" und "natürliche" Risiken in der Geschichte der Arbeitsmedizin', in Hamburger Stiftung für Sozialgeschichte (Hrsg.), *Arbeitsschutz und Umweltgeschichte* (Cologne: Volksblatt, 1990), 109 et passim.
49. Christian Rothe, *Erkrankungen von Chemiearbeitern und die Entwicklung der Berufskrankheitenverordnung von 1925* (Diss. med. Frankfurt/M., 1987); Wolfgang Hien, *Chemische Industrie und Krebs: Zur Soziologie des wissenschaftlichen und sozialen Umgangs mit arbeitsbedingten Krebserkankungen in Deutschland* (Bremerhaven: Wirtschaftsverlag, 1994).
50. Theodor Sommerfeld, *Entwurf einer Liste der gewerblichen Gifte* (Jena, 1908); *idem*, with Richard Fischer, *Liste der gewerblichen Gifte* (Jena, 1912); the history of this socially reformative institution, which was founded following international congresses on insurance and hygiene, remains to be written.

9

Housewives as Home Safety Managers: The Changing Perception of the Home as a Place of Hazard and Risk, 1870–1940

Joel A. Tarr and Mark Tebeau

'Like the poor and taxes, the home hazards will be with us always.'
K.H. Hamilton, *Illustrated World,* 1918.

'We should be the "safety managers" of our homes.'
Ethel M. Hanson, *Fourteenth National Safety Congress,* 1925.

'There are no accidents, just poor injury prevention.'
Ronald Smothers, *New York Times,* 26 May, 1993.

Introduction

The last decade has seen the appearance of a number of works dealing with the evolving conception of the home in American history. Combining social and architectural analysis, these studies focus not only on changing building styles and home layouts and decoration, but also on alterations in family structure and especially the place of women in relationship to home and family.[1] Within this context, the concept of the home as a location for the occurrence of accidents is especially interesting because it raises issues relating to control over and management of the home environment as well as responsibility for accident prevention (or 'injury control' in today's parlance) within the home.

This chapter focuses on five major themes involved in the history of home accidents – the evolution of the safety movement in the United States; the discovery of risk within the home and the place of home safety in the national safety movement; the role of women in home safety; and the unsuccessful organizational attempts of the National Safety Council and the National Red Cross to control home accidents from 1914 to 1940.

The identification of the home as a locale where serious accidents might occur directly challenged the idea that the home was a 'haven'. The concept of the home as a refuge from a ruthless and chaotic world was primarily a creation of the Victorian period. By the 1850s, spokespersons for the American middle class were arguing that the family was the basis for an ideal society and that it would provide durability and stability to the social order. As Clifford E. Clark notes, the function of the home was to 'be a refuge from the outside world, a fortress designed to protect, nurture, and strengthen the individuals within'.[2] The idea of the home as a retreat from the cares and dangers of the world received articulation for at least a century and would later serve as an important rationale for enhancing home safety.

Linked in with the concept of the home as haven was the idea of the home as women's 'sphere'. During the nineteenth century, increasing separation occurred between residence and work, with men often going off to labour in office and industry. Women, meanwhile, remained behind to raise families and to provide the emotional and physical support enabling men to labour in the ruthless and materialistic outside world of work. Women, it was argued, were 'best suited, both biologically and emotionally' to provide stability against the shocks of the marketplace and the world of business, remaining in charge of family and of home.[3] Even the coming of modern technology, as Ruth Schwartz Cowan has argued, reduced the chores and functions of men within the household, but increased the housewife's responsibilities and work-load.[4]

If the home was to furnish an idealistic and peaceful environment, however, it needed to be a place where risk could be avoided. And this meant attempting to protect against accident occurrence. The home, therefore, had to be neatly rather than chaotically organized, with furniture in its proper place, clutter removed, slippery floors and stairways carpeted, dangerous materials and tools out of the reach of children, and family members protected from hot stoves and other dangerous kitchen devices. Fire, especially, was to be guarded against, and here women were expected to worry about the potential for conflagration from fireplaces, stoves, and various lighting devices. Once electrical technology began to enter the home, primarily after 1900, bringing with it many concerns as well as benefits, women were also expected to ensure its safe use, protecting against shock hazards and other possible accidents.

In order to be responsible for providing a risk-free home, women had to take on the role of home managers. While a number of nineteenth-century authors wrote about the need for good household management, it was Catharine Beecher's numerous books and articles that presented one of the earliest and fullest pictures of the housewife as manager. Attempting to 'redeem woman's profession from dishonour' and to demonstrate that women could 'find self-respect within their traditional sphere', Beecher asserted the managerial role of the housewife in the home, protecting her family against danger and risk within a framework of Christian principles.[5]

Beecher emphasized that in order to become effective, women were required to become efficient and skilled managers, making housework into a 'scientific study' and utilizing the newest technology. Their domestic and managerial responsibilities included the rearing of children and nurturing their health, ensuring that food and drink were healthful and well prepared, cleaning the house and keeping it in an orderly way, and protecting against disease and ill-health. Beecher also recognized the important role of accidents in the household. In her classic study, *A Treatise on Domestic Economy*, published in 1841, she included a chapter 'On Accidents and Antidotes'.[6] In this chapter, rather than discussing accident prevention ('safety'), she accepted the inevitability of home accidents and provided 'antidotes' for a range of household mishaps from choking to burns to poisoning.[7] As will be dealt with later, the field of home economics, which strongly emphasized the concept of the woman as home 'manager' and as a user of the insights of science and the tools of technology, further developed the link between the role of women as home-makers and accident prevention.

Accidents and Safety in Industry and in the Home

The idea of accidents as 'preventable', however, as Bill Luckin has noted, is a relatively new one. When 'nature' is viewed as threatening, he writes, accidents are often seen as inevitable, but when 'nature' is demystified and secularized, accidents are regarded as preventable.[8] The movement for accident reduction in American society occurred in the context of a social change that made individuals increasingly intolerant of accepting injuries that they did not believe were their responsibility. Evidence for this attitude change, writes Randolph E. Bergstrom, is provided by the explosion of personal injury suits in the courts of cities such as Boston and New York in the late nineteenth and early twentieth centuries. In 1870, for instance, injury suits composed only 41 per cent of torts filed in New York courts, but by 1910 they had grown to 82 per cent. Work injury suits comprised the highest number filed, followed by injuries incurred from the city's sidewalks and streets and from the city's buildings. In fact, the number of cases that resulted from residence and business-place accidents increased twenty-fold.[9] Since the New York population was increasingly a renting population (87.9 per cent in 1910), accidents that might have previously been handled privately now entered into the public realm.[10] That people turned increasingly to the courts for relief from injuries stemming from accidents reflected a belief that they could and should be prevented.[11]

The first accidents to be attacked by an organized safety movement were industrial accidents. In the late nineteenth century, America had the highest work-related death rate of any industrialized nation. The most dangerous occupation was coal mining. From 1900 to 1906, the average yearly death toll in US coal mines was 33.5 per 10,000 workers; this compared with 20.6 per 10,000 for Prussia, 12.9 for Great Britain, and only 9.1 for France. Railroading was almost as hazardous, and worker fatalities per 10,000 workers reached a high of 28 in 1904, with 3,632 men being killed.[12] In 1917, there were 11,338 fatal industrial accidents and 1,363,080 non-fatal accidents.[13] In the context of a modernizing nation, oriented towards a belief in scientific ideas and a faith in technology, and concerned with concepts such as efficiency and conservation, accidents on such a massive scale became increasingly unacceptable to both elites and the wider public. The safety movement that began in industry in the first decades of the twentieth century – that is, a movement with a national organizational presence – is a logical component of what Robert H. Wiebe calls 'The Search for Order' of the Progressive period.[14]

The major factors driving the industrial safety movement were media exposé and various investigations, such as that of Crystal Eastman, *Work Accidents and the Law* (a contribution to the six-volume investigation, *The Pittsburgh Survey*), which aroused public opinion about industrial work conditions.[15] In addition, the growing body of litigation based upon common-law negligence doctrine and the realization by major corporations such as US Steel that industrial accidents were costly and reduced the efficient operation of their firms played important roles.[16] Growing awareness of the magnitude of the industrial accident problem produced a broad-based reform movement, grounded in some of the largest and most dangerous industries in the nation – agricultural machinery, coal, iron and steel, and railroading.[17] Thus, a major concern of the Progressive period – the efficient use of resources – came into play, as human and natural resources were both seen as endangered and in need of protection.[18]

Beginning in 1907, a number of elements combined to give impetus to the safety movement. In that year, the American Institute of Social Science directed the first national safety exhibition, held at the Museum of Natural History in New York; four years later, in 1911, the American Museum of Safety, funded largely by steel executives and designed to educate employees and employers about safety, was incorporated in New York State.[19] In 1907 also, the Association of Iron and Steel Electrical Engineers was founded, and from its beginnings strongly promoted factory safety. In 1912 it sponsored the First Co-operative Safety Congress (held in Milwaukee), and out of this conference a committee was appointed to form a 'National Organization for the Promotion of Safety to Human Life...'. Initially called the National Council for Industrial Safety, in 1914 it was renamed the National Safety Council (NSC).[20] By 1917, the NSC had grown into a major national organization with 3,300 members, focusing primarily on the promotion of industrial safety.[21] Eventually, it would broaden its efforts to include safety in other areas of American society, becoming the nation's leading safety organization.

The drive for home safety and its emergence as an organized movement was closely related to the movement for industrial accident prevention. Widespread concern over home hazards that involved public health factors, however, pre-dated the industrial safety movement. In the late nineteenth century, for instance, sanitarians, health reformers, and 'sanitary scientists' attempted to alert housewives to new dangers lurking in the home from faulty domestic plumbing – plumbing that could lead to the formation of 'sewer gas' and 'germs', and the consequent outbreak of 'house diseases'. It was the housewife's responsibility, noted the advice books, to keep the home sanctuary free from such threats to health.[22]

While the risk from exposure to house diseases differed in character from the risk from accidents, they both identified a responsible figure in the home whose task it was to guard against hazard. And the responsible figure in most of such situations was the housewife rather than the husband. As one leading sanitarian maintained, 'the men of the house come and go', while 'the women are conversant with every nook of the dwelling, from basement to roof, and on their knowledge, wisdom, and skill the physician rests his hopes'.[23] In a different sense, the perception of risk in either case involved a warning that the home was not inviolate as a sanctuary, and that without proper watchfulness and care by the housewife or 'home manager', danger could creep in.[24]

Anthropologists such as Mary Douglas and Clifford Geertz have maintained that a perception of risk is usually dependent upon a social representation that can be defined as a culturally conditioned way of viewing the world.[25] The timing of the movements for domestic hygiene and for the elimination of home accidents, and the number of analogies between the two movements, suggests that they were related to a set of larger cultural constructs. At the turn of the century, these concepts were identified with the growth of the middle class and the development of modernism, and especially to the belief that science and technology could produce purposeful and beneficial change.

The first major safety journal to publicly express concern over risk within the home as well as the workplace was the magazine of the fire insurance industry, *Insurance Engineering*, first published in 1901, and renamed *Safety Engineering* in 1913. Focusing on the danger from fires, in 1912 *Insurance Engineering* began presenting articles on home fire safety. Warning that '"Safety First" is as important in the home as elsewhere', it presented rules for fire safety, warned about the dangers from gas leakage and electrical fire hazards, and commented that home fire danger was greatest in a period of economic depression because of fires that were deliberately set in order to collect insurance.[26]

The National Safety Council recognized home safety as a relatively important concern at its first organizing meeting. The organization's biweekly magazine, *National Safety News*, and the proceedings of its National Safety Congresses, however, reveal that it held a much lower priority than did industrial safety. The first report of the 'Home Safety Committee', for instance, formed in 1915, and chaired by a man who also headed the Fire Prevention Committee, emphasized the need to preach home accident prevention not only to reduce children's accidents, especially involving fire, but also to influence them so that when they became 'the workmen and the executives' of the future, they would preach 'accident prevention in the business and industrial world'.[27] The consciousness that the home itself was an important locale for accidents, however, received scant attention, thus reflecting, as one founder of the safety movement later commented, that home safety was the 'step-child of the safety movement'.[28]

Women and the Safety Movement

The role that women should play in the safety movement and particularly their relationship to home safety was redefined as the movement matured. Even though, as has been noted, women were early recognized as being dominant in their 'separate sphere' – the home – the safety movement initially found it difficult to provide them with a significant role in regard to accident prevention. In February of 1917, for instance, *Safety Engineering* published an article entitled 'For "The Man on the Job" At Home – Cause and Prevention of Household Accidents'. Complaining that the 'cause and prevention of household accidents' had been neglected, the article maintained that 'carelessness or thoughtlessness' were, as in industry, the main cause of household accidents. Among these accidents, it found those involving electrical appliances, the use of gasoline, tainted food, falls, cuts, and burns to be most common. While women were not completely neglected in the article, the assumption was that they had no special role or responsibility and that men would make the essential safety decisions.[29]

Within the growing safety movement there was clearly ambivalence concerning women's role in a field still primarily oriented towards male-dominated industry. A 1915 *Safety Engineering* editorial reflected this attitude when it noted the spread of women's suffrage across the nation, and then asked the rhetorical question:[30]

> Why are women not more prominent now in the several problems relating to our social ills? Why, for instance, do we hardly hear of them in the safety movement? Is anyone more affected by our high accident ratio than the women? Is it not a fact that as in war it is woman who suffers when father, husband, brother, or son, is killed or incapacitated by an accident? Is it not a fact also that woman's sphere and influence place her in a peculiarly advantageous position in relation to the inoculating of safety habits in the coming generation, a question fundamental to substantial accident reduction and to our continued leadership in industry and commerce?

In actuality, women in the Progressive period were deeply involved in reform activities of various types, especially those relating to welfare, public health and sanitation in the city ('municipal housekeeping'). The absence of women from the safety movement during its beginning years can best be explained by the movement's early focus on major industries such as steel and railroads that largely employed men. Most middle-class women had as their 'primary daily experience ... the home', while men were concerned with making a living and with business.[31] Thus, a clear perception of gender difference in focus existed. By emphasizing the special responsibility of women to develop a safety consciousness on the part of the males in their families, *Safety Engineering* minimized the extent to which women were exposed to risk at home.[32]

Two years later, however, in 1917, the journal broadened its appeal, running two editorials concerning women entitled

'Housewives and Home Hazards'. Focusing on the danger of fires, it bemoaned the fact that fire fighting was seen as a man's job and noted that the 'housewife's responsibility should be considered ... [since] housewives are the ones to prevent fires in the homes'. The article observed that fire could mean the loss of home and children, and that women should be educated in fire prevention because of both their presence at home during the day and their involvement in everyday matters that involved fire hazards.[33]

By 1918, the National Safety Council had organized a 'Women's Session', devoted to the 'interests of the employers of women'. The session reflected the large war-time involvement of women in industry as well as a growing awareness of home hazards.[34] Speakers in this session focused evenly on women's industrial and home experiences in regard to safety. In the most thorough home safety presentation at an NSC meeting to that time, H.W. Forster, General Manager of the Independence Bureau in Philadelphia, noted the contradiction between the common view of the 'haven of safety which the home constitutes' and the high accident rate that existed there. Forster listed the chief home accident causes, naming falls, mechanical failures, burns and shock from electrical equipment, cuts from edged tools, gas, fire, and poisons. He emphasized the special responsibility of women to remove hazardous situations and to prevent family members from taking risks. Even though 'Women in War Industries' was one of the major themes of the session, NSC male spokesmen emphasized that while woman's 'sphere of active influence in safety work covers the whole field ..., safety in the home and safety instruction' were her special province.[35] Such a position emphasized that while women may have played a valuable role in the war, their true place was in the home.

The end of the war resulted in the sharp diminution of the number of women in industry and the question of woman's role in the safety movement surfaced anew. At the end of 1919, the chairman of the 'Women in Industry Section', Tracy Copp, led a move to have eighteen national women's organizations join with the NSC in organizing public safety in the nation's communities and schools. Copp wrote, 'Now that women have finished the war work in which they displayed such constant courage and skill, they are seeking some social task which is worthy of their ability and which will grip their interest as the war work did. We believe accident prevention offers this field of activity, and the toll of deaths among children alone should arouse every public spirited woman to action'.[36] An editorial accompanying the article commented that while 'the women of the country ... have played almost no part in this movement', the time had come for the safety movement to spread beyond industry and into the community at large and to enlist the 'two great groups heretofore left untouched – the women in the homes and the children in the schools'.[37] The movement beyond industrial safety to a broader concern with safety in public places and in the home reflected both the normal tendencies of bureaucracies to expand and a realization on the part of the organization's officers that safety was a concern throughout society rather than in industry alone.[38] In addition, the greater activism of the safety movement undoubtedly involved the harnessing of moral energy that had been evident both in Progressive Movement reforms such as child labour legislation and food and drug inspection and in American involvement in World War I.[39] Because of its heavy dependence on volunteerism, in order to expand the safety movement the National Safety Council attempted to enlist members from many areas of society and to include both men and women.

Home Economics and Home Safety

Historians writing during the last generation have documented societal discrimination against women and the belief that they should be restricted to a 'separate sphere' of activity, usually in the home. The profession of home economics, however, which developed during the late nineteenth and early twentieth centuries, was intended to be women's domain and to provide co-equal status with men. Ideas such as those that called on women to emphasize planning, system, and order in the home can be traced to the writings of Catharine Beecher, but most students of the modern home economics movement agree that it emerged in the late nineteenth century.[40] Although the movement's leaders differed on elements of strategy, they agreed that the home and the larger society were intertwined. That is, the rhetoric of home economics moved away from the separate sphere argument without relinquishing the concept that the home was women's domain. And, they argued, in this domain women trained in the 'science' of home economics would bring scientific principles to home management. Or, as Ellen H. Richards, the movement's pre-eminent leader noted, 'HOME ECONOMICS STANDS FOR: The ideal home life for today unhampered by the traditions of the past. The utilization of all the resources of modern science to improve the home life'.[41] Thus, home economics, like other change-oriented new professions of the time, relied upon scientific rationalism and the doctrine of efficiency to establish its authority.[42]

As the home economics movement grew, a national structure

evolved, beginning with the holding of the first Lake Placid, New York, Conference on Home Economics in 1899, followed by formation of the American Home Economics Association in 1908. With a largely female constituency that included high school teachers, journalists, and academics, the home economics movement spread rapidly throughout American society. By 1916, 17,778 students were enrolled in home economics courses at 195 colleges and universities; in addition, in 1917, another 27,000 students attended 450 home economics extension courses.[43]

The concept of 'efficiency' strongly influenced the home economy movement during the century's first decades. The Progressive era experienced an efficiency craze likened by historian Samuel Haber to a 'secular Great Awakening'.[44] Many women believed that efficiency would emancipate them from the home's burdens and elevate them to a status of home scientific managers, putting home work on a par with men's work outside the home.[45] By the second decade of the new century, Taylorist efficiency zeal and the nineteenth-century gender ideology of 'separate spheres' had coalesced in the home economics movement to form a reform agenda that fitted with Progressive efforts to create a more orderly society.[46]

Given its emphasis on management and efficiency, the involvement of home economics in the home safety movement is understandable. David E. Nye observes that home economics spokeswomen 'sought to emulate in the home the work of engineers in the factory', reconceptualizing the home as a 'management site controlled by women ... a domestic factory that produced healthy and happy citizens'.[47] Like any up-to-date factory, the modern home needed to be equipped with the latest in production technology: running water and sewerage, central heating, telephones, and, most of all, electricity, to provide both light and power for various appliances such as vacuum cleaners, dish-washing machines, washing machines, electric stoves, refrigerators, and toasters.

In order to publicize the link between home safety and home management, in 1929 the National Bureau of Casualty and Surety Underwriters offered a graduate fellowship of $1,000 for a 'study of home safety as an index of good home management'.[48] The announcement noted that just as 'efficiency' was linked to industrial and traffic safety, so would home safety prove to be a vital aspect of 'a well-managed home'. The fellowship could be used in a Ph.D. programme in a university with a 'properly qualified home economics department', and was to be directed by an advisory committee containing representatives of the American Home

Economics Association, the NSC, and the National Organization for Public Health Nursing.[49]

Gertrude Zurrer, a Chicago resident, was the first winner of the safety fellowship. She chose to pursue her studies at the University of Chicago under the direction of Edith Abbot, a former Hull House resident who had become a professor of social economy and dean at the University's School of Social Service Administration.[50] At the nineteenth NSC Safety Congress, Zurrer discussed the rationale and plan for her study, noting the absence both of statistics and of research in the field. Zurrer's approach involved linking home accidents to social problems. 'But we all know where perhaps most accidents happen. (That is just it perhaps; we have no figures to show.)', she said. 'It is where the woman must leave her children and go to the factory, or where she has a very large family, or where she is a foreigner. These women do not go to the clubs'.[51]

Zurrer's comments highlight the tension that existed between social workers concerned with larger questions of social welfare and home economists primarily oriented towards preventing problems from emerging in the new consumer-oriented economy.[52] By the 1920s, home economists had begun to find considerable corporate employment. Jobs in business organizations seemed natural to home economists who described their profession as the 'business of housekeeping' or the 'profession of housework'.[53] Corporations, however, did not typically hire women as efficiency experts, but rather to help sell consumer goods and assuage societal fears about new electrically-powered technologies. Women's business roles, therefore, usually related to the home and not to the factory. And home economists encouraged this division of labour, reconceptualizing the home in terms of Taylorism and also as a centre of consumption over which women had power.[54]

Advocating that women exercise discretion and care in their household consumption, home economists ushered in the rapidly developing consumer society. They broke with past traditions of household architecture that prized individual taste and style and suggested an alternative vision for middle-class homelife which emphasized planning, efficiency, and safety. Christine Frederick, whose books included *The New Housekeeping* and *Household Engineering: Scientific Management in the Home*, summed up the multifaceted role of the modern mother: 'Today the woman in the home is called upon to be an executive as well as a manual labourer. Just to be a good worker and keep on working until you drop is not sufficient – or efficient either. The more planning, the more brains, the more management a woman puts into her housework, the less friction and the less nervous energy she will have to expend'.[55] Heroic mother Lillian Gilbreth provided the model, advocating a home designed in a minimalist style and free of clutter to aid with mother's efficiency.[56] Thus, despite the belief that women could be professionals and scientific managers, the message of home economists was surprisingly similar to that found in the writings of nineteenth-century pioneers like Catharine Beecher, oriented around the notion of the home as a place of perfectibility and social salvation.[57]

The language of both the home economics movement and the home safety movement resides within debates about feminism in the early twentieth century. The two sides of the janus-face of feminism discovered by Nancy Cott appear strongly within both movements.[58] In the realm of home economics, spokespersons like Charlotte Perkins Gilman envisioned that women's housework would become an upgraded type of work done professionally in the home. She argued that the rationalization and removal of many domestic chores from the home would free women from the burdens of domesticity and allow the home to be run more efficiently.[59] The dominant strand of home economics therefore retained the conceptualization of the home as woman's domain, even if professionally managed. The rhetoric of the home safety movement resembles this strain most closely. Safety experts argued that women should manage the home from their position within the home. They did not discard the notion of domesticity; rather, they supplemented it with the professional ethos of the new emerging and consumer-oriented middle class.

Specifying the Risks

As the 'safety' community grew more conscious in the 1920s that the home contained considerable hazards, attempts were made by various 'experts' and spokespeople to specify what those risks might be and how they might be mitigated. Of the variety of items that came to be commonly identified as 'home hazards', three will be discussed here: fire, technology, and falls. Of the three, the first and third can be defined as 'traditional' hazards while the second was strongly linked with the concept of the modern home. All were marked by a combination of an environmental and a behavioural approach, although in each case women were acknowledged to be the most responsible parties for accident prevention.

(i) *Fire*

America has always had a higher rate of fires than most European countries and American cities such as Baltimore, Boston, Chicago, New York, Philadelphia, Pittsburgh, and San Francisco experienced massive fires in the nineteenth and early twentieth centuries.[60] Home fires had not been a special matter of concern by fire authorities, but the advent of the home safety movement now caused a more intense look at the individual residence. As in other matters of home safety, there had been earlier warnings about the phenomena. In 1841, for instance, Beecher cautioned her readers about the hazards of the hearth fire: 'When fires are covered, at night, care should be taken that no coal of fire adheres to a broom or brush used for sweeping the hearth. All combustionable articles should be removed to a distance from the fireplace, lest a spark should fly out and set them on fire'.[61] If not careful with fire, came messages from household advisers, then one courted disaster.

The insurance industry, as much as any other agency in America, was responsible for increasing the awareness, institutions, and technology needed to fight fires. As the industry gained strength, insurers helped lead the campaign for more professional and technologically advanced fire protection as well as for fire codes and fireproofing. Much of the effort of the industry and of reformers in the nineteenth century focused on improving water delivery systems, forming professional municipal fire companies to replace volunteer companies, persuading municipalities to purchase improved firefighting technology and fire alarm systems, and pressuring city councils to approve new fire codes.

Home fires began receiving increased attention early in the twentieth century. *Insurance Engineering* and its successor, *Safety Engineering*, published a column called 'Residence Fires', which related details of fires, their causes, and total losses. In terms of protection, they warned of unsafe practices such as using inflammable liquids for cleaning purposes or a lack of care with matches. They also advocated collaboration between architects and fire insurers to design and build fire-resistant homes.[62]

The National Board of Fire Underwriters launched a magazine in 1917 entitled *Safeguarding America Against Fire* (*SAAF*), and in 1923 it devoted nearly an entire issue to home fire prevention. In an editorial the Board noted the 'strange fact ... that men will provide factories and offices with elaborate systems of exit and life-saving devices to protect employees from fire, and then will erect homes to shelter their own families without a single precaution for saving their lives in a similar emergency'.[63] The *SAAF* regularly ranked the causes of home fires that caused the most financial loss, with defective flues, roof sparks from chimneys, stoves, furnaces and boilers, electrical wiring, and matches and smoking, as the highest.[64]

The *SAAF* insisted, however, that a large majority of fires were preventable, and blamed inattention and carelessness for 75 per cent of the 15,000 annual fire-related deaths, half of which were in the home. This emphasis on behavioural causes was the same as nineteenth-century explanations. The 1875 *Household Cyclopaedia*, for instance, maintained that 'nine-tenths of the number [of conflagrations] originate in carelessness and inattention'.[65] What was different in the twentieth century was the development of a body of expertise about fire prevention that emphasized the use of new fireproof materials and of structural techniques such as fire breaks and dual exits. The fire insurance industry urged home builders and owners to demand that contractors, architects, and electricians use the newest fire-prevention technologies and materials in construction and fully abide by fire codes.[66] This information slowly penetrated the NSC.[67]

Speakers at NSC Safety Congresses and articles on safety continued to place the largest responsibility for fire prevention on the housewife. It was her responsibility to prevent carelessness with matches, to avoid the use of inflammable cleaning fluids, to stop the misuse of kerosene lamps, gas stoves and flatirons, to avoid the piling up of oily rags and clothing, and to be vigilant for excessive wear of electrical wires.[68] Good home management, emphasized *Safety Engineering*, remained the key to fire prevention, with new tools such as improved fire extinguishers and respirators provided by science and technology making her job easier.[69] In 1922, as a reminder to parents, and especially to housewives, the *SAAF* published a 'Home Inspection Blank for Schoolchildren', really intended for parents, which posed 26 questions about common home fire hazards including: 'Do you keep your matches away from heat and out of the reach of children? Do you ever keep or use gasoline [*sic*] in the home? Do you use electric pressing irons?'[70] Hopefully, the children and the list would remind parents, and especially housewives, of their responsibilities in regard to fire prevention.

(ii) *Technology*

A major characteristic of the changing American home in the late nineteenth and early twentieth centuries was its increasing dependence on technology and technological networks, many involving the use of electricity. Ruth Schwartz Cowan has described the manner in which the industrial revolution of the nineteenth century, which provided the material conditions making possible the establishment of separate spheres, was followed by a twentieth-century technological revolution that 'eventually would serve to undermine the very ideology that lay at their base'.[71] The operative word in Cowan's quote for this essay is 'eventually', because turn-of-the-century technologists and engineers believed that women needed to go through a series of learning stages in regard to the use of home technology based upon assumptions about their capacity to comprehend the new systems and their hazards.

The new technological improvements, such as electricity and the telephone, like older systems like water and sewerage, were linked to a network that existed outside of the home. These connections were often thought to be hazardous. As David Handlin observes, 'Every utility that entered or was part of the home at some time was thought to be a source of danger'. Americans feared gas and electric lines not only because of their fire potential but also because 'they suspected that they emitted noxious fumes or rays'.[72] Just as housewives as well as men worried over the seepage of deadly sewer gas into homes, so they viewed the even more difficult-to-comprehend qualities of electricity with 'fear and trembling'.[73]

Engineers and technicians often believed women to be ignorant of the new household technologies.[74] In her book, *When Old Technologies Were New: Thinking About Electric Communication in the Late Nineteenth Century*, Carolyn Marvin notes that turn-of-the-century electrical journals pictured women as incapable of comprehending or appreciating the new energy source. 'Endless stories of women's unpreparedness and incapacity in a world of technical expertise', she writes, 'time and again demonstrated the reassuring conclusion that women would always depend on male prowess to conquer the world for them'. Women who had attained technological knowledge and power were held to have gone astray. The need, therefore, was for male 'experts' to contain the hazards of the dangerous technology.[75]

As electricity increasingly entered urban homes and moved from an elite prerogative to middle-class commonplace, the proliferation of electrical appliances and the desire of manufacturers to develop mass markets forced a reconceptualization of women's technological skills. Housewives had to become knowledgeable about electricity if they were to avoid shocks and other electrical accidents. It was incumbent on the housewife to become an 'amateur electrician', with an understanding of 'the proper care of electrical household appliances'. She had to be able to change a fuse, understand the functions of the sewerage system, and of gas stoves and heaters, and not be dependent on the 'experts' for all contingencies.[76] Education was one way to acquire such knowledge. *Good Housekeeping Magazine*, for instance, published a number of articles on the 'ABC of electricity for housekeepers', as well as furnishing bulletins and sponsoring courses in the schools to instruct 'women in the proper and the safe use and care of appliances and equipment in their home'.[77] Such education would also be tied, as will be discussed later in the chapter, to the growing home economics movement. In addition, the magazine established the Good Housekeeping Institute to test and approve electrical appliances.

But would education alone be sufficient to reduce home accidents involving electricity? Public utilities were anxious to emphasize electricity's inherent safety in order to increase electricity use and to stimulate the purchase of appliances.[78] A 'few simple precautions', promised the Wisconsin Public Service Corporation's safety engineer, would keep electricity 'no more hazardous than many other tools or materials used in everyday home life'.[79] In the 1920s, the National Electric Light Association, the public utility industry's trade association, created a 'Women's Committee' and an 'Accident Prevention Committee' to forward 'safety work for women in the electrical industry'. The function of the so-called 'utility women' was to 'inform themselves on the use of electricity in the home, the best methods of rendering service and courtesy to the customer, and ... [to train] themselves in safety practice'. In order to emphasize that electricity was much safer than the older household technologies it was replacing, the Association published a pamphlet entitled 'Common Sense', that laid down ten 'simple rules' regarding safe use of electricity.[80] 'Common Sense', however, as one women safety expert emphasized, was not always enough, and knowledge and education were also required.[81]

If the hazards of electricity were to be controlled, performance standards would have to be established. The Bureau of Standards, created by Congress in 1901 to systematize and regularize national standards for use in science, engineering, manufacturing, commerce and education, took the lead in this matter.[82] Much of the Bureau's work related to electricity and gas provision as well as to standards for various materials such as paints, textiles and inks. In 1915 it produced its first circular written for the consumer – Circular 55, dealing with 'Measurements for the household' – and describing the operation of common household measuring devices such as scales, gas, water and electric meters, and clocks, and how to use them in planning and buying a house. Two years later, in 1917, the Bureau issued a second publication concerning household materials – Circular 70 – designed 'to make scientific results available for those with little or no technical training'.[83]

Most significant for home safety, however, was the Bureau's issue in 1918 of Circular 75 – 'Safety in the Household' – prepared, according to the introduction, because of the increase in hazards 'in modern times from the service of gas and electricity and the use of such dangerous articles as matches, volatile oils, poisons, and the like'. The Circular drew on safety code data gathered by the Bureau's divisions, and covered electrical and lighting hazards, gas, fire and chemical hazards, and other miscellaneous home accidents such as falls, cuts and burns. The public enthusiastically greeted these circulars, and they became 'best sellers', thus testifying to the public's appetite for useful information on hazards and risks.[84]

Throughout the 1920s, electrical utilities touted the safety of electrical appliances, especially as compared with past energy and lighting technologies. They especially emphasized the manner in which they would end the drudgery of housework and provide increased standards of cleanliness and health in the home.[85] In the 1920s, electrification of the domestic market accelerated, as electrical utilities and corporations such as General Electric and Westinghouse developed their appliance lines.[86] Appliances such as electric ranges, refrigerators, and radios now joined the irons, fans and vacuum cleaners that had been available before World War I. Electricity, promised the industry's admen, was safe and liberating, fitting in well with modern society.[87]

(iii) *Falls*

Most safety experts acknowledged that falls were the commonest form of home accidents. They were recognized as a very old problem – 'the law of gravity has been taking its toll of life and limb throughout the centuries ... our troubles really began with a fall in the Garden of Eden. Since that day falls have been our most serious accident hazard'.[88] Some of the causes of falls were relatively easy to identify: 'The shaky step-ladder, the favourite rocking chair, the wobbly straight chair are stepping stones to death and to the hospital'. Solutions also seemed mostly commonsensical: get a good step-ladder, take care in the bathtub, sprinkle salt on the icy walk in the winter, avoid polished floors, and teach the children to put their toys away.[89] The housewife, acting as safety manager, was clearly responsible for eliminating these accident-producing conditions. In comparison with accidents from other causes, the cause of falls seemed simple to understand. And yet, their very simplicity made them illustrative of the difficulties of reducing home accidents.

One of the basic problems was statistical. When speakers at the NSC Safety Councils or writers on safety spoke of falls, they often differed or were unclear about the number of people who were yearly injured or killed by falls or how the falls occurred. They agreed that the falls were largely 'not spectacular', and that 'the human element seems to contribute more than any other circumstances'.[90] Structural factors were also believed to be partially responsible, although their actual share was unclear. As one North Carolina study reported, falls were caused by:

> poor illumination, loose or broken treads, badly spaced treads, or by obstructions left on the stairway. In addition, North Carolina women and children fall in bath tubs, out of beds, from ladders, from porches and windows, [and] from vehicles, trees and platforms.

Some of these falls may not have 'been preventable', observed the speaker, but the larger number were 'due to inherent faults in mechanical construction or to personal carelessness'.[91]

By 1929, more information became available when the NSC began publishing its statistical compilation, *Accident Facts*. It did not, however, go very far beyond the earlier generalizations, and frequently observed that data on falls was hard to obtain.[92] In the absence of comprehensive statistics, the NSC used data sets compiled by various authorities such as insurance companies or local and state reports, with results that were sometimes confusing. Estimates, for instance, concerning the number of deaths that resulted from falls ranged from one-third to almost half of home accident fatalities. There was general agreement, however, that the aged, and especially women, were more susceptible to injuries or death from falls.[93]

Most speakers who discussed falls at the National Safety Congresses were not 'experts' in either human behaviour or construction and design. Recommendations followed commonsensical principles. Women were advised to follow good managerial practices, keeping rugs from slippery surfaces, removing toys from walkways, and providing for good lighting. Speakers frequently recommended that a good small step-ladder be available in the home. It was not until 1938, for example, that an architect made a presentation on falls, arguing that both architects and builders had an obligation to consider that particular risk. In a presentation much more specific than those of other speakers on falls, he emphasized the safety advantages of 'modern styles' compared to those of the 'architectural styles of yesteryear'. Specifically, he noted the need for care in locating steps and stairs, the necessity of adequate lighting, and the availability of new and safer materials such as rubber-backed rugs.[94]

This presentation highlighted the extent to which falls, the commonest form of home accidents, were relatively devoid of research and expertise. Even today one scholar notes that there is 'No comparable [to automobile safety] interest or financial support ... available for studies of falls in the built environment', with steps and stairs continuing to be the most 'dangerous element' in the American home.[95]

Priority Setting Through Statistics

The broadening of the safety movement to include the home as well as industry received considerable impetus from the statistical work conducted by the NSC and by various insurance companies.[96] Since public health statistics were often considered unreliable, beginning in 1921 the Council began collecting its own accident statistics. It prepared a standard accident report form and distributed it among cities of over 25,000 in population. The data were supplied by its membership – by 1921, the Council had established local councils in about forty cities – and by local governments, especially municipal and county coroners.[97] Public safety, especially involving ʾutomobile accidents, was increasingly becoming a matter of social concern, as media publicity and statistics revealed a growing number of automobile-related deaths and injuries. The statistical work of these local councils included the daily compilation of statistics on all accidents, analysis of the statistics to reveal causation, and use of the statistics for publicity purposes.[98] Beginning in 1927, the reporting of home accident statistics became a regular feature of the *National Safety News*. In 1929, when the NSC began publishing *Accident Facts*, home accident statistics received their own section.

Insurance companies were also important in the improvement of the statistical accident record and early players in the home safety movement. Before state and public health officials began to identify home accidents as distinct from accidents of other types, insurance companies had marked the home as a perilous place. By the late nineteenth century, the business of insurance underwriting was separated into three distinct areas: life contracts, fire contracts, and liability contracts. Generally, life insurance companies offered policies which insured individuals; fire underwriters insured property from fire losses (perhaps the most common of all accidents and one of the most severe), while liability contracts developed in the late nineteenth century for use in industries to protect employers and property owners from suits brought by injured workers and people injured on their premises.[99]

The first company to do a considerable amount of accident insurance underwriting was Aetna, which began operating in this area about 1890. Up to 1913, Aetna offered only industrial accident insurance. In that year, however, the company began offering a policy which diverged dramatically from the traditional accident policies offered by life insurance companies. Rather than targeting individuals who might have an accident, this broad-based liability policy – 'combined residence insurance' – protected home-owners from calamities of all sorts related to the home.[100] The insurance joined several different types of liability into a single policy: accident, water damage or explosion, glass breakage, and burglary.[101] This policy reflected Aetna's point about risk in the unsafe home. As the company's in-house publication, *The Aetna Agency Edition,* noted in 1913, 'We only wish (the business man) were as safe as he feels [at home]. Not a day passes but we have it most unpleasantly brought to our attention that the home is no sure isle of safety'.[102]

Like other policies offered by life insurance companies, accident policies were directed at individuals who faced substantial financial loss because of misfortune. A 1913 Aetna marketing magazine, for instance, portrayed a giant moose-head trophy lying across a home office desk and noted that:

> A few minutes before the man whose office is shown in this picture reached his desk this 200-pound trophy fell from its place on the wall. Had he been seated at his desk his accident insurance policy in the AETNA would have meant $30,000 to his estate. The exceptional character of this narrow escape but emphasizes the fact that the lives of most men are full of hazards, against the results of which accident insurance alone can afford any protection.

The article specifically identified merchants, manufacturers, bankers, lawyers, and doctors as those most susceptible to 'loss of income' from accidents.[103] Following Aetna, New York's Metropolitan Life began offering an accident policy in 1921.[104] Agents were encouraged to target those who had already purchased life insurance policies or men working in certain occupations.[105]

The marketing literature of both Aetna and Metropolitan became more articulate about the causes of accidents as they gathered accident statistics. Metropolitan pioneered in using accident statistics in their advertising, noting that 15 per cent of all accidents occurred in the home.[106] Such campaigns clearly identified the home as a place of hazard and encouraged middle-class men to protect themselves from the consequences of such accidents, but without specifying how to eliminate the hazards.

The idea that the home was hazardous, however, was not easy to establish given the long-standing ideal of the home as haven.[107] In the 1920s, the NSC continued to give its highest priority to industrial accidents, while placing public accidents, which essentially meant accidents involving the automobile, as a second cause. Home safety remained a distant third as a matter of concern and focus. W.H. Cameron, the National Safety Council Managing Director, reflected these priorities, commenting in an article in the *Annals of the American Academy of Political and Social Science* that there were only 'two divisions of the safety problem – industrial and public', completely overlooking home accidents.[108] Ironically, in the same year, 1926, at the fifteenth Safety Congress, the NSC held its first full session devoted to home safety.[109]

A major reason for home safety's low ranking was a lack of sources for funding. Normally an NSC 'section' represented a particular type of industry – automotive section, chemical section, cement section, marine section, metals section – and industry members provided funding for that section's activities. Membership on the NSC Executive Committee also came primarily from industry, although a few representatives of insurance companies and local and governmental safety groups were included. As Lew Palmer of the New York Equitable Life Assurance Company, an early promoter of home safety, acknowledged in 1930, the NSC had 'not devised any practical revenue from the home safety side of accident prevention. It has to pay its own way. We can't take the money that we have coming from industry and turn it all over to home safety...'.[110]

It is also possible that the industry-dominated NSC leadership saw home safety as 'women's work' – that is, since the National Safety Council was an organization that had developed out of concern over factory safety (a male-dominated world), and since it had largely a male membership, it believed that the home was woman's domain and responsibility. Thus, it played down the priority of home safety by denying it a separate Home Safety Section (sections constituted the major divisions of the NSC), and at its annual congresses it usually combined home safety with 'school safety' or other such issues, or made it part of a separate 'Women's Session'.[111] That discussion of the issue often took place in such a gender-identified separate session emphasized the extent to which home safety was considered women's responsibility.

Middle- and upper-class women involved in home safety shared this attitude. Speaking in 1929 before the General Federation of Woman's Clubs, Arvilla Miller warned that home accident statistics indicated that the time of looking at 'the home as the haven of rest, security and protection against the stresses of the world outside' had come to an end. She maintained that 'serious study, followed by organized effort', was necessary to cope with the problem, and as an action model she pointed to the NSC, founded by 'far-seeing men' who had recognized the scope of the industrial accident problem. Home accidents, she argued, called for the 'women of America' to take similar action through their women's clubs. Thus, a nationwide movement could begin, leading to the appointment of a Home Safety Committee in every women's club and the consequent great reduction of home accidents. Under Federation leadership, she concluded, a day would arrive 'when every woman may rightfully lay claim to the title, *safety director in the home*'.[112]

The optimism expressed by Miller in her speech was not widely shared. Throughout the talks delivered at the home accident sessions of the National Safety Congresses, and in journal articles published in the late 1920s and the 1930s, writers on home safety complained about their inability to define the home accident problem, the difficulty of obtaining 'facts', and the need for extensive research. Safety experts noted that not only was information unknown or difficult to obtain, but also that victims were not forthcoming about the circumstances of their misfortune. Speakers at the home safety sessions of the Safety Congresses, often representing middle-class women's clubs, occasionally raised class and ethnic issues, mentioning the poor and immigrants as responsible for a major number of accidents and also for maintaining secrecy about them. Katherine Fisher, the Director of the Good Housekeeping Institute, expressed the belief that poor women were less receptive to the safety messages than middle-class women:[113]

> Homes in which hazardous conditions are most frequently found are usually homes on 'the other side of the tracks.' These are the kind of homes in which it is most difficult to offset ignorance of hazardous conditions by teaching women through our safety educational work. Women in such homes ... are not 'exposed' to safety education .... They are seldom members of women's clubs, parent-teachers'

associations, or other community organizations, because they have little time and less inclination for the serious activities of such groups.

Other speakers, and not necessarily women, expressed similar sentiments, noting that most accidents occurred in the homes of immigrants or of the 'poorly housed ... people who are not easily reached in group life and [who] do not have ... organizations that can be easily made accessible'.[114]

Speaking in 1929 at the eighteenth National Safety Congress, Jane Addams of Hull House agreed that the poor and recent immigrants were most likely to be accident victims: 'I am sure if you will make an investigation', she commented, 'the children of working mothers will be found to head the list of those maimed and injured and killed.' Addams argued, however, in contrast to many safety experts at the time, that poor housing conditions not poor management produced home accidents – factors such as inadequate lighting, the lack of roof guards, and the absence of playgrounds, as well as women required to work rather than caring for their families. She called on the NSC to do for home safety what it had done for industrial safety and made three specific recommendations as a way to reach that goal: that corporations provide mother's pensions so they could stay at home to guard their children; that construction companies build improved housing, with children's safety in mind; and that schools add safety education to domestic science classes.[115] On the eve of the Great Depression, none of these recommendations was taken seriously by the NSC membership.

The Red Cross Enters the Field

The continued growth of home accidents in the 1930s, and the NSC's lack of success in reducing them, resulted in the entry of the National Red Cross into the home accident field. Organized in 1881 by Clara Barton, the original purpose of the Red Cross was to engage in disaster relief activity. In the first decades of the twentieth century, it concentrated on first-aid and life-saving, and actively participated in World War I providing troop services. In the 1920s, the Red Cross shifted its focus to the provision of emergency care for accident victims and accident prevention. Although it had a professional organization and a federal charter, the Red Cross was largely staffed by a corps of trained volunteers in local chapters.[116] By building co-operative networks with groups such as the Boy and Girl Scouts, the Federation of Boys Clubs of America, the International Association of Police Chiefs, and various state health and highway departments, the Red Cross greatly extended its influence.

In the late summer of 1935, after examination of home safety programmes in several cities, Red Cross Vice-Chairman James L. Fieser issued a detailed memorandum projecting a Home and Farm Accident Prevention Program. He proposed to base the Home and Farm Accident Prevention Programs in local chapters run by committees with wide community representation. The steps he outlined included study of the accident problem, community education, service to the individual home and home inspection, publication of results, work with co-operative agencies, and first-aid instruction. Fieser confidently predicted that by 'attaining these objectives, the ultimate goal – the reduction of accidents – will be realized'.[117]

The Red Cross was an opportunistic mission-oriented organization, with a strong sense of territoriality.[118] In a meeting with National Safety Council officials, Robert Bondy, new director of the Red Cross programme, assured the NSC that his organization would not attempt to duplicate any NSC functions, such as the nation-wide collection of accident statistics. However, when an NSC official proposed that the Red Cross finance a joint accident prevention project utilizing the NSC research and statistical knowledge, Bondy opposed the plan. In a revealing letter to Fieser, Bondy laid out his objections:[119]

> We must keep in touch with the Safety Council. We must avoid duplication of what they are doing. We must use their specialized and skilled service where possible, but I do not consider it timely to undertake any joint projects at this time or any significant expenditure of money for their materials. Our own program will become so much bigger than anything the Safety Council has undertaken, that it is important to avoid having the tail wag the dog.

Clearly the Red Cross believed that the home accident field represented a niche where they could greatly enhance their stature. In September 1935, Admiral Cary T. Grayson, the Red Cross National Chairman, wrote a letter about the new effort to Mabel T. Boardman, the previous long-time Red Cross Chair, and approvingly reported that 'one of our people' had said that the new home and highway activity would 'mark a new epoch in Red Cross affairs', providing an 'entree to the American home that has not otherwise been possible'.[120]

The Red Cross strategy to combat home accidents involved great amounts of publicity and education, but little research. In an internal memorandum, Vice-Chair Fieser outlined this strategy:[121]

> The accident prevention program of the American Red Cross is exclusively and strictly educational. It employs no technical safety

> experts. It has no laboratories for the testing of safety devices. It does not undertake to speak with authority in the safety field ... it does not participate in the promotion of safety legislation. It simply interests its Chapters in organizing special efforts for the more general recognition by householders and farmers of common accident hazards that exist in their homes and on their farms, with suggestions for eliminating or preventing them.

A 'nation-wide Home Inspection Campaign' launched the programme, and over 26 million home inspection forms, as well as window cards, were distributed in the schools. Within several months after the programme had begun, 2,500 of the 3,710 Red Cross chapters had appointed a Home and Farm Accident Prevention Chairman. Radio programmes and newspaper articles on safety were sponsored, and 'action pictures', showing home accident injuries, were published in the newspapers.[122] Red Cross officials persuaded President Franklin D. Roosevelt to call a National Accident Conference, held on 18 December, 1935. Secretary of Commerce Daniel C. Roper served as conference director and Admiral Grayson was the presiding officer and first speaker.[123]

Underlying the Red Cross strategy was a belief that people needed to be educated about risk in order to reduce accidents. Writing in the *Red Cross Courier,* Fieser commented that the 'public's point of view is sick':[124]

> A few hundred lives in danger on a sinking vessel causes feverish interest and concern yet this same public attaches little significance to the almost unbelievable fact that each year, for the past five, an average of more than 30,000 men, women and children were burned to death, blown to pieces, electrocuted, poisoned, drowned and killed by falls in the one spot supposedly safer than any other – the home!

In his keynote address at the National Accident Conference in 1935, Grayson repeated the old behavioural argument – that the accident toll 'was created and caused by people themselves, and the solution lay in self-education and self-discipline'.[125] This strategy, as in earlier prognoses of the home accident problem, of necessity involved the 'home-maker' or the woman in the home. As Irma Gene Nevins, National Director of the Red Cross Accident Prevention Service wrote in 1947, 'Prevention of accidents in the home is largely the responsibility of the home-maker – and much depends up-on [*sic*] her ability to keep the house in order and in good repair', as well as properly supervising children.[126]

Thus, traditional ideas about home accident prevention involving changing people's behaviour and women as home safety managers dominated the Red Cross strategy. But even though it had a widespread network of local chapters and distributed great quantities of accident prevention materials, the Red Cross programme did not go well, and reports from the local chapters to the central headquarters indicated a widespread sense of frustration.[127] By the late 1930s, the Red Cross was faced with the decision either to get out of the home accident field or to alter its basic strategy. The option chosen was to modify the accident programme and to combine it with the organization's successful First Aid and Water Safety, an action taken on 1 July, 1939. In 1941, the Red Cross began offering formal classes in accident prevention, awarding certificates upon completion in a manner similar to that provided in first-aid and water safety.[128] This strategy appeared more satisfactory than the previous less-structured approach, but Red Cross officials had been forced to realize that a victory over home accidents was, at best, slow and uncertain.[129] Although it maintained its involvement in the home accident field, the Red Cross never dominated it in the manner that it had originally expected.

Conclusions

The years between 1907 and 1941 were years of both success and relative failure for those in the field of safety. The major successes were achieved in the areas of 'work' or workplace accidents, as industrial mortality and morbidity declined at a fairly steady pace from the highs reached early in the century.[130] These gains were largely a result of intensive safety campaigns, improvements in work conditions and medical care, adoption of protective devices for machinery, and a shorter work week, cutting the industrial fatigue that was often a factor in industrial accidents. Home accidents, on the other hand, remained extremely high, averaging about 30,000 per year from 1928 to 1956. The campaign against home accidents may be accounted partially successful in that only accidents from falls appeared to advance faster than population growth, but these accounted for about half of all home accident deaths. Elderly people over 65 and children and infants under five were the most vulnerable. Fire was the next highest cause, with about 16 per cent of the total, while the remainder scattered among factors such as poisons, fire-arms, and household appliances: all of these categories stabilized at about the same rate in the 1930s.[131]

The persistence of and even increases in home accidents during the first half of the century suggest that the home accident problem was much more complex than either the NSC or the Red Cross realized, and not especially responsive to a strategy based on changing human behaviour and modifying the environment through publicity, educational campaigns, and safety check-lists.[132] One approach to comprehending its complexity is to focus on the differences between the home and the factory. The factory was ideally a structured environment with a workforce whose discipline was directed by individuals (foremen) charged with management responsibility and where machines set the pace of work. Once industrial managers stopped believing that accidents were largely the worker's fault and understood that production gains could be achieved and liability reduced with safety measures, industrial accidents dropped sharply.[133] And media-aroused public outrage over the volume of industrial accidents in the Progressive period also pressured industrial leaders to make safety improvements.

In the home, however, as with the automobile, discipline was difficult to enforce, especially with children. Home furniture and decorative arrangements were often haphazard, dictated as much by fashion as by a rational attempt to reduce danger. For all of the period under consideration, most safety organizations considered the housewife to be the responsible figure or 'home manager' – the equivalent of the factory manager or foreman. In addition, the home had been touted as a 'haven' from the hazards of the world and hence was difficult to consider as involving danger, especially given that, as a place, it was the environment most familiar to people. Oftentimes responsibility for a home accident lay with a family member, leading either to concealment or to a reluctance to demand change. And, unlike factory safety, which had been partially driven by society's moral outrage at industrial accidents, except in the case of landlord malfeasance, home accidents could not generate an equivalent amount of social anger.[134]

By 1940, those involved in the safety movement recognized that the home was, in reality, still a 'separate sphere', and that tactics that had successfully reduced accidents in industry would not work in the home.[135] The 1950s and 1960s, however, witnessed a revolution in the area of accident prevention as accidents became the domain of public health investigators. In 1940 only the beginnings of this shift to 'injury control' were visible.[136] Some of the problems with home accident control probably lay in the absence of financing for investigation and the lack of serious research into causation. The task was complicated, however, by the belief that the 'home safety problem' was really not one problem but a multitude of problems, each requiring a different solution. Home accidents were considered especially obdurate because of the difficulty in obtaining information, causing behavioural change, and making environmental improvements. The sanctity and privacy of the home were hard to breach. But perhaps the factor that would prove most difficult in the search for a solution was the fact, as one NSC safety congress speaker observed, 'it is not the unusual condition or the new implement that brings about accidental injuries in or about ... homes. It is the condition people have gotten accustomed to that causes the majority of accidents'.[137] In short, people still regarded the home as a haven where the safeguards that they erected in the outside world of the street and the factory could be disregarded.[138]

Acknowledgements

We would like to thank Julian Waller, MD, for inviting us to deliver a version of this chapter in a session on the history of injury control at the American Public Health Association Annual Meeting in 1994, and Leslie Fisher of the New York State Department of Health for sharing with us his manuscript, 'Public Health Protection – Then and Now'. Our thanks also to John Burnham for his great helpfulness in sharing his ideas about accidents and accident prevention and his many suggestions on sources; and to Maurine Greenwald for helpful comments.

Notes

1. See, for instance, Clifford Edward Clark, Jr, *The American Family Home, 1800–1960* (Chapel Hill: University of North Carolina Press, 1986), David P. Handlin, *The American Home: Architecture and Society 1815–1915* (Boston: Little Brown and Co., 1979), Dolores Hayden, *The Grand Domestic Revolution: A History of Feminist Designs for American Homes, Neighbourhoods, and Cities* (Cambridge, MA: MIT Press, 1985), Gwendolyn Wright, *Moralism and the Model Home: Domestic Architecture and Cultural Conflict in Chicago 1873–1913* (Chicago: University of Chicago Press, 1980), and *idem*, *Building The Dream: A Social History of Housing in America* (Cambridge, MA: MIT Press, 1981).
2. Clark, *op.cit.* (ref. 1), 29.
3. Charles R. King, *Children's Health in America: A History* (New York: Twayne Publishers, 1993), 47.
4. Ruth Schwartz Cowan, *More Work for Mother: The Ironies of Household Technology from the Open Hearth to the Microwave* (New York: Basic Books, 1983); Clark, *op.cit.* (ref. 1), 29.
5. Susan Strasser, *Never Done: A History of American Housework* (New York: Pantheon Books, 1982), 185.
6. Catharine E. Beecher, *A Treatise on Domestic Economy, For the Use of*

Young Ladies At Home and At School (Boston: Marsh, Capen, Lyon, and Webb, 1841. Reprinted, New York: Source Book Press, 1870), 245–50; Strasser, *op.cit.* (ref. 5), 57–8.

7. In a section of a separate chapter, Beecher did give advice about procedures in case of fire in the home or stable. See Beecher, *ibid.*, 372. In the revised edition of this book, published in 1869, she transferred the problem of house fires to the chapter on 'Accidents and Antidotes'. This volume also discussed the problem of carbon monoxide poisoning, produced by using airtight stoves in sealed rooms. See also Strasser, *op.cit.* (ref. 5), 57–8.
8. 'Accidents, Disasters and Cities', *Urban History*, xx (1993), 5–18.
9. Randolph E. Bergstrom, *Courting Danger: Injury and Law in New York City, 1870–1910* (Ithaca: Cornell University Press, 1992), 21–3.
10. *Ibid.*, 158.
11. *Ibid.*, 167–96.
12. Carl Gersuny, *Work Hazards and Industrial Conflict* (Hanover, New Hampshire: University Press of New England, 1981), 20. The total number killed was 4,534, in 1907.
13. Harold U. Faulkner, *The Decline of Laissez Faire 1897–1917*, Vol. vii, *The Economic History of the United States* (New York: Rinehart & Co., 1951), 277.
14. Robert H. Wiebe, *The Search for Order 1877–1920* (New York: Hill and Wang, 1967). See, also, the contribution by Arthur F. McEvoy to this volume.
15. (New York: Russell Sage Foundation, 1910). Bergstrom, *op.cit.* (ref. 9), 48–50, explores some of the difficulties in securing accurate work accident statistics for the period 1870–1910.
16. State passage of workmen's compensation laws in the beginning of the century altered liability for workplace accidents, historically based on the common-law negligence doctrine. See Price V. Fishback, 'Liability Rules and Accident Prevention in the Workplace: Empirical Evidence From The Early Twentieth Century', *Journal of Legal Studies*, xvi (1987), 306.
17. There is no comprehensive study of the American safety movement, but see the following sources for insights into its beginnings: William Graebner, *Coal-Mining Safety in the Progressive Period: The Political Economy of Reform* (Lexington: University Press of Kentucky, 1976), 156–7; Lew W. Palmer, 'History of the Safety Movement', *Annals of the American Academy of Political and Social Science*, cxxiii (1926), 9–19 (this entire volume of *The Annals* is devoted to 'Industrial Safety'). For a discussion of accidents in the railroad industry, see Walter Licht, *Working for the Railroad* (Princeton: Princeton University Press, 1983), 181–201, and Steven W. Usselman, 'The Lure of Technology and the Appeal of Order: Railroad Safety Regulation in Nineteenth Century America', *Business and Economic History*, xxi (1992), 290–9. A study by Mark Aldrich of American industrial safety is forthcoming.

18. Graebner, *op.cit.* (ref. 17), 158–60; Daniel M. Berman, *Death on the Job: Occupational Health and Safety Struggles in the United States* (New York: Monthly Review Press, 1978), 77.
19. Daniel Nelson, *Managers and Workers: Origins of the New Factory System in the United States 1880–1920* (Madison: University of Wisconsin Press, 1975), 32.
20. See *Proceedings of the First Co-Operative Safety Congress, Held Under the Auspices of Iron and Steel Electrical Engineers* (Milwaukee, Wisconsin, 30 Sept. – 5 Oct., 1912); Palmer, *op.cit.* (ref. 17),10–13. In addition, in 1912 the American Mine Safety Association was formed. The National Safety Council absorbed the organization in 1915.
21. Faulkner, *op.cit.* (ref. 13), 277–8; and Graebner, *op.cit.* (ref. 17).
22. Nancy Tomes, 'The Private Side of Public Health: Sanitary Science, Domestic Hygiene, and the Germ Theory, 1870–1900', *Bulletin of the History of Medicine*, lxiv (1990), 509–39.
23. Quoted in *ibid.*, 528.
24. *Ibid.*, 511–13. See p. 528 for hygiene in home and responsibility of women.
25. Clifford Geertz, *Local Knowledge: Further Essays in Interpretive Anthropology* (New York: Basic Books, 1983), 19–35; Mary Douglas and Aaron Wildavsky, *Risk and Culture: An Essay on the Selection of Technical and Environmental Dangers* (Berkeley: University of California Press, 1982).
26. 'Rules for Safety', *Insurance Engineer*, xxiv (Nov. 1912), 269; 'Gas-Electric Peril in Homes', *Safety Engineering* [henceforth *SE*], xxix (1915), 217–18; 'The Fight Against Fire', *SE*, xxx (1915), 284.
27. 'Report of the Home Safety Committee', *Proceeding of the National Safety Council* [henceforth, *Proceedings, NSC*], Detroit, 1916, 30–2.
28. See Lew R. Palmer, 'Report on the National Safety Council's Special Committee on Home Safety', in *Transactions of the Twenty-Eighth National Safety Council* (1939), copy found in the Papers of the Children's Bureau, Dept of Labour, National Archives.
29. 'For "The Man on the Job" At Home – Cause and Prevention of Household Accidents', *SE*, xxxiii (1917), 103.
30. 'Universal Suffrage and University Safety', *SE*, xxix (1915), 222.
31. See Maureen A. Flanagan, 'Gender and Urban Political Reform: The City Club and Woman's City Club of Chicago in the Progressive Era', *American Historical Review*, xcv (1990), 1032–50.
32. In 1914, at the NSC Third Safety Congress, the famous journalist Ida M. Tarbell addressed the 'Economic Session' of the conference on safety, but paid attention almost entirely to safety and men in industry. See 'Economics Session', Third Safety Congress, *Proceedings, NSC* (Chicago, 1914), 119–25.
33. 'Housewives and Home Hazards', *SE*, xxxiii (1917), 303–04.
34. In 1919, at the Eighth Safety Congress, a 'Woman's Section' was

organized. See 'Organization of a Women's Section' *Proceedings*, NSC Eighth Safety Congress, 1919, 1412–16.

35. H.S. Forster, 'Safety in the Home', *Proceedings*, Seventh Safety Congress, 1918, 447–52. The comment was made by NSC President David Van Schaack, who called the session to order.
36. 'Women in Industry Section Invites National Women's Organizations to Cooperate in Public Safety', *National Safety News* [henceforth *NSN*], 312 (1 Dec., 1919), 1–2.
37. C.W. Price, 'Safety a Part of Community Life', *NSN*, 312 (1 Dec., 1919), 3.
38. 'Public places' referred primarily to the streets and the new hazards presented by the proliferation of the automobile.
39. 'Plans for Public Safety Campaigns in Great Demand', *NSN*, 314 (15 Dec., 1919), 1–2; 'Outline of a Public Safety Plan', *ibid.*, 2, 4.
40. Kathryn Kish Sklar, *Catharine Beecher: A Study in American Domesticity* (New York: W. W. Norton, 1973); Strasser, *op.cit.* (ref. 5), 188–9.
41. Quoted in Strasser, *op.cit.* (ref. 5), 210.
42. On this point see Glenna Matthews, *'Just a Housewife:' The Rise and Fall of Domesticity in America* (New York: Oxford University Press, 1987) and Margaret W. Rossiter, *Women Scientists in America: Struggles and Strategies to 1940* (Baltimore: Johns Hopkins University Press, 1982).
43. Matthews, *op.cit.* (ref. 42), chapter 6, 'The Housewife and the Home Economist', 145 ff., especially 152–8; Strasser, *op.cit.* (ref. 5), 206; Rossiter, *op.cit.* (ref. 42), 276–7.
44. Samuel Haber, *Efficiency and Uplift: Scientific Management in the Progressive Era, 1890–1920* (Chicago: University of Chicago Press, 1964), ix. See also Wiebe, *op.cit.* (ref. 14).
45. On how technological change held out the promise of emancipation see Cowan, *op.cit.* (ref. 4) and Hayden, *op.cit.* (ref. 1).
46. Although few monographs have focused directly on the home economics movement, many excellent discussions of the movement exist. See, for instance, Matthews, *op.cit.* (ref. 42); Rossiter, *op.cit.* (ref. 42); and Strasser, *op.cit.* (ref. 5).
47. David E. Nye, *Electrifying America: Social Meanings of a New Technology* (Cambridge, MA: MIT Press, 1992), 252.
48. This was the seventh graduate fellowship in the field of safety education offered by the National Bureau of Casualty and Surety Underwriters. See announcement, 'A Fellowship in Home Safety', in Papers of the Children's Bureau, National Archives; 'Bureau Offers Fellowship in Home Safety', *NSN*, xxi (1930), 26.
49. The fellowship was first announced in 1929 but there were few applicants. The fellowship was won by a Miss Gertrude Zurrer, who pursued her studies at the University of Chicago. She presented her research plan at the Nineteenth National Safety Congress, but never finished her graduate degree.

50. For a discussion of Edith Abbot's career as an academic and a social reformer, see Robyn Muncy, *Creating a Female Dominion in American Reform 1890–1935* (New York: Oxford University Press, 1991), 69–92.
51. See Gertrude Zurrer, 'The National Bureau's Study of Home Accidents', *Proceedings, Nineteenth Safety Congress*, xix (1930), 232–7; see, also, Frances L. Swain, 'Teaching Home Safety Through Good Home Management', *Proceedings, Twentieth Safety Congress*, xx (1931), 182–6.
52. Daniel J. Walkowitz, 'The Making of a Feminine Professional Identity: Social Workers in the 1920s', *American Historical Review*, xcv (1990), 1051–75.
53. Strasser, *op.cit.* (ref. 5), 212.
54. Bertha June Richardson wrote *The Woman Who Spends: A Study of Her Economic Function* (Boston: Whitcomb & Barrows, 1904). See also Nye, *op.cit.* (ref. 47), chapter 6.
55. Christine Frederick, *Household Engineering: Scientific Management in the Home* (Chicago: American School of Home Economics, 1920), 69; quoted from Strasser, *op.cit.* (ref. 5), 214. See also Christine Frederick, *The New Housekeeping: Efficiency Studies in Home Management* (Garden City, N.Y.: Doubleday Page, 1913).
56. Rossiter, *op.cit.* (ref. 42), 259.
57. Matthews, *op.cit.* (ref. 42), 153.
58. Nancy Cott, *The Grounding of Modern Feminism* (New Haven: Yale University Press, 1987).
59. Hayden, *op.cit.* (ref. 1), 194–5.
60. On the role of fire in American life see Margaret Hindle Hazen and Robert M. Hazen, *Keepers of the Flame: The Role of Fire In American Culture, 1775 – 1925* (Princeton: Princeton University Press, 1992); Christine Meisner Rosen, *The Limits of Power: Great Fires and the Process of City Growth in America* (New York: Cambridge University Press, 1986).
61. Beecher, *op.cit.* (ref. 6), 299.
62. 'Architecture and Fire Insurance', *Insurance Engineering*, xii, no. 3 (1907), 235.
63. *Safeguarding America Against Fire*, vi, no. 5 (May 1923), 2.
64. *Ibid.*, 3.
65. Alexander Hamilton, *Household Cyclopaedia of Practical Receipts and Daily Wants* (Springfield: W. J. Holland, 1875), 390–1. Quoted in Hazen and Hazen, *op.cit.* (ref. 60), 115.
66. George P. Hodges, 'Home Is Worth Guarding Against Fire', *NSN*, xxi (1930), 108–10, 149.
67. NSC speakers frequently cited inaccurate statistics concerning fire deaths, failing to distinguish between home and industrial fire deaths. See Walter Forrester, *Twelfth Safety Congress*, 862; Paxton Mendelsohn, *Fifteenth Safety Congress*, 185; Gertrude Zurrer,

Twentieth Safety Congress, 196; and R. B. Criswell, *Twenty-third Annual Safety Congress*, 84–6.

68. Experts from the fire underwriters seldom spoke at National Safety Congresses and speakers discussing fire there appeared to be unaware of their research.
69. K.G. Martin, 'The Housewife As A Fire Preventionist: Fire Dangers in Apartment-House Homes From a Woman's Point of View', *SE*, xxviii (1924), 353–8; Paxton Mendelsohn, 'Home Fires and Their Causes', *NSC Proceedings*, Fifteenth Congress (1926), 185–91. Men also were assigned responsibilities for home fire prevention such as ensuring the safety of wiring and keeping the basement unlittered. See Hodges, *op.cit.* (ref. 66), 109–10, 149.
70. National Board of Fire Underwriters, 'Home Inspection Blank for Schoolchildren', *Safeguarding America Against Fire*, v, no. 1 (1922), 1–4.
71. Cowan, *op.cit.* (ref. 4), 66–70.
72. Handlin, *op.cit.* (ref. 1), 455.
73. Tomes, *op.cit.* (ref. 22), 538; C.H. Claudy, 'Electrical Invasion of the Home', *Scientific American*, cxv (2 Dec., 1916), 502–3.
74. It is worth noting, however, that in the late nineteenth century women were expected to be capable of understanding domestic hygiene and the scientific information involved; men, however, usually assumed the responsibility for the plumbing and structure. See Tomes, *op.cit.* (ref. 22), 514, 527–8. For a modern discussion of women and technology see Jan Zimmerman (ed.), *The Technological Woman: Interfacing with Tomorrow* (New York: Praeger, 1983).
75. Carolyn Marvin, *When Old Technologies Were New: Thinking About Electric Communication in the Late Nineteenth Century* (New York: Oxford University Press, 1988), 22–31; Strasser, *op.cit.* (ref. 5), 73–6.
76. Bertha Winter Mahoney, 'As The Home Keeper Sees It', *NSC Proceedings*, Sixteenth Congress, xvi (1927), 138–40.
77. Katherine A. Fisher, 'Making Household Equipment Safe to Use', *NSC Proceedings*, Eighteenth Congress, xviii (1929), 300–6. Katherine Fisher was Director of the Good Housekeeping Institute and a frequent participant in NSC affairs.
78. Nye, *op.cit.* (ref. 47), 259–77; Mark H. Rose, *Cities of Light and Heat: Domesticating Gas and Electricity in Urban America* (University Park, PA: Pennsylvania State University Press, 1995), 107–9, 139–46.
79. James A. Ryan, 'Efficient Slaves of Intelligent Masters', *NSN*, xx (1929), 116, 126; Nye, *op.cit.* (ref. 47), 276–80.
80. Esther Rockey, 'First Aid to Home Accidents', *NSC Proceedings*, Twentieth Congress, xx (1932), 186–90.
81. Gertrude Zurrer, 'The Welfare Agencies and Home Safety', *NSC Proceedings*, Twentieth Congress, xx (1932), 195.
82. Rexmond C. Cochrane, *Measures for Progress: A History of the National*

Bureau of Standards (Washington: National Bureau of Standards, 1966), 43.

83. *Ibid.*, 137.
84. *Ibid.*, 137–8. A consolidated edition of the three circulars appeared in 1918 as 'Measurements, materials, and safety for the household'.
85. Katherine Fisher, 'Safety Begins at Home', *NSC Proceedings*, Twenty-Fourth Congress, xxiv (1935), 113; Zella Patterson, 'The Safe Use and Care of Household Appliances', *NSC Proceedings*, Twenty-Seventh Congress, xxvii (1938), 145–7; and Rose *op.cit.* (ref. 78), 511–25.
86. Nye, *op.cit.* (ref. 47), 266–77; and Harold Platt, *The Electric City: Energy and the Growth of the Chicago Area, 1880–1930* (Chicago: University of Chicago Press, 1991), 236–44.
87. Ruth Cowan (*op.cit.*, ref. 4) has argued that technology created 'More Work for Mother' but Strasser (*op.cit.*, ref. 5, 78–84) observes that women actually welcomed electricity and electrical appliances because it relieved them of 'backbreaking labour'. Claude Fischer has suggested that the telephone, rather than changing the lifestyles of women, was fitted by women into their daily routines. See Claude S. Fischer, *America Calling: A Social History of the Telephone to 1940* (Berkeley: University of California Press, 1992), 268–72.
88. The first quoted section comes from H. Walter Forster, 'Accident Prevention in the Home', *Twelfth Safety Congress, Transactions*, xii (1923), 861, the second from NSC, *Accident Facts, 1936* (Chicago: NSC, 1937), 10.
89. H.S. Forster, 'Safety in the Home', *Transactions, Seventh Safety Congress* (1918), 447–9; A.A. Mowbray, 'Hazards in the Home', *Hygeia*, iv (1926), 618; and Elsie Thomas Culver, 'Home May Be Sweet But Is It Safe?', *NSN*, xxi (1930), 79–80.
90. Mrs Edward M. Land, 'Safety Program of the General Federation of Women's Clubs', *Transactions, Nineteenth Safety Congress* (1930), 240–1; and William C. Knoelk, 'The Schools Responsibility for Home Safety', *Transactions, Twenty-Fifth Safety Congress* (1936), 135.
91. Land, 'Safety Program', 241.
92. For instance, the 1932 edition of *Accident Facts* noted that, 'Due to lack of data, it is impossible to classify home fatalities accurately according to type of accident and age of victim.'
93. 'Is There Any New Way of Getting Hurt?', *NSN*, xxi (1930), 40, 96; and *Accident Facts* (1937), 16–17. A 1929 compilation by the Travellers Insurance Company identified home falls as being involved in one out of three home injuries, with falls on stairs being the most common accident followed by falls on level floors with rugs and then bathtub and shower falls.
94. John R. Fugard, 'Safety in the Home', *Transactions, Silver Jubilee Safety Congress* (1938), 143–4.
95. John Templer, *The Staircase: Studies of Hazards, Falls, and Safer Design* (Cambridge, MA: MIT Press, 1992), Vol. 1, 1–23.

96. For NSC and statistics, see Frederick S. Crum, 'How We Die from Accidents in Careless America', *NSN*, iv, no. 4 (1912), 17–18. See, also, Lucian W. Chaney, 'The Need for More Definite Analysis of Accident Causes', *Annals of the American Academy*, cciii (1926), 40–5. See, also, John Burnham, 'How the Discovery of Accidental Childhood Poisoning Contributed to the Development of Environmentalism in the United States', *Environmental History Review*, 19 (1995), 57–82. In the 1930s, the American Red Cross developed an accident prevention programme.
97. 'Report of the Statistical Committee', *Proceedings*, Eighth Safety Congress, 1004–7; Frederick S. Crum, 'Report of Committee on Statistics', *Proceedings*, Ninth Safety Congress, 1920, 321–7; and 'To the Stranger in Our Midst', *NSN*, iv (1921), 3.
98. 'Outline of a Public Safety Plan', *NSN*, no. 314 (1919), 2, 4; 'What the Local Councils Did in 1921', *NSN*, iv (Oct. 1921), 25; and Julian H. Harvey, 'Organizing a Local Safety Council', *Annals of the American Academy*, cxxiii (1927), 32–3. See also Lew R. Palmer, 'Report of the NSC's Special Committee on Home Safety', *Transactions of the Twenty-Eighth National Safety Council*, ii (1939), 133–4.
99. Life insurance companies sometimes offered liability coverage through specific divisions to comply with state laws which demanded that the capital of life and fire insurance policies be invested separately.
100. 'Combination Residence Insurance', *The Aetna Agency Edition*, ii, no. 9 (June 1913), 296. It is important to note that this policy did not cover loss by fire. There had long been a separation of business between fire and life insurance companies. It is unclear if this informal organizing practice ever became codified. As a consequence, liability insurance, which was usually underwritten by corporations dedicated to writing life insurance, could not be built into fire insurance policies.
101. *Ibid.*, 296.
102. 'Safe at Home', *The Aetna Agency Edition*, ii, no. 5 (February 1913), 231. By the 1910s, Aetna had paid over $10 million in claims on its 'Accident and Health Policy'.
103. 'Aetna-ized', *The Aetna Agency Edition*, ii, no. 7 (April 1913), 265.
104. See, for instance, any of the early issues of *The Accident and Health Monitor* which is cited below. A fairly substantial literature exists which discusses Metropolitan Life and its programmes of social welfare. See, for instance, Marquis James, *The Metropolitan Life: A Study in Business Growth* (New York: Viking, 1947); or, more recently, Angel Kwolek-Folland, 'Gender, Self, and Work in the Life Insurance Industry, 1880–1930', in Ava Baron (ed.), *Work Engendered: Toward a New History of American Labour* (Ithaca, N.Y.: Cornell University Press, 1991).
105. *The Accident and Health Monitor*, no. 14 (11 March, 1922); *ibid.*, no. 17 (1 April, 1922). The company discouraged agents from offering such policies to women.

106. *Ibid.*, no. 68 (21 July, 1923).
107. For instance, see H.W. Forster, 'Safety in the Home', *Proceedings*, Seventh Safety Congress (1918), 447; and comments of C.M. Talbert, chair, 'Public Safety Section', NSC: 'I had rather thought that home was a fairly safe place .... I always felt that when I got behind my own doors, I was at least safe from the dangers that follow me through the daily work.' *Proceedings*, Ninth Safety Congress (1920), 385.
108. W.H. Cameron, 'Organizing for Safety Nationally', *Annals of the American Academy*, cxxii (1926), 2.
109. Mrs James N. Downey, 'Home Safety', *NSC*, Fifteenth Safety Congress, xv (1926), 167–92. Other papers in the session dealt with the economic costs of accidents, accidents and the family, accidents in the hospital, and home fires.
110. NSC, *Transactions, Nineteenth Safety Congress* (1930), 246–7; see, also, Palmer, *op.cit.* (ref. 28), 133–5. The NSC was funded by member dues, contributions, and by the sale of materials. Today it also does consulting on safety matters.
111. The complaint that home safety was 'the step-child of the safety movement' was echoed approximately fifteen years later at the Twenty-Eighth National Safety Congress. Lew R. Palmer, Chairman of the NSC Special Committee on Home Safety, protested about the lack of a stand-alone Home Safety Section in the Council. See Palmer, *op.cit.* (ref. 28), 133–4. See, also, Rosamond Losh, 'Home Accidents Are *Preventable*', *NSN*, xviii (1928), 18, 88.
112. Mrs D. Edwin (Arvilla) Miller, 'Home Safety in the Community', *NSN*, xx (1929), 93–4, 134. Italics added.
113. Katherine Fisher, 'A Man's Job', *NSN*, xxxvi (1937), 40. Fisher also argued that men should get involved in home safety because 'safety in the factory begins at home'.
114. Fred Rosseland, 'Getting the Women to Help in Better Home Safety', *Transactions, Fifteenth Safety Congress* (1926), 183–4, and E. Williams Corn, 'Most Accidents Occur in Homes of Poorly Housed', *ibid.*, 189; Bernice Neuberger, 'Developing a Community Program for Home Safety', *Transactions, Sixteenth Safety Council* (1927), 131–2.
115. Jane Addams, 'What Accidents Mean to the Community', *Transactions, Eighteenth Safety Congress* (1929), 295–8. Addams expressed surprise at the number of home accidents. For a discussion of the relationship between crowding and accidents see Molly Ladd-Taylor, *Mother-Work: Women, Child Welfare, and the State, 1890–1930* (Urbana: University of Illinois Press, 1994), 28–9.
116. Estelle Rebec and Gustave R. Gaedderet, 'The History of the American National Red Cross', Vol. vii: 'The Development of First Aid, Life Saving, Water Safety and Accident Prevention' (Washington, D.C.: The American National Red Cross, 1950, unpublished), 36–73.

117. Vice-Chairman [James L. Fieser] to Staff Members, 'Status and Fall Plans of the Home and Farm Accident Prevention Program', G.I. Letter #12, 20 Aug., 1935, Red Cross Archives, Washington, D.C.
118. Rebec and Gaedderet, *op.cit.* (ref. 116), 63.
119. Quoted in *ibid.*, 97.
120. Cary T. Grayson to Mabel T. Boardman, 14 Sept., 1935, Red Cross Archives.
121. James L. Fieser to Staff Members, 21 July, 1936, Red Cross Archives.
122. The Chairman [Cary T. Grayson] to Chapter Chairmen, 7 Sept., 1935, C.S. 625–H.H.–1, Red Cross Archives; American National Red Cross, 'Home and Farm Accident Prevention', in *Annual Report* (1936), 103–4; and Rosemary L. Lilie, 'Home and Farm Accident Prevention in the Midwest', *Red Cross Courier* (April 1936), 10, 27.
123. James L. Fieser to Daniel C. Roper, 26 Nov., 1935, Fieser to The President [FDR], 26 Nov., 1935, and Franklin D. Roosevelt to Fieser, 3 Dec., 1935, Red Cross Archives. The Red Cross had played an important role in providing first-aid training and life-saving training to various Depression-era federal programmes such as the CWA, the FERA, and the CCC. Rebec and Gaedderet, *op.cit.* (ref. 116), 76–81.
124. 'Home and Farm Accident Prevention: A New Nation-Wide Program Initiated by the Red Cross', *Red Cross Courier* (Oct. 1935), 9.
125. Rebec and Gaedderet, *op.cit.* (ref. 116), 97. In an internal memo to Chapter Chairmen, Grayson noted that 'hazards and bad habits' caused accidents. See The Chairman [Cary T. Grayson] to Chapter Chairmen, 7 Sept., 1935, C.S. 625–H.H.–1, Red Cross Archives.
126. Irma Gene Nevins, 'Is Your Home Free of Hazards', *Red Cross Courier* (May 1947), 8.
127. The NSC had supposedly taken some satisfaction at the Red Cross's inability to mount an effective campaign against home accidents. John Melpolder, the 'Consultant' to the Program, reported that the NSC's attitude was: 'There are a lot of agencies that dabble in this field, but they get out of it as soon as they've gotten some publicity out of it, and have done more harm than good.' Melpolder to James L. Fieser, 11 Sept., 1937, Red Cross Archives.
128. John Melpolder had replaced Robert Bondy as head of the programme in 1937. In that year he wrote to Fieser, 'the Red Cross, by common consent, has preempted the home and farm accident prevention field. Now what are we going to do with it or, rather, in it?' However, he 'retired' in 1939. See John Melpolder to Fieser, 18 Nov., 1937, Red Cross Archives; 'Accident Prevention and First Aid Consolidated', *Red Cross Courier* (June 1939).
129. Norman H. Davis to Chapter Chairmen, 30 Sept., 1941, Red Cross Archives.
130. The subject of automobile safety was of great interest during these years and attracted attention that might have been directed to home safety. In the 1920s, it became a major concern of the NSC. See Joel

W. Eastman, *Styling vs. Safety: The American Automobile Industry and the Development of Automotive Safety, 1900–1966* (New York: University Press of America, 1984).

131. William Haddon, Jr, Edward A. Suchman, and David Klein, *Accident Research: Methods and Approaches* (New York: Harper & Row, 1964), 30–6. Deaths from motor vehicle accidents rose in absolute numbers but actually declined by a measure of death rate per 100 million vehicle miles. Pedestrian deaths rose to a peak in 1937, but then steadily decreased thereafter. I. Jay in Home Accident Prevention: *American Journal of Public Health,* xlii (1952). Brightman *et al.*, 'Mortality Statistics as a Direction Finder', 842. Safety experts believed that advancing automobile safety was more difficult than factory safety because of the need to apply discipline to both driver and pedestrian. In addition, existing road and street systems, built for different types of vehicles travelling at lower speeds, raised the accident potential. Traffic safety engineering, influenced by ideas derived from scientific management, advanced as a field in these decades, developing a variety of technologies to provide signals and controls. The main emphasis in accident prevention, however, fixated on driver behaviour and traffic controls. By the mid-1920s, agitation over rising numbers of automobile injuries and deaths caused many states to pass laws dealing with licensing, speeding, penalties and safe driving conditions.
132. One speaker at the Sixteenth NSC Congress (1926) had anguished that the home accident problem was 'insurmountable'. See Joel D. Hunter, 'What Accidents Mean to the United Charities', *NSC Proceedings,* Sixteenth Congress, xvi (1926), 126.
133. Nelson, *op.cit.* (ref. 19), 30–3.
134. We are indebted to David Hounshell for this observation.
135. Richard W. Thrush, 'Home Safety Activities of Selected National Groups: The American Red Cross', *NSC Proceedings*, Twenty-Ninth Safety Congress, xxix (1940), 183.
136. See Julian A. Waller, 'Reflections on a Half century of Injury Control', *American Journal of Public Health,* lxxxiv (1994), 664–70; and Haddon *et al., op.cit.* (ref. 131).
137. Land, *op.cit.* (ref. 90), 242; Knoelk, *op.cit.* (ref. 90), 131; and Brightman *et al., op.cit.* (ref. 131), 843.
138. See, for instance, Paul Slovic, Baruch Fischhoff and Sarah Lichtenstein, 'Facts and Fears: Understanding Perceived Risk', in R.C. Schwing and W.A. Albers, Jr (eds), *Societal Risk Assessment: How Safe is Safe Enough?* (New York: Plenum Press, 1980), 181–214.

10

War on the Roads: Traffic Accidents and Social Tension in Britain, 1939–45

Bill Luckin

It is unwise to be over-dogmatic about collective mentalities during any historical epoch. But there can be little doubt that, by the mid-1930s, an increase in radical pacifism together with a growing body of anxiety-ridden popular literature confirmed that very large numbers of Britons had become convinced of the inevitability of war.[1] Within this terrifying collective psychic scenario, it was aerial bombardment or poison gas attack, or both, that were expected to reduce the great cities of Britain to ruin in astonishingly short periods of time. These fears and projections locked into and were reactivated by memories of Zeppelins, Gotha bombers and mass slaughter in the trenches.[2] There was, moreover, no clear divide between fevered visions of 'future war' and the 'rational' planning for 'real' conflict in which governments, civil servants and the military had been engaged since the late 1920s. A dialectical relationship had grown up between policy-making and fictional extrapolation from the 'hard facts of science'. Powerful interest groups – particularly those pressing the claims of a generously funded and prestigious Air Force – capitalized on fear of bombs and gas, and writers, film-makers and magazine editors improvised on expert assessments of the nature of the 'next war' to produce ever more devastating depictions of the 'death of civilization'.[3]

Those responsible after 1925 for devising a blue-print for civil or 'passive' defence were no less obsessively haunted by catastrophist obsessions. Quantitative estimates became ever more alarmist and were used as a basis for arguing that, compared with the Great War, vastly increased loads of bombs would be dropped in ever more concentrated periods of time, with a minimum estimated death-toll of 50 fatalities per ton.[4] In the aftermath of such onslaughts, the Army and specially trained police units would need to be deployed to control panic-stricken flight from key centres of industrial production. Mass looting and rioting would degenerate into anarchistic or communistic assaults on the forces of law and order. Water, electricity and sanitation systems would be blasted into extinction, allowing killer infections to return to claim huge numbers of lives. Medical resources would be massively over-stretched.[5]

The precise operation of lighting restrictions – already known as the 'black-out' during the First World War[6] – in minimizing the effects of aerial bombardment divided and confused defence experts throughout the 1920s and early 1930s. Such measures were widely believed to have a debilitating effect on morale and war production. (Winston Churchill, who had gained valuable first-hand ministerial experience of the over-bureaucratization of work and leisure during the First World War, strongly supported this view, although, by 1940, he would be outmanoeuvred by 'military' and 'civil defence' elements within the War Cabinet.)[7] There was doubt, also, as to whether a total black-out would obscure the targets that were meant to be obscured: 'the bomber', as Baldwin had lamented in a much-quoted phrase in 1932, would 'always get through'.[8] Yet by the mid-1930s, scientific experiment, increasing international tension and ever more horrific predictions of the damage that would be inflicted by systematic bombing, had convinced those responsible for the planning and co-ordination of air-raid precautions, that Britain had no alternative but to commit herself to rigorous lighting regulations. The fact that the Germans had undertaken a large-scale black-out exercise in Berlin in 1935 also played its part.[9] Semi-secret black-out experiments were undertaken in a number of British towns between 1936 and 1938 and, by the outbreak of war, a highly complex administrative structure had evolved. It was directed by Sir John Anderson at the Home Office who, since the 1920s, had played a dominant role in departmental thinking on civil defence.[10] (Anderson had also been involved in preventive planning for the expected collapse of law and order during the General Strike in 1926, and the containment of 'terrorism' in India between 1932 and 1937.)[11]

When the black-out was finally brought into operation in the early autumn of 1939, the impact was profound. According to Terence O'Brien, the stoic official historian of civil defence during the Second World War:

> The black-out, imposed on the whole of the country on 1st September, transformed conditions of life more thoroughly than any other single feature of the war. The historian, incapable of describing it may be allowed recourse to the statement that it had to be seen (or experienced) to be believed. It made all movement by pedestrians or vehicles on the roads after dark a matter at least of difficulty and frequently of danger; subjected all work in factories, offices and shops to new physical and mental strain; seriously hampered all railway and dock operations; conferred on each citizen

> an additional responsibility for the public safety, and gave him in his own home a new and often unwelcome sense of isolation. It clearly (as had long been foreseen) set the authorities difficult problems in balancing strategical advantages with disadvantages.[12]

The gravest of these disadvantages were undoubtedly experienced by road users, and particularly pedestrians. Eight thousand people perished on the roads in 1939; eight and a half thousand in 1940; and nine thousand in 1941.[13] A downward trend only started to establish itself in 1942, and this would in time reduce traffic accidents during the immediate post-war years to levels lower than any experienced since the mid-1920s. But this improvement owed less to reductions in the severity of the black-out than to a dramatic cut-back – from about 2 million to around 800,000 – between 1939 and 1942 in the number of private cars on the roads. (There was also a somewhat surprising decrease – from about 3 million to about 2.5 million – in all other types of vehicles.)[14] Petrol rationing and slowly improving driver expertise undoubtedly played a more significant role in saving lives than minor 'concessions' such as a reduction in the speed limit in built-up areas and extensions of summer time.

Yet, in one sense, the road crisis of 1939–41 was no more than an exaggeratedly savage version of what had become normal throughout the preceding decade. In 1930, 1933 and 1934, fatalities on the roads had risen above 7,000 and at no time had injuries numbered fewer than 200,000 a year.[15] This class-inflected 'slaughter on the roads' had precipitated a vociferous national debate. The major participants were a rampantly pro-car lobby, dominated by the Society of Motor Manufacturers and Traders (SMMT), a moderate road safety organization – the National Safety First Campaign – and a radical 'neo-Luddite' pressure group, the Pedestrians' Association.[16] By 1940 greatly expanded car-ownership together with the semi-official doctrine that motorized transport had been central to the continuation of economic recovery, had significantly undermined the root-and-branch 'anti-motorism' championed by the Pedestrians' Association. It was now claimed by government, the motoring organizations and 'moderate' road safety activists that it was naïve pedestrian fallibility rather than bad driving which frequently determined the severity of road traffic accidents. This, certainly, was the view underlying the emergent 'human factors' orthodoxy legitimated by the influential Alness Committee on Road Safety which reported just before the outbreak of hostilities. According to this interpretation, motorists must make every effort to adjust to the demands of war and the 'comprehensive' black-out. But even more crucial was the role of pedestrians and their readiness to adapt to the disciplines of a fully and irreversibly 'mechanized' civilization.[17] Without a scintilla of irony, the Minister of Transport, Captain Euan

Wallace, stated in January 1940 that safety campaigns would be directed 'chiefly to helping the pedestrian because he [*sic*] was the worst sufferer, under black-out conditions [and] it lay in his hands to make the greatest contribution to safety'.[18]

Given pre-war, vehicle-related levels of death and injury, this broadly pro-motorist ideology implied nothing less than an emergency programme in social re-education. Already by the mid-1930s Britain had become a highly motorized society. In 1900 nearly 9,000 fatalities had been attributed to 'traditional' accidental causes – burning, scalding, explosions, drowning and domestic falls. Yet by 1930 nearly 7,000 people were dying on the roads, no fewer than twice as many as the combined death-toll from the now declining categories of burns and drowning. Whether assessed according to deaths per head of population, per vehicle or per thousand of miles of road, the British record was a disturbing one. True, Germany, and to a lesser extent the United States, were also experiencing heavy road casualties. But fatalities in Britain by 1939 had reached the exceptionally high figure of 24 per 10,000 vehicles. As for vehicle-related injuries, these seemed to be even more frequent in Britain than elsewhere. In 1939, the figure per 10,000 miles of road reached nearly 13,000 – marginally higher than that for accident-prone Germany and four times worse than for the United States.[19]

In terms of specific, vulnerable groups, child fatalities had reached crisis proportions during the 1930s. As *Table 1* implies, the disruption of war, mass evacuation, and the black-out probably contributed to an increase in mortality which would continue until 1946. Within the sphere of official propaganda and rhetoric, child deaths loomed large. In May 1941 there occurred 'an all-time high record in the number of children killed. No fewer than ... 166 ... or over 5 every day'.[20] Among adult pedestrians, the elderly were profoundly disoriented by the watery light disseminated by side-lights or, following modifications to the regulations, from a single heavily masked headlamp. Whether stepping out from behind a bus or parked car, walking down pitch-black city streets, or attempting to cross too close to what seemed to be slowly moving vehicles: in all these circumstances failure to adjust to a greatly reduced field of vision and a much shorter reaction-time frequently proved fatal. Those over the age of fifty were particularly at risk in built-up areas, where traffic densities were at their highest, but it was also imperative to be on one's guard on twisting and unlit country roads and lanes.[21] Despite repeated pleas for care, the elderly continued to be killed and injured in large numbers, and in May 1940 they represented 75 per cent of all adult pedestrian fatalities. (The ratio in favour of males was eight to two.)[22]

Those driving or riding any form of vehicle were much better protected: and this, more than anything else, fuelled public criticism of civilian car-owners and allegedly irresponsible and under-trained service personnel.[23] The number of private car-owners who died on the roads remained both stable and low before, during and after the black-out. Motor cyclists, however – and this was the golden age of motor cycling – became significantly more vulnerable than drivers of private cars. Bicyclists fared rather better: too many were dying, but the adverse conditions of the early war years failed to trigger any dramatic upsurge in either fatalities or injuries.

Table 1: Road Fatalities 1938–1950

	Children	Adults	Motorists	Motor Cyclists	Adult Cyclists
1938	870	2176	339	989	1196
1939	850	3647	385	1064	1190
1940	972	3742	339	1148	1158
1941	1231	3550	386	1287	1124
1942	1112	2538	306	821	931
1943	993	2065	281	537	938
1944	1134	2180	360	540	984
1945	1053	1549	310	484	752
1946	828	1661	266	649	675
1947	767	1613	278	664	688
1948	834	1534	221	505	679
1949	746	1560	312	675	707
1950	674	1579	321	935	679

Royal Society for the Prevention of Accidents, *Road Accident Statistics 1938–54* (London: n.d.), 1–4.

In terms of the temporal and spatial distribution of death and injury, *Table 2* confirms that there was a decisive war-time movement towards more accidents occurring during 'hours of darkness'. (In terms of absolute numbers, however, relative traffic flows continued to ensure that day-time casualties predominated.) Locational and environmental differentials were more complex. A comparison of eight urban areas during the autumn and early winter of 1938 and 1939 revealed wide disparities and suggested that pre-existing patterns of traffic movement, public awareness and education campaigns, as well as policing and sentencing policies, had all played a part.[24] Thus in Gateshead and Salford low levels of road accidents remained low; the same was true of Bolton. In Leeds, where the number of pre-war fatalities had been high, there was only a small increase. But in Manchester, Birmingham and Newcastle upward movements were registered: 36 to 90, 49 to 89 and 13 to 30 respectively. And in Glasgow, deaths on the road spiralled from 44 to 143 between September and December 1939. Nearly all of these deaths were of pedestrians: 51 were killed on Saturday nights; and approximately 30 'may have been drunk'.[25] Pubs, 'road-houses', and the alleged social irresponsibility of the 'brewing interest', developed into foci for increasingly animated debate.[26]

Table 2: Average Daily Number of Fatalities 1938–1950

	Total	Darkness	Daylight
1938	18.1	–	–
1939	22.7	–	–
1940	23.5	11.5	12.0
1941	25.1	9.9	15.2
1942	19.0	6.9	12.1
1943	15.9	5.4	12.1
1944	17.5	5.4	12.1
1945	14.4	3.7	10.5
1946	13.9	4.6	9.3
1947	13.4	4.1	9.3
1948	12.3	4.1	8.2
1949	13.1	4.4	8.7
1950	13.7	4.9	8.8

Royal Society for the Prevention of Accidents, *Road Accident Statistics 1938–54* (London: n.d.), 6.

The figures for London confirmed the extent to which the elderly had become the unwitting civilian victims of the total black-out. Comparing September–December 1938 with the same months a year later, a Metropolitan Police report concluded that for those aged 55–64 and 65–74, the increase in road fatalities had been from 25 to 91 and 26 to 88 respectively.[27] Even more than the very young, therefore, those over 50 showed a tragic inability to adjust to civil defence measures that had been devised to protect them against the supposedly civilization-destroying bombs of the Luftwaffe. Little wonder that critics demanded assurances that the 'comprehensive' black-out really did serve the best interests of non-combatant – and particularly non-combatant urban – populations. Policy-makers, they insisted, had been over-influenced by the 'bomb' and 'gas' scares of the 1920s and early 1930s, and were therefore guilty of a potentially catastrophic miscalculation.

Nor did the statistics for road injuries provide compensating grounds for optimism. One of the biggest shocks of the early months of the war was the terrible severity of so many non-fatal, vehicle-related accidents. During this 'national emergency of the roads', a correspondent informed *The Times* in 1939 'no fewer than 18,000 people [in December] have been seriously injured'.[28] The gravity of non-fatal mishaps continued to generate anxiety: in 1941, when the volume of traffic had been greatly reduced as a result of petrol rationing, one injured person out of every 22 was still failing to recover. The comparable pre-war figure had been one out of 39.[29]

At the peak of the 'accident crisis' between September 1939 and January 1940, the arithmetic of death and injury provided the backcloth for a tense debate on three fronts: the nature and efficacy of the black-out regulations; the balance between the policies and rival jurisdictions of the military and the civil government; and the role of motorized transport in peace and war. The larger public, however, remained uninvolved. During the 1930s, the Pedestrians' Association had sought to publicize the isolation and numbing shock experienced by the seriously injured and by the families of the dead. Now that fatalities were moving rapidly upwards and road safety belatedly gaining extensive coverage in press, Parliament and on the radio, those most directly affected by the carnage might have been expected to express anger and opposition to the black-out. But this was not the case, and the social 'invisibility' of victims and families remained very nearly as absolute as it had been during peace-time. Lord Cecil of Chelwood – pacifist, staunch believer in the inevitability of mass destruction from aerial bombardment and chairman of both the League of Nations Union and the Pedestrians' Association – articulated his own uncompromising prognosis:

> The people who are killed or suffer are scattered all over the country. They are poor people, for the most part. They have no means, or very little means, of defending themselves.... The little efforts that are made by the pedestrian societies and so on are hampered by want of funds, by the fact that there is no great commercial interest in the safety of the roads, that all the commercial interests involved are in favour of no interference with the motors ... which might impede the profits of those who live by the motor trade.[30]

Detailed analysis of these 'scattered' tragedies might help to define a social history of the road accident in twentieth-century Britain, but no more than an outline account can be attempted here. It is self-evident that such occurrences were – as, indeed, they still are – sudden, isolated and isolating experiences.[31] Yet, under wartime conditions, the mix of externally enforced patterns of self-control, combined with the intermittent mental and physical disorientation associated with total conflict, served to distract attention away from every form of individual or 'selfish' 'problem'.[32] Furthermore, the very existence of a black-out that had been belatedly and hurriedly brought into operation redoubled public fears of sudden and horrifically effective bombing by the Luftwaffe.[33] Civilian 'slaughter' came to be perceived as a short-term cost which had to be stoically endured. For some, however, the burden was undoubtedly heavier than for others. The authorities continued to insist that the 'human factors' model was being even-handedly applied to drivers and pedestrians alike, but in reality, it was the non-driver who was unceasingly urged to acknowledge the necessity for 'adjustment' and 're-education'.

If the victims of road accidents remained largely 'silent' and 'invisible', in Parliament a small number of MPs began to criticize the government over the extent and technical detail of the black-out. None was more cogently outspoken than J. C. Wedgwood, one-time Liberal, ex-Labour Chancellor of the Duchy of Lancaster and an unpredictable and highly individualistic member of the Independent Labour Party.[34] Wedgwood's critique went much further than objections tabled by members who pleaded for more and better road-signs, extensions of summer-time and the abolition of the black-out in far-flung and 'non-strategic' rural areas. In a crucial debate in January 1940, Wedgwood traced the regulations directly back to the 'bomb' and 'gas' obsessions of the early 1930s:

> When the evacuation and the black-out were decided on, everybody thought we were going to be bombed immediately, and not merely bombed as we were in the last war but bombed so disastrously that the whole centre of the Empire would be untenable. The estimates that were made of the results of one bombing raid were ... in the nature of 200,000 casualties .... They made a mistake. I think everyone agrees that they made a mistake.[35]

Wedgwood went on to argue that, had the 'lessons' of Barcelona and Helsinki been properly absorbed, the government would not have 'evacuated all those people, [and] gone to the enormous expense of ARP. [They] would not have insisted on the black-out'. Nor was he convinced that the policy had proven itself in commonsensical, strategic terms: '[the Germans] have to come far further than we do: and they are short of petrol ... we have as much as we want ... [but] their petrol was used up in Poland'. Like many of his contemporaries, Wedgwood believed that Hitler was not yet ready to commit the Luftwaffe to a large-scale assault on London or any other urban centre. Economic exigency dictated that the Germans must not 'bomb us unless we bomb them'. And, even if there were to be a radical change of emphasis, the 'comprehensive' black-out might still not do what it was expected to do.[36]

> Suppose it were conceivable that one bombing raid by Germany could kill 200,000 in London. How many less would be killed if they raid us (a) in daylight, when they can see or (b) in moonlight, when

> they can see, or, (c) when all they can see is a subdued light which, by following the course of the Thames, they will know is London?[37]

How did the government respond to these criticisms of major strands of its war and defence policies, expressed, as they now frequently were, in the rhetoric of 'saving lives on the roads'? In attempting to answer this question, two points need to be borne in mind. First, every party to the dispute was operating in a military and logistic vacuum: what the Luftwaffe would actually do in late 1940 and 1941 was not known to those who participated in the debate in late 1939 and early 1940. Secondly, those who argued that thousands of pedestrians must not be sacrificed on the altar of the black-out might well have been presented by their governmental opponents as 'soft' and 'appeasing' advocates of a negotiated peace. In reality, official spokesmen resisted impugning the motives of those who called for radical modifications to the lighting regulations, emphasizing instead the overwhelming and long-proven strategic centrality of the civil defence system as a whole. In so doing, they sought to outmanoeuvre their critics by studiously avoiding the contagious rhetoric of 'slaughter' and 'carnage', while simultaneously reinforcing public apathy in relation to a major and potentially catastrophic social problem.[38]

Replying to his critics, and to Wedgwood, in particular, Sir John Anderson accentuated the certitudes of black-out ideology and steered round the dilemma of associated human and social costs. He argued that absolute, or near-absolute darkness over great centres of population would prevent enemy planes from identifying primary targets. The strategy would also cut back on the volume of successfully aimed bombs and minimize the damage done by others that were randomly or wholly unaimed. In terms of visibility from the air, the regulations would render cities and large towns much less easy to pick out, with smaller centres of population taking on the scale and patina of villages, and villages disappearing altogether from the bomber's view.[39] Yet massively more significant to Anderson than these practical and potentially life-saving considerations were the symbolic and morale-boosting aspects of the measures. 'Consider the position in Germany', he warned. 'All the evidence goes to show that the black-out in Germany is even more complete than in this country, even in parts of Germany far removed from the frontier. The Germans are a methodical, systematic, careful people. They have not imposed on themselves the self-denial that is involved in a complete black-out for reasons that they do not regard as fully justified'.[40] Anderson was convinced that the Luftwaffe would seek to destroy Britain's military and industrial war effort and undermine the 'national will to resist'. But, even if this did not occur, the 'discipline' of the black-out would still serve to reinforce rather than undermine morale and 'war-readiness'. Viewed from this perspective, deaths and injuries on the roads were of subsidiary importance: the price would quite simply have to be paid. The alternative, and one which had haunted policy-makers ever since the end of the Great War, was of an abjectly demoralized urban population, bombed out of house, home and sanity, wandering the streets, looting, and threatening every tenet of social and state control.[41]

Opposition in the Commons, which had peaked during the initial period of crisis between September 1939 and January 1940, subsided as national unity asserted itself and the possibility of a negotiated peace receded. The monthly statistics of death and injury on the roads fell, and rose and fell again throughout 1940 and 1941. But there would be no further full-dress debate in the Commons.

In the Lords it was more like business as usual. More outspoken than MPs and less shackled by the dictates of party discipline and the agreement not to disagree, peers confronted the road accident crisis both as a national emergency and as the continuation of an intolerable pre-war dilemma, reaching back to the shelved recommendations of the Alness report.[42] Any historian seeking confirmation of the continuing centrality of the Upper House in relation to social policy during the first half of the twentieth century, need look no further than the large-scale debates on the road traffic crisis between 1939 and 1941.[43] Peers represented a microcosm of a Britain of 'progressive motorists' and 'Luddite pedestrians', and gave voice to attitudes which the government would have preferred to see suppressed. Militant representatives of the 'speed at all costs' brigade mingled with traditionalist non-drivers and backwoods aristocrats who despised and lampooned every form of motorized transport. Debate was spiced by anecdote as peers attempted to reassert moral, patrician control over the gross social indiscipline implied by this unprecedented chaos on the roads.

The vehemently patriotic car-enthusiast, Lord Sandhurst, recounted how he had tried to persuade a policeman to arrest a driver who had jumped the lights in west London:

> Last night, as I was going home, I went from Gloucester Road tube station and reached Cromwell Road, which I was just going to cross, the lights being in my favour, when a car came up and went straight across the lights without stopping. It turned round and, still against the lights, proceeded to come back. There was a policeman standing on the corner just beside me and I said to him: 'Why the deuce do you not stop that car?' In a very leisurely manner, when I repeated my question, he went over and waved a light at the car and stopped it. Then, in a very gentle tone, he said: 'Do you realize that you

crossed against the lights?' The fellow said: 'Oh, did I? There are so many things to look at that I did not see them'.[44]

The adamantly pedestrian Lord Newton claimed that he 'intervened in this debate because I have a very strong personal interest in the question, having myself been knocked down four times by motor cars. I seldom leave my home without anticipating gloomily that the fifth and final accident may take place'.[45]

'Speed', in the view of Lord Cecil, constituted 'a very great social evil',[46] while Lord Snell, for the government, warned that the country must 'regain the sense of sacredness of individual life ... I sometimes think that the animals, and especially dogs, are acquiring a traffic sense almost more quickly than some human beings'.[47] Other speakers detected an insidious relationship between a lack of 'charity' on the roads and the 'soullessness' of totalitarianism. 'I sometimes wonder', mused the Bishop of Worcester, 'whether, unconsciously, we are being infected with that totalitarian philosophy which cares nothing for human personality. I sometimes wonder whether the continued spectacle of suffering may not be dimming the pity and compassion which we normally feel'.[48] Later, in 1945, the Archbishop of York would make precisely the same point. 'Of late years', he said, 'we have increasingly disregarded the values of the life of the individual. I think it is because we have become apathetic about the value of the individual that we tolerate this terrible death and casualty roll which goes on day by day on our roads'.[49] Less 'anti-pedestrian' than the Commons, and more sympathetic to the plight of non-drivers, most speakers in the Lords nevertheless depicted both parties as prodigals, who must be reminded of the great and enduring ethical certitudes: death on the roads in wartime Britain symbolized social atomism and insubordination.

When, much later, in 1944, the peers again debated road safety, the traumas of 1939–41 had receded amid the heady but still half-suppressed euphoria of 'total' victory. Comparisons were nevertheless still made between the 'waste' of life on the roads and the 'slaughter' of the battlefield. Lord Samuel told the House that the 'number of people killed and wounded (in the war) was no fewer than 370,000. On the roads during the war the number of people killed and injured was 588,000 – 50 per cent more than all those who have been killed and wounded in those terrible campaigns on land, on sea and in the air'.[50] Since significant increases in car-ownership were predicted for the post-war period, steps clearly had to be taken to reduce the 'carnage'. But how could or should this be done? Would responsibility for road accidents continue to be identified in terms of the 'guilty' and 'immoral' pedestrian and/or motorist, with the pedestrian bearing a heavier burden of guilt? Or would other variables – the state of roads and traffic signs, and the individual technical condition of the individual vehicle – be incorporated into a new orthodoxy? Addressing the Lords in summer, 1944, Lord Leathers, the Minister for War Transport, hinted at a change in official attitude. 'The problem is indeed partly psychological', he stated, 'a human problem, and partly physical, a problem of machines and their roads; of segregation of different types of traffic; even of curves and frictions'.[51]

But despite superficial modifications, there would be no immediate transformation, as the 'road traffic problem' modulated slowly and circuitously into the more positive ideology of 'road safety'. Initiatives by the Ministries of War Transport and Transport during the later years of the war had, in this sense, reasserted rather than reversed the position of the Alness Committee: human, rather than vehicular or road systems, shortcomings were still to be given maximum emphasis and publicity, by means of campaigns backed by the government and the Royal Society for the Prevention of Accidents (RoSPA).[52] Yet, despite continuing clashes between RoSPA and the now much less influential Pedestrians' Association, the relationship between drivers and non-drivers entered a phase of greater stability. Automotive systems of transport were more than a generation and a half old; car-ownership had become progressively more egalitarian; a once startling and fear-inducing technology had finally established itself within the realm of the totally familiar. It might be scant comfort but if you were knocked down in post-war Britain, it was much more likely than in 1935 or during the black-out that you would be killed or injured by a social coequal than by a social superior. Road accidents, like driving, had been dramatically democratized.[53]

It was only in the year of the Coronation in 1953 that the House of Commons again devoted a major debate to the road traffic accident question. The views and values expressed at that time threw light back onto the extraordinary happenings of 1939–41 in the same way in which the black-out had revealed in the starkest possible detail the tragedy of the 1930s. The debate also illuminated once again why, in war and peace, the traffic accident had remained so under-politicized and why the experience of such traumatic events had only rarely been shared outside the individual family and the hospital ward: why, in other words, public accidents had been largely excluded from public discourse and debate.

By the early 1950s, then, open or subterranean conflict between private motorists and pedestrians had receded. But the framework within which the notion of 'road safety' was beginning to replace the 'road traffic problem' continued to be dominated by the 'human factors model'. Within that paradigm blame and recrimination were giving way to growing consensus over the complexities governing relationships between men, women, vehicles and the larger urban and rural environments.[54] It was as if, in its first full moment of social and cultural acceptance, the motor car had been shorn of its most blatantly 'moral' – and 'immoral' – attributes. There were still 'miscreants' on the roads – in the early 1950s these were depicted as youthful motor-cyclists, who antisocially refused to wear crash-helmets. But such culprits were now categorized less in terms of 'immorality' or 'wickedness' than as individuals and groups to be psychologically and sociologically monitored and 'converted'. This drive towards 'social normalization' was reinforced by a greater readiness to perceive drivers, pedestrians and roads in their own distinctive environmental, technological and systemic terms. During the 1930s and 1940s, and particularly in the worldview championed by the Pedestrians' Association, the motor car had been repeatedly compared to a railway locomotive: a deadly machine, characterized exclusively by its capacity for uncontrolled speed, which must be segregated, as railway engines had been, from those whom it might irreparably damage. Segregation was by no means absent from the dominant discourse of the 1950s but now it was formulated in a positive rather than cataclysmic manner: the speed of cars must be matched by adequate road systems and thus be technologically neutralized. Simultaneously, drivers and pedestrians, subjected to more ambitious and psychologically shocking advertising campaigns, were to be alerted to the ever-threatening spectre of user fallibility.[55] The 'human factors' model, inherited from the Alness Committee, had largely defined the road traffic debate for more than a decade. Now, in a period of transition, 'morality' began to be replaced by 'system'. At the same time, parliamentarians pressed for motorways to cope with rapidly increasing numbers of cars and lorries and for the regular monitoring of the roadworthiness of every vehicle on the highway.[56] Such pleas were rejected on the grounds of economy, excessive interventionism and bureaucratic unwieldiness.[57] But a climate had been created in which technological inadequacy – and, after that, speed, drunken driving and the absence of passenger restraint – would come, reluctantly, to be acknowledged as determinants of death and injury. The 'human factors' model would remain – as it remains today – dominant, but a space had been provisionally created for quite differently nuanced constructions of road safety.[58]

Lest all this smacks too much of historical progressivism, there is a need to focus on backward as well as forward connections. In 1953, as in the years of the black-out, it was war and warfare which dominated debate of what was now once more perceived as an unprecedented 'crisis on the roads'. (In reality, as George Strauss, a veteran of immediate post-black-out attempts to increase the efficiency of public road education programmes, pointed out, the statistical record was much better than at any time since the 1920s.)[59] The point of reference was now Korea and the frequently cited fact that the daily toll on the roads was higher than that of entire actions in which the British contingent had become involved in that theatre.[60] In the early 1950s, as in the early 1940s, the languages of conflict and nationalism combined to create a discourse heavily skewed towards post-eugenic concern with 'economy' and 'national waste'. Simultaneously, these images of warfare – in a style reminiscent of Susan Sontag's delineation of metaphorical representations of cancer – continued to be over-insistently transposed onto the victim of the road accident.[61]

To conclude that the Second World War was bad for British pedestrians may be less banal than it seems. Death and injury on the roads during the 1930s had revealed a fragile technological system neither fully comprehended nor legislatively controlled by a government, which, despite its claims to care for the 'ordinary man', shaped its policies predominantly in the interests of the affluent and the moderately well-off – and hence in favour of the car-owning classes. It was this tendency, together with a law enforcement system which only rarely punished individuals in their role as car-owners, that had first generated the social construction of a 'road traffic problem' during the later 1920s.[62] The wartime conditions in which the crisis became ever more severe were heavily, though not exclusively, determined by the black-out. Legitimated by shared public and official terror of the consequences of mass bombing, the full spectrum of lighting regulations was only rarely opposed by those most directly threatened or affected by it. Like the great majority of injured combatants, those who experienced serious wartime accidents on the roads suffered silently and stoically.

It may nevertheless be tempting to seek to counterfactualize political and social processes in such a way as to show that interwar 'fear of the bomber' – and of poison gas – were 'wrong' or 'mistaken': and that, *pari passu*, the government ought not to have been seduced into introducing so far-reaching a system of social control. But does this make for good history and can it convincingly account for the beliefs, motivations and actions of the politicians, civil servants, drivers and pedestrians who have been described in this chapter? Mass bombing in Britain during the Second World War killed 50,000 and injured 60,000 more.[63] Given this volume of wartime civilian casualties, any allegedly 'exaggerated' fear of the destructiveness of aerial bombardment can only have been deeply and commonsensically rooted in a collective yearning for survival. All that was missing, in other words, from terrifying popular representations of 'future war' during the 1920s and 1930s were unknowable details of massively more sophisticated explosives and bomb delivery systems, whereby ever larger numbers of people would be exterminated, or subjected to extreme physical or psychic threat. Collective nightmare had jumped forward a decade but had failed (as, logically, it must) to incorporate the 'future' detail of mass bombardment: Dresden, Hiroshima, Vietnam, Cambodia, Baghdad. Retrospectively, each of these episodes would simultaneously make real and legitimate the wilder shores of 'fantasy' that had been morbidly summoned up and elaborated during the 1920s and 1930s.

As for the 'comprehensive' black-out, it is hardly worthwhile to attempt to calculate how many additional city-dwellers might have been killed, or pedestrians saved, had the regulations been less intrusively or rigorously applied. Such measures clearly had more to do with social discipline and 'war readiness' than the protection of unfortunately dispensable non-combatants.[64] Each party to the global conflict was deeply aware of what had to be done to protect the integrity and operational efficiency of a modern warfare state.

Concerned with a unique and bizarre series of events – when the 'car' came briefly to appear as threatening as the 'gun' – this essay has been deliberately skewed towards official discourses and the ways in which the 'war on the roads' was simultaneously justified and deplored by the government and an 'ethical' opposition. Class-inflected conflict had been perennially present on the roads of Britain throughout the 1930s, with public debate suffused by images of needless death and mutilation. When war was finally declared, and the black-out brought into operation, this rhetorical repertoire fused with analogous visions of an 'ultimate' and unprecedentedly destructive world conflict. The extent to which so intensely charged a cultural climate, and the policy debates located within it, may have recontextualized and reshaped the individual 'moment of the accident' itself, raises different and complex sets of historical questions.[65] If we are to develop a historiographically convincing reconstruction of the reactions, beliefs and attitudes of those injured in or bereaved by death in road traffic accidents – in both war and peace – we shall need to listen attentively to legal documents, police and insurance records, newspaper reports and taped interviews.

Acknowledgement

Many thanks to Roger Cooter for help with an earlier draft of this chapter.

Notes

1. Anti-war feelings have been anatomized by Martin Ceadel in *Pacifism in Britain: The Defining of a Faith* (Oxford: Oxford University Press, 1989). The same author has traced connections between 'morbid fantasy' and the 'realities' of war in 'Popular Fiction and the Next War 1918–1939', in Frank Gloversmith (ed.), *Class, Culture and Social Change: A New View of the 1930's* (Brighton: Harvester Press, 1980), 161–84. Invaluable contextual information is contained in Valentine Cunningham, *British Writers of the Thirties* (Oxford:

Oxford University Press, 1988), 155–210. Anti-air raid precautions are exhaustively – and at times exhaustingly – described by Terence O'Brien in *Civil Defence* (London: HMSO, 1955).

2. Major interpretations of the transmission of ideas and obsessions between the two world wars are presented in Paul Fussell, *The Great War and Modern Memory* (Oxford: Oxford University Press, 1975) and Modris Eksteins, *The Rites of Spring: The Great War and the Birth of the Modern Age* (London: Bantam Press, 1989). What 'really' happened in terms of bombing is chronicled in Llwellyn Woodward, *Great Britain and the War of 1914–1918* (London: Methuen, 1967), chs 2 and 3. Official interwar dread of annihilation from the air is documented in Uri Bialer, *The Shadow of the Bomber: The Fear of Air Attack in British Politics* (London: Royal Historical Society, 1980). A more overtly social and cultural approach to some of these issues is provided in David Edgerton, *England and the Aeroplane: An Essay on a Militant and Technological Nation* (London: Macmillan, 1991) and Paul Fussell, *Wartime: Understanding and Behaviour in the Second World War* (Oxford: Oxford University Press, 1989), 13–18.
3. This theme is contextualized in I.F. Clarke, *Voices Prophesying War, 1763–1984* (Oxford: Oxford University Press, 1966) and *idem*, *The Pattern of Expectation: 1644–2001* (New York: Basic Books, 1979). See, also, W. Warren Wager, *Terminal Visions: The Literature of Last Things* (Bloomington: University of Indiana Press, 1982). Rosalind Williams depicts equally extreme, imagined 'subterranean' fears during the late nineteenth century in *Notes on the Underground: An Essay on Technology, Society and the Imagination* (Cambridge, Mass.: MIT Press, 1990). Spencer R. Weart's *Nuclear Fear: A History of Images* (Cambridge, Mass.: Harvard University Press, 1988) assesses comparable anxieties and mentalities in the mid- and late twentieth century.
4. The best short accounts of interwar 'death-toll' theory are to be found in Richard M. Titmuss, *Problems of Social Policy* (London: HMSO, 1955), ch.1; A.J.P. Taylor, *English History 1914–45* (Oxford: Oxford University Press, 1965), 535–6; and Barry D. Powers, *Strategy Without Slide-Rule: British Air Strategy, 1914–1939* (London: Croom Helm, 1976), 50–5 and 122–3.
5. Titmuss states that in September 1938 the 'medical director of one well-known London clinic thought it was "clear to everyone that there must be an immediate inundation with cases of neurosis on the declaration of war – and certainly after the first air raid"'. Titmuss, *op.cit.* (ref. 4), 5.
6. The relationship between the black-out and road traffic accidents during the First World War is touched on by Arthur Marwick in *The Deluge: British Society and the First World War* (London: Macmillan, 1965), 136–8.
7. Churchill's short-lived and unsuccessful opposition to the 'comprehensive' black-out is documented in Public Records Office (PRO) War Cabinet 55 (39) 12, 466–7, 21 October, 1939: CAB

73/16 C.L.R. (39), 6 November, 1939; and War Cabinet 121 (39) 3 December 21 1939. ('It was important ... to pay regard to the general gloom caused by the black-out which exhausted the strength of the people for making the resistance which would be required as the war proceeded.' [488])

8. This passionate appeal-cum-lament is in *Parl. Deb.*, 5th ser., Vol. 270, 630–8 (10 November, 1932). The background is analysed in R.K. Middlemas and J. Barnes, *Baldwin: A Biography* (London: Weidenfeld and Nicolson, 1969), chs 27 and 28.
9. O'Brien, *op.cit.* (ref. 1), 91.
10. The immediate pre-war planning period is thoroughly covered by O'Brien, *ibid.*, 166–230.
11. A somewhat sycophantic account of his career as a whole is supplied by J. Wheeler-Bennett in *John Anderson: Viscount Waverley* (London: Macmillan, 1962). But Charles Loch Mowat believed Anderson to be 'perhaps the ablest of a distinguished generation of civil servants': C.L. Mowat, *Britain Between the Wars 1918–1940* (London: Methuen, 1955), 295.
12. O'Brien, *op.cit.* (ref. 1), 319–20. There is as yet no social history of the black-out. But relevant material may be found in Angus Calder, *The People's War* (London: Jonathan Cape, 1969), ch. 4: Tom Harrisson, *Living Through the Blitz* (London: Collins, 1976); and Robert Hewison, *Under Siege: Literary Life in London 1939–45* (London: Methuen, 1977), chs 1 and 2. Among contemporary accounts Henry Green, *Caught* (London: Hogarth Press, 1943) and William Sansom, *Westminster at War* (London: Faber and Faber, 1947), are particularly illuminating.
13. Royal Society for the Prevention of Accidents (RoSPA), *Road Accident Statistics 1938–54* (London: n.d.), 1.
14. William Plowden, *The Motor Car and Politics 1896–1970* (London: The Bodley Head, 1971), Appendix B, 456.
15. *Road Accident Bulletin*, 17 November, 1943, 1–8.
16. Interactions and conflicts between these bodies are described by Plowden, *op.cit.* (ref. 14), *passim.*
17. *Select Committee on Prevention of Road Accidents. Report and Evidence*, British Parliamentary Papers (PP), 1937–8: XXIII and 1938–9: II. From a large array of contemporary opinion of this type see, also, PRO: MT 34/354, *Standing Interdepartmental Committee on Road Accidents*, 'Report on Special Study of Fatal Road Accidents in Selected Areas during March 1940', 3 ('The principal cause of accidents, both in daylight and in darkness is lack of care or error of judgement on the part of the pedestrian...'); and PRO: MT 24/355, 'Road Accidents in Wartime', 7 February 22 1943.
18. *The Times*, 30 January, 1940.
19. PRO: MT 34/356, 'House of Lords Select Committee Memorandum submitted on behalf of the Minister of Transport' (n.d. but probably

1939).

20. PRO: MT 34/355, 'Committee on Road Safety in War ... Note by RoSPA', 28 January, 1942. See, also, 'Road Accidents in Wartime' (ref. 17), 4.
21. In his *Saville* (Harmondsworth: Penguin Books, 1978), David Storey writes of the hero's father: 'He had been coming home from work one morning, while it was still dark, riding down one of the many lanes that led from the pit to the village, when he had seen the lights of two cyclists coming towards him and had already turned tiredly to ride between them before he realized they were the heavily shaded headlights of a car.... He had broken both his legs, an arm, and had damaged several ribs.' (68) My thanks to Malcolm Pittock for drawing my attention to this passage.
22. PRO: MT 34/354, *Standing Interdepartmental Committee*, 'Note by Secretary on "Pedestrian Accidents"', 1 May, 1940.
23. This was a controversial issue in Parliament. See, for example, *Parl. Deb.*, 5th ser., Vol. 356, 500 (27 January, 1940). Gordon White, member for Birkenhead, East: *Parl. Deb. (HL)*, 5th ser., Vol. 118, 911–26 (26 March, 1941); and *ibid.*, Vol. 119, 75–7 (23 April, 1941).
24. Over-leniency in the courts had long been condemned. See PRO: MT 34/356, 'Response to Criticism of Ministry of Transport by Lord Reading' (Memorandum by A.V.T. Robinson); PRO: MT 34/355, 'Memorandum to Road Safety Committee from the Pedestrians' Association', 11 November, 1941; and Plowden, *op.cit.* (ref. 14), 253, 267–8 and 283. See, also, for background to this topic, Clive Emsley, '"Mother, What Did Policemen Do When There Weren't Any Motors?" The Law, the Police and the Regulation of Motor Traffic in England, 1900–1939', *Historical Journal*, xxxvi (1993), 357–82.
25. On Manchester, Salford, Leeds, Newcastle and Birmingham see PRO: MT 34/352, 'Road Fatalities: Comparisons of four Months, 1938 and 1939' (Memorandum by F. Cook), 25 January, 1940. For Bolton see *Chief Constable's Annual Report to the Watch Committee*, 1941, 11. The Glasgow experience is outlined in PRO: MT 34/352, 'Investigation into Causes of Road Accidents' (Memorandum by F. Cook), 26 January, 1940: and *ibid.*, 'Road Accidents', 5 February, 1940.
26. A British Medical Association committee had reported on the subject in summer, 1935 – see *British Medical Journal: Supplement*, 27 July, 1935, 57. During the war-time road crisis the 'lay', 'anti-alcohol' position was eloquently and ironically stated by Viscountess Astor, *Parl. Deb.*, 5th ser., Vol. 356, 527–32 (23 January, 1940). The 'modern', medical approach, emphasizing the depressive effects of drinking on performance and reaction-time was summarized by Dr Edith Summerskill, *ibid.*, 526–7. See, also, PRO: MT 34/354, 'Alcohol and Road Accidents', Memorandum, 1 May, 1940.

27. PRO: MT 34/352, 'Press Conference held at Ministry of Information. Monday, January 29, 1940'. Transcript.
28. Lord Lamington, *The Times*, 15 December, 1939.
29. *Parl. Deb.*, 5th ser., Vol. 120, 317–18 (21 October, 1941). The Bishop of Westminster. See, also, 'Road Accidents in Wartime'. 'The number of persons injured in the years immediately before the war remained fairly constant at 226,000. [Non-fatal] accidents were thereafter fewer but more deadly [*sic*] than they were before the war.' (5)
30. *Parl. Deb. (HL)*, 5th ser., Vol. 120, 327 (21 October, 1941).
31. There is no social history of the car accident but highly pertinent material is presented in Wolfgang Schivelbusch, *The Railway Journey: The Industrialization of Time and Space in the Nineteenth Century* (Leamington Spa: Berg, 1977), 129–49 and in a little-known and eccentric faction by Ilya Ehrenburg, *The Life and Times of an Automobile*, trs. Joachim Neugroschel (New York: Urizen Books, 1976).
32. This point was persuasively made by Lord Hampton in *Parl. Deb. (HL)*, 5th ser., Vol. 120, 327 (21 October, 1941).
33. According to A.J.P. Taylor, A.R.P. measures may have been suddenly and tardily introduced precisely in order to underscore the necessity for immediate and absolute 'war readiness': Taylor, *op.cit.* (ref. 4), 538. J.C. Wedgwood made a rather different, though complementary, observation when he wrote that 'gas masks and A.R.P. were solely invented by the government in order to terrify the old women of this country into welcoming our strong silent Prime Minister on his return from supping with the devil': C.V. Wedgwood, *The Last of the Radicals: Josiah Wedgwood M.P.* (London: Jonathan Cape, 1951), 231–2.
34. See the inevitably partisan 'family biography' cited above (ref. 33) and the more measured entry by the same author in the *Dictionary of National Biography 1941–50* (London: Oxford University Press, 1959), 941–3.
35. *Parl. Deb.*, 5th ser., Vol. 356, 534 (23 January, 1940).
36. *Ibid.*, 535–6.
37. *Ibid.*, 536.
38. Public disinterest was widely noted. See *Parl. Deb.*, 5th ser., Vol. 356, 485 (23 January, 1940), Captain Euan Wallace, Minister of Transport; *Parl. Deb. (HL)*, 5th ser., Vol. 120, 321 (21 October, 1941), The Bishop of Worcester; and *ibid.*, 331, Lord Newton.
39. *Parl. Deb.*, 5th ser., Vol. 356, 542–5 (23 January, 1940).
40. *Ibid.*, 548.
41. Comparative analysis of civil defence is central to historical evaluation of the kinds of points canvassed by Anderson and his opponents: but the literature on the topic is extremely limited. See, however, the titles cited in R.J. Overy, *The Air War 1939–1945* (London: Europa Publications, 1980), 24–5. For comparisons between London and Paris there are the comments of Oliver

Simmonds, member for Duddeston, Birmingham in *Parl. Deb.*, 5th ser., Vol. 356, 524 (23 January, 1940). On the very early development of 'anti-gas' 'practices' in Japan see the tantalizing snippet in Yukio Mishima, *The Sea of Fertility*, trs. Michael Gallagher *et al.* (Harmondsworth: Penguin Books, 1985), 482.

42. The 'non-party' and 'non-partisan' nature of the peers' wartime debates on the road traffic crisis were retrospectively confirmed by Lord Elton, *Parl. Deb. (HL)*, 5th ser., Vol. 137, 1110 (21 November, 1945).
43. This is a dimension that could be revealingly investigated in the context of the debate generated by Paul Addison in *The Road to 1945* (London: Jonathan Cape, 1975). See, also, Harold L. Smith (ed.), *War and Social Change* (Manchester: Manchester University Press, 1986).
44. *Parl. Deb. (HL)*, 5th ser., Vol. 115, 149 (6 December, 1939).
45. *Idem*, Vol. 118, 473 (25 February, 1941).
46. *Ibid.*, 466.
47. *Ibid.*, 482.
48. *Parl. Deb. (HL)*, 5th ser., Vol. 120, 321 (21 October, 1941).
49. *Idem*, Vol. 137, 1093 (21 November, 1945).
50. *Idem*, Vol. 132, 1152 (26 July, 1944). When the speech was made, the position was broadly as stated. But the period between D-Day and Armistice saw a massive increase in casualties. By the end of the war, nearly 265,000 members of the British armed forces had been killed, and 227,000 injured. See *History of the Second World War: Statistical Digest of the War* (London: HMSO, 1951. Reprinted with corrections, 1975), Table 14.1. I am grateful to David Edgerton for clarifying this point.
51. *Parl. Deb. (HL)*, 5th ser., Vol. 132, 1165 (26 July, 1944).
52. *Parl. Deb.*, 5th ser., Vol. 518, 1207–8 (28 July, 1953).
53. And, as the youthful James Callaghan pointed out in 1953, car-drivers were now also more likely to be killed or injured by *other* car-drivers. *Ibid.*, 1119.
54. An important early study of this type had been Alker Tripp, *Town Planning and Road Traffic* (London: Edward Arnold, 1943). Tripp had been Assistant Commissioner of Police for the Metropolis.
55. See Alan Irwin, *Risk and Control of Technology: Public Policies for Road Traffic Safety in Britain and the United States* (Manchester: Manchester University Press, 1985), ch. 5.
56. *Parl. Deb.*, 5th ser., Vol. 518, 1122 (28 July, 1953), James Callaghan.
57. *Ibid.*, 1218, response on behalf of the government by Sir Hugh Lucas-Tooth, Under-Secretary of State at the Home Office.
58. Irwin, *op.cit.* (ref. 55), Part 3.
59. *Parl. Deb.*, 5th ser., Vol. 518, 1205 (28 July, 1953). See, also, the comments of Godfrey Nicholson, member for Farnham, *ibid.*, 1150–1.

60. *Ibid.*, 1155, John Snow, member for Lichfield and Tamworth. By this stage RoSPA had turned to the dramatization of the road accident problem in terms of 'unacceptable comparabilities'. It was claimed that during any 'typical' year, 'everybody' in Bolton would be 'killed' or 'injured' on the roads; that the entire population of Rye would be 'decimated'; and the 'equivalent' of a children's Saturday Cinema Club wiped out. There were similarities here with wartime imagery and the representations deployed by critics of the government between 1939 and 1941.
61. Susan Sontag, *Illness as Metaphor and AIDS and its Metaphors* (Harmondsworth: Penguin Books, 1991).
62. This broadly relativistic approach, which also emphasizes the roles of scape-goating and moral panic, is presented in an extreme form in J.P. Gusfield, *The Culture of Public Problems: Drinking-Driving and the Symbolic Order* (Chicago: University of Chicago Press, 1984).
63. Basil Collier, *The Defence of the United Kingdom* (London: HMSO, 1957), Appendix L, 528.
64. This position was buttressed by the official contention that the 'general public' would be unnecessarily alarmed by even minor modifications to the black-out and would consequently 'turn against' an 'irresponsible' government. See PRO: CAB 73/16, *Ministerial Committee on Lighting Restrictions: First Report*, 67, November 1939; and PRO: CAB 73/22, *Committee on Black-Out Restrictions*, Memorandum, 1 August, 1944.
65. On this issue see Bill Luckin, 'Accidents, Disasters and Cities', *Urban History*, 20 (1993), 5–18 and the chapter by Roger Cooter in this volume.

Bibliography – Selected Secondary Sources

Accidents and Health: The Responsibilities of Medicine and Education. Report of Proceedings of the Convention held at the Royal College of Surgeons of Edinburgh on Monday and Tuesday 6 and 7 April, 1970. Edinburgh: The Medical Commission on Accident Prevention, 1970.

Accident Facts. Chicago: National Safety Council, 1988 (1st edn 1921).

Aldrich, Mark. 'Preventing "The Needless Peril of the Coal Mine": The Bureau of Mines and the Campaign Against Coal Mine Explosions, 1910–1940', *Technology and Culture,* 36 (1995), 483–518.

Arnold, Lorna. *Windscale, 1957: Anatomy of a Nuclear Accident.* Basingstoke: Macmillan, 1992; 2nd edn 1995.

Baker, C.W. and W. Chapman (eds). *Man and Society in Disaster.* New York: Basic Books, 1962.

Baker, Susan P. 'Injuries in America: A National Disaster'. In Russell C. Maulitz (ed.), *Unnatural Causes: The Three Leading Killer Diseases in America.* New Brunswick, N.J.: Rutgers University Press, 1989, 135–46.

Baker, Susan P., B. O'Neill and R.S. Karpf. *The Injury Fact Book.* Lexington, Mass.: D.C. Health, 1984.

Barkun, Michael. *Disaster and The Millennium.* New Haven/London: Yale University Press, 1974.

Barton, Allen H. *Communities in Disaster: A Sociological Analysis of Collective Stress Situations.* New York: Doubleday, 1969.

————. *Social Organization Under Stress: A Sociological Review of Disaster Studies.* Washington: National Academy of Sciences–National Research Council, 1963.

Bartrip, Peter. 'Accidents and Ill-Health: The Hidden Wages of The Workplace', *Social History of Medicine,* 3 (1990), 291–6.

————. *Workmen's Compensation in Twentieth-Century Britain.* Aldershot: Avebury, 1987.

———— and P.T. Fenn. 'The Measurement of Safety: Factory Accident Statistics in Victorian and Edwardian Britain', *Historical Research,* 63 (1990), 58–72.

———— and S.B. Burman. *The Wounded Soldiers of Industry: Industrial Compensation Policy, 1833–1897.* Oxford: Clarendon Press, 1983.

Bayer, Ronald (ed.). *The Health and Safety of Workers: Case Studies in the Politics of Professional Responsibility.* New York: Oxford University Press, 1988.

Beck, Ulrich. *Risk Society: Towards a New Modernity*, trs. Mark Ritter, with introduction by Scott Lash and Brian Wynne. London: Sage, 1992.

Benson, John. 'English Coal-miners' Trade-union Accident Funds, 1850–1900', *Economic History Review*, 28 (1975), 401–12.

Bergstrom, Randolph E. *Courting Danger: Injury and Law in New York City, 1870–1910.* Ithaca: Cornell University Press, 1992.

Berkowitz, Edward D. *Disabled Policy: America's Programs For The Handicapped.* Cambridge: Cambridge University Press, 1987.

Berman, Daniel M. *Death On The Job: Occupational Health And Safety Struggles in the United States.* New York: Monthly Review Press, 1987.

Bolderson, Helen. 'The Origins of the Disabled Persons Employment Quota and its Symbolic Significance', *Journal of Social Policy*, 9 (1980), 169–86.

Bourriau, Jannine (ed.). *Understanding Catastrophe.* Cambridge: Cambridge University Press, 1992.

Brandt, Allen M. 'Exploring the Dangerous Trades', *Reviews in American History*, 17 (1989), 101–7.

Bryant, E. *Natural Hazards.* Cambridge: Cambridge University Press, 1991.

Burnham, John C. 'Why Did the Infants and Toddlers Die Shifts in Americans' Ideas of Responsibility for Accidents – From Blaming Mom to Engineering', *Journal of Social History*, 29 (1996), 817–38.

Burton, I., *et al. The Environment as Hazard.* New York: Oxford University Press, 1978.

Caplan, Eric Michael. 'Trains, Brains and Sprains: Railway Spine and the Origins of Psychoneuroses', *Bulletin of the History of Medicine*, 69 (1995), 378–419.

Castel, Robert. 'From Dangerousness to Risk'. In Graham Burchell, Colin Jones and P. Miller (eds), *The Foucault Effect: Studies In Governmentality.* London: Harvester/Wheatsheaf, 1991, 281–98.

Carson, W.G. 'Hostage to History: Some Aspects of Occupational Health and Safety in Historical Perspective'. In Breen Creighton and Neil Gunningham (eds), *The Industrial Relations of Occupational Health and Safety.* Sydney: Croom Helm, 1985.

Cliff, Kenneth Stephenson. *Accidents: Causes, Prevention and Services.* London: Croom Helm, 1984.

Cooter, Roger. 'Die medizinische "Entdeckung" van Unfallen und die

Industrialisierung Medizinischer Sozialbeziehungen in Großbritannien um die Jahrhundertwende'. In Dietrich Milles (ed.), *Gesundheitsrisiken, Industriegesellschaft und Soziale Sicherungen in der Geschichte.* Bremerhaven: Wirtschaftsverlag NW, 1993, 85–100.

————. 'Bones of Contention? Orthodox Medicine and the Mystery of the Bone-setter's Craft'. In W.F. Bynum and Roy Porter (eds), *Medical Fringe and Medical Orthodoxy, 1750–1850.* London: Croom Helm, 1987, 158–73.

————. *Surgery and Society in Peace and War: Orthopaedics and the Organization of Modern Medicine, 1880–1948.* London: Macmillan, 1993.

———— and John Pickstone, 'From Dispensary to Hospital: Medicine, Community and Workplace in Ancoats, 1828–1948', *Manchester Region History Review,* 7 (1993), 73–84.

Covello, V.T. and J. Mumpower. 'Risk Analysis and Risk Management: An Historical Perspective', *Risk Analysis,* 5 (1985), 103–20.

Craven, P. 'The Meaning of Misadventure: The Baptiste Creek Railway Disaster of 1854, and Its Aftermath'. In Roger Hall *et al.* (eds), *Patterns of the Past: Interpreting Ontario's History.* Toronto: Dundurn, 1988, 108–28.

Cullen, Michael J. *The Statistical Movement in Early Victorian Britain: The Foundations of Empirical Social Science.* Hassocks, Sussex: Harvester, 1975.

Curran, Daniel J. *Dead Laws for Dead Men: The Politics of Federal Coal Mine Health and Safety Legislation.* Pittsburgh: University of Pittsburgh Press, 1993.

Curson, Peter. 'Introduction'. In John I. Clarke *et al.* (eds), *Population and Disaster.* Oxford: Blackwell, 1989, 1–23.

Cvetkovich, George and Timothy C. Earle. 'Environmental Hazards and the Public', *Journal of Social Issues,* 48 (1992), 1–20.

Dake, Karl. 'Myths of Nature: Culture and the Social Construction of Risk', *Journal of Social Issues,* 48 (1992), 21–37.

Daston, Lorraine J. 'The Domestication of Risk: Mathematical Probability and Insurance 1650–1830'. In Lorenz Kruger *et al.* (eds), *The Probabilistic Revolution.* Vol. 1: *Ideas in History.* Cambridge, MA: MIT Press, 1987, 237–60.

Defert, Daniel. '"Popular Life" and Insurance Technology'. In Graham Burchell, Colin Jones and P. Miller (eds), *The Foucault Effect: Studies In Governmentality.* London: Harvester/Wheatsheaf, 1991, 211–34.

Derickson, Alan. *Workers' Health, Workers' Democracy: The Western Miners' Struggle, 1891–1925.* Ithaca, N.Y.: Cornell University Press, 1988.

Dinsdale, W.A. *History of Accident Insurance in Great Britain.* London: Stone & Cox, 1954.

Disasters: The Journal of Disaster Studies and Management. 1976 – current.

Douglas, Mary. *Purity and Danger: An Analysis of the Concepts of Pollution and Taboo.* London: Routledge, 1966.

————. 'Environments at Risk'. In her *Implicit Meanings: Essays in Anthropology.* London: Routledge, 1975, 230–48.

————. *Risk Acceptability According to the Social Sciences.* New York: Russell Sage Foundation, 1985.

————.'Risk as a Forensic Resource', *Daedalus*, 119 (1990), 1–16.

———— and A. Wildavsky. *Risk and Culture: An Essay on the Selection of Technological and Environmental Dangers.* Berkeley: University of California Press, 1982.

Duckham, Helen and Baron. *Great Pit Disasters: Great Britain, 1700 to the Present Day.* Newton Abbot: David & Charles, 1973.

Eastman, Joel W. *Styling vs. Safety: The American Automobile Industry and the Development of Automotive Safety, 1900–1966.* New York: University Press of America, 1964.

Eijndhaven, Jose van and Peter Groenemegen. 'The Construction of Expert Advice on Health Risks', *Social Studies of Science*, 21 (1991), 257–78.

Elliot, Gil. *Twentieth Century Book of the Dead.* London: Allen Lane, 1972.

Eyler, J.M. *Victorian Social Medicine: The Ideas and Methods of William Farr.* Baltimore: Johns Hopkins University Press, 1979.

Ewald, Francois. 'Insurance and Risk'. In Graham Burchell, Colin Jones and P. Miller (eds), *The Foucault Effect: Studies In Governmentality.* London: Harvester/Wheatsheaf, 1991, 197–210.

Ewald, Francois. *L'etat Providence.* Paris: Grasset, 1986.

Figlio, Karl. 'How Does Illness Mediate Social Relations? Workmen's Compensation and Medico-legal Practices, 1890–1940'. In Peter Wright and A. Treacher (eds), *The Problem of Medical Knowledge.* Edinburgh: Edinburgh University Press, 1982, 174–224.

————.'What is an Accident?' In Paul Weindling (ed.), *The Social History of Occupational Health.* London: Croom Helm, 1985, 180–206.

Fischer-Homberger, Esther. *Die Traumatische Neurose. Vom Somatischen Zum Sozialen Leiden.* Berne: Hans Huber, 1975.

Foreman-Peck, James. 'Death on the Roads: Changing National Responses To Motor Accidents'. In Theo Barker (ed.), *The Economic and Social Effects of the Spread of Motor Vehicles*. London: Macmillan, 1987, 264–90.

Froggatt, Peter and J.A. Smiley. 'The Concept of Accident Proneness: A Review', *British Journal of Industrial Medicine*, 24 (1964), 1–12.

Garb, S. and E. Eng. *Disaster Handbook*. New York: Springer, 1969.

Gersuny, Carl. *Work Hazards and Industrial Conflict*. Hanover, N.H.: University Press of New England, 1981.

Gevitz, Norman. '"Helps for Suddain Accidents": Stephen Bradwell and the Origin of the First Aid Guide', *Bulletin of the History of Medicine*, 67 (1993), 51–73.

Giddens, Anthony. *The Nation State and Violence*. Cambridge: Cambridge University Press, 1985.

————. *The Consequences of Modernity*. Stanford: Stanford University Press, 1990.

Gillespie, Richard. 'Accounting for Lead Poisoning: The Medical Politics of Occupational Health', *Social History*, 15 (1990), 303–31.

Graebner, William. *Coal-Mining Safety in the Progressive Period: The Political Economy of Reform*. Lexington: University of Kentucky Press, 1976.

Green, Judith. 'Accidents and the Risk Society'. In Roger Burrows *et al.* (eds), *A Sociology of Health Promotion and the New Public Health*. London: Routledge, 1995.

————. 'The Medico-legal Production of Fatal Accidents', *Sociology of Health and Illness*, 14 (1992), 373–89.

————. 'Some Problems in the Development of a Sociology of Accidents'. In Sue Scott *et al.* (eds), *Private Risks and Public Dangers*, Explorations in Sociology No. 43. Aldershot: Avebury, 1992, 19–33.

Greenwood, Major *et al.* 'Deaths by Violence, 1837–1937', *Journal of the Royal Statistical Society*, 104, Pt 2 (1941), 146–63 and (discussion) 163–71.

Gusfield, Joseph R. *The Culture of Public Problems: Drinking-Driving and the Symbolic Order*. Chicago: Chicago University Press, 1981.

Guy, Chester C. 'The Railroad Surgeon. His Associations, His Hospitals, His Past, His Present', *Industrial Medicine and Surgery*, 32 (1963), 351–60.

Hacking, Ian. *The Emergence of Probability: A Philosophical Study of Early Ideas About Probability, Induction and Statistical Inference*. Cambridge: Cambridge University Press, 1975.

————. *The Taming of Chance*. Cambridge: Cambridge University Press, 1990.

Haddon, William Jr *et al. Accident Research: Methods and Approaches*. New York: Harper & Row, 1964.

Hadfield, Robert L. *Sea-toll of Our Time: A Chronicle of Maritime Disaster During the Last Thirty Years*. London: H.F. & G. Witherby, 1930.

Hair, P.E.H. 'Accidental Death and Suicide in Shropshire, 1780–1809', *Transactions of the Shropshire Archaeological Society*, 59 (1972), 63–75.

————. 'Deaths from Violence in Britain: A Tentative Secular Survey', *Population Studies*, 25 (1971), 5–24.

————. 'Mortality from Violence in British Coal-Mines, 1800–50', *Economic History Review*, 21 (1968), 545–61.

————. 'Measuring the Blood on the Coal: The Use and Abuse of Medical Statistics', *Medical Historian*, No. 2 (1989), 3–10.

Hamilton, James A.B. *British Railway Accidents of the Twentieth Century*. London: Allen & Unwin, 1967.

Hanawalt, Barbara. 'Childrearing Among the Lower Classes of Late Medieval England', *Journal of Interdisciplinary History*, 8 (1977), 1–22.

————. *Growing Up In Medieval London: The Experience of Childhood in History*. New York: Oxford University Press, 1993.

————. *The Ties That Bound: Peasant Families in Medieval England*. Bloomington: Indiana University Press, 1986.

————. 'Violent Death in Fourteenth and Fifteenth Century England', *Comparative Studies in Society and History*, 18 (1976), 297–320.

Harrington, Michael. *The Accidental Century*. Baltimore: Penguin, 1966.

Harrison, Barbara. '"Some of them gets lead poisoned": Occupational Lead Exposure In Women, 1880–1914', *Social History of Medicine*, 2 (1989), 171–95.

Hazen, Margaret H. and Robert M. Hazen. *Keepers of the Flame: The Role Of Fire In American Culture, 1775–1925*. Princeton: Princeton University Press, 1992.

Hazlett, T. Lyle and William W. Hummel. *Industrial Medicine in Western Pennsylvania, 1850–1950*. Pittsburgh: University of Pittsburgh Press, 1957.

Health and Safety Executive. *One Hundred Fatal Accidents in Construction*. London: HMSO, 1978.

Heinrich, H.W. *Industrial Accidents Prevention: A Scientific Approach*. New York: McGraw-Hill, 1931; 3rd edn 1950.

Iskrant, Albert P. and Paul V. Joliet. *Accidents and Homicide*. Cambridge, MA: Harvard University Press, 1968.

Jennings, Humphrey. *Pandaemonium, 1660–1886: The Coming of the Machine as Seen by Contemporary Observers*, edited by Mary-Lou Jennings and Charles Madge. London: Andre Deutsch, 1985.

Johnson, B.B. and V.T. Covello. *The Social and Cultural Construction of Risk.* Dordrecht: Reidel, 1987.

Jones, Eric L. 'The Reduction of Fire Damages in Southern England, 1650–1850', *Post-Medieval Archaeology*, 2 (1968), 140–9.

———— and J.L. Anderson. 'Natural Disasters and the Historical Response', *Australian Economic History Review*, 28 (1988), 3–20.

———— *et al. A Gazetteer of English Urban Fire Disasters 1500–1800.* Historical Geography Research Series No. 13 (Norwich, 1984).

Jones, Helen. 'Employers' Welfare Schemes and Industrial Relations in Inter-War Britain', *Business History*, 25 (1983), 61–75.

Journal of Risk and Uncertainty, 1985–current. (Interdisciplinary 'analysis of risk-bearing behavior and decision making under uncertainty'.)

Kartman, Ben and Leonard Brown (eds). *Disaster* [Accounts of American disasters]. New York: Pellegrine & Cudahy, 1948.

Keller, Thomas. 'Railway Spine Revisited: Traumatic Neurosis or Neurotrauma?', *Journal of the History of Medicine and Allied Sciences*, 50 (1995), 507–24.

Kessler, Henry Howard. *Accidental Injuries: The Medico-legal Aspects of Workmen's Compensation and Public Liability.* Philadelphia: Lea & Febiger, 1931; 2nd edn 1941.

Kipling, M.D. and A. Gow. 'Legislation and Accident Prevention: A Historical Review', *Medical History*, 10 (1966), 400–4.

Krimsky, Sheldon and D. Golding (eds). *Social Theories of Risk.* London/New York: Praeger, 1992.

Krohn, Wolfgang and Georg Krucken. *Riskante Technologien: Reflexion Und Regulation.* Frankfurt: Suhrkamp, 1993.

Kruger, Lorenz, L.J. *et al.* (eds). *The Probabilistic Revolution.* Cambridge, MA: MIT Press, 1987. 2 volumes.

Landes, David S. 'What Room For Accident In History? Explaining Big Changes By Small Events', *Economic History Review*, 47 (1994), 637–56.

Lane, Roger. *Violent Death In The City: Suicide, Accident, And Murder in Nineteenth-century Philadelphia.* Cambridge, MA: Harvard University Press, 1979.

Le Gall, Yvon. *Historie des Accidents du Travail.* Nantes: L'Université des Nantes, 1982.

Levidow, Les. 'Nuclear Accidents By Design', *Science as Culture,* No. 9 (1990), 99–109.

————. 'De-reifying Risk', *Science as Culture,* No. 20 (1994), 440–56.

Licht, Walter. *Working for the Railroad.* Princeton: Princeton University Press, 1983.

Lloyd, Geoffrey. 'Introduction: Understanding Catastrophe'. In Jannine Bourriau (ed.), *Understanding Catastrophe.* Cambridge: Cambridge University Press, 1992, 1–4.

Luckin, Bill. 'Accidents, Disasters and Cities', *Urban History,* 20 (1993), 5–18.

————. *Pollution and Control: A Social History of The Thames in the Nineteenth Century.* Bristol/Boston: Hilger, 1986.

————. *Questions of Power: Electricity and Environment in Inter-war Britain.* Manchester: Manchester University Press, 1990.

Luhmann, Niklas. 'Technology, Environment and Social Risk: A Systems Perspective', *Industrial Crisis Quarterly,* 4 (1990), 223–31.

Mallalieu, W.C. 'Joseph Chamberlain and Workmen's Compensation', *Journal of Economic History,* 10 (1950), 45–57.

Masters, Dexter. *The Accident.* London: Faber, [1955] 1985.

Micale, Mark S. and Paul Lerner (eds), *Traumatic Pasts: Studies in History, Psychiatry and Trauma in the Modern Age.* Forthcoming.

Milles, Dietrich (ed.). *Gesundheitsrisiken, Industriegesellschaft und Soziale Sicherungen in der Geschichte.* Bremerhaven: Wirtschaftsverlag NW, 1993.

Munts, Raymond. *Bargaining for Health: Labor Unions, Health Insurance, And Medical Care.* Madison, Wisconsin: University of Wisconsin Press, 1967.

Myers, Charles S. *The Use of Gruesome and Humorous Propaganda for Accident Prevention.* London: National Institute of Industrial Psychology, *c.*1936.

Nash, J.R. *Darkest Hours: A Narrative Encyclopedia of World-Wide Disasters.* Chicago: Nelson-Hall, 1976.

Nelkin, Dorothy (ed.). *The Language of Risk.* Beverly Hills: Sage, 1985.

———— and Michael S. Brown. *Workers At Risk: Voices from the Workplace.* Chicago: Chicago University Press, 1984.

———— and M. Pollak. 'Problems and Procedures in the Regulation of Technological Risk'. In R.C. Schwing and W.A. Albers (eds), *Societal Risk Assessment. How Safe is Safe Enough?*. New York: Plenum Press, 1980, 233–48.

Nichols, Theo. 'On the Analysis of Size Effects and "Accidents"', *Industrial Relations Journal*, 20 (1989), 62–5.

————. 'Industrial Injuries in British Manufacturing Industry and Cyclical Effects: Continuities and Discontinuities in Industrial Injury Research', *Sociological Review*, 39 (1991), 131–9.

Nuffield Provincial Hospitals' Trust. *Casualty Services and Their Setting: A Study in Medical Care.* Oxford: Oxford University Press, 1960.

Perrow, Charles. *Normal Accidents: Living with High-Risk Technologies.* New York: Basic Books, 1984.

Pick, Daniel. *War Machine: The Rationalisation of Slaughter in the Modern Age.* New Haven: Yale University Press, 1993.

Pickstone, John V. *Medicine in Industrial Society: A History Of Hospital Development In Manchester and Its Region, 1752–1946.* Manchester: Manchester University Press, 1985.

Porter, Theodore M. *The Rise of Statistical Thinking 1820–1900.* Princeton, N.J.: Princeton University Press, 1980.

————. *Trust in Numbers: The Pursuit of Objectivity in Science and Public Life.* Princeton, N.J.: Princeton University Press, 1995.

Plowden, William. *The Motor Car and Politics in Britain, 1896–1970.* Harmondsworth: Penguin, 1973.

Rabinbach, Anson. *The Human Motor: Energy, Fatigue and the Origins of Modernity.* Berkeley: University of California Press, 1992.

————. 'Social Knowledge, Social Risk, and the Politics of Industrial Accidents in Germany and France'. In Dietrich Rueschemeyer and Theda Skocpol (eds), *States, Social Knowledge, and the Origins of Modern Social Policies.* Princeton, N.J.: Princeton University Press, 1996, 48–89.

Rolt, Lionel T.C. *Red for Danger: A History of Railway Accidents and Railway Safety.* 4th edn, Newton Abbot: David and Charles, 1982.

Rosenberg, Mark L. 'Violence Is a Public Health Problem'. In Russell C. Maulitz (ed.), *Unnatural Causes: The Three Leading Killer Diseases In America.* New Brunswick, N.J.: Rutgers University Press, 1989, 147–68.

Rosner, David and Gerald Markowitz. *Deadly Dust: Silicosis And The Politics Of Occupational Disease In Twentieth Century America.* Princeton: Princeton University Press, 1991.

——— (eds). *Dying for Work: Workers' Safety and Health in Twentieth-century America.* Bloomington: Indiana University Press, 1987.

———. 'The Early Movement for Occupational Safety and Health, 1900–1917'. In J.W. Leavitt and R.L. Numbers (eds), *Sickness and Health in America: Readings in the History of Medicine and Public Health.* 2nd edn, Madison, Wisconsin: University of Wisconsin Press, 1985, 507–21.

Sayer, J.H. 'Accidental Death, Past and Present', *Medical Press,* 238 (1957), 551–3.

Rule, John. *The Experience of Labour in Eighteenth-Century Industry.* London: Croom Helm, 1981.

———. *The Labouring Classes in Early Industrial England, 1750–1850.* London: Longman, 1986.

Sagan, Scott D. *The Limits of Safety: Organizations, Accidents and Nuclear Weapons.* Princeton, N.J.: Princeton University Press, 1993.

Schivelbusch, Wolfgang. *The Railway Journey: The Industrialization of Time and Space in the 19th Century.* Leamington Spa: Berg, 1986.

Schwing, R.C. and W.A. Albers, Jr (eds). *Societal Risk Assessment: How Safe is Safe Enough?* New York: Plenum Press, 1980.

Scott, Rachel. *Muscle and Blood.* New York: Dutton & Co., 1974.

Scott, Sue *et al.* (eds). *Private Risks and Public Dangers,* Explorations in Sociology No. 43. Aldershot: Avebury, 1992.

Shires, G. Tom. 'Care of the Injured in America: Organizational and Physiological Considerations'. In Russell C. Maulitz (ed.), *Unnatural Causes: The Three Leading Killer Diseases in America.* New Brunswick, N.J.: Rutgers University Press, 1989, 169–82.

Siegelbaum, Lewis. 'Industrial Accidents and Their Prevention in the Interwar Period'. In William O. McCagg and Lewis Siegelbaum (eds), *The Disabled in the Soviet Union.* Pittsburgh: University of Pittsburgh Press, 1989, 85–117.

Smith, Keith. *Environmental Hazards: Assessing Risk and Reducing Disaster.* London: Routledge, 1991.

Smith, Roger and Brian Wynne (eds). *Expert Evidence: Interpreting Science in the Law.* London: Routledge, 1989.

Stone, Deborah. *The Disabled State.* Philadelphia: Temple University Press, 1984.

Templer, John. *The Staircase: Studies of Hazards, Falls and Safer Design.* Cambridge, MA: MIT Press, 1992.

Thomas, Keith. *Man and the Natural World: Changing Attitudes in England 1500–1800.* London: Allen Lane, 1983.

————. *Religion and the Decline of Magic: Studies in Popular Beliefs in Sixteenth- and Seventeenth-century England.* Harmondsworth: Penguin, 1973.

Tombs, S. 'Safety, Statistics and Business Cycles: A Response to [T.] Nichols', *Sociological Review*, 40 (1992), 132–45.

Tucker, Eric. *Administering Danger in the Workplace: The Law and Politics of Occupational Health and Safety Regulation in Ontario, 1850–1914.* Toronto: University of Toronto Press, 1990.

Usselman, Steven W. 'The Lure of Technology and The Appeal of Order: Railroad Safety Regulation in Nineteenth-century America', *Business and Economic History*, 21 (1992), 290–9.

Wagar, W. Warren. *Terminal Visions: The Literature of Last Things.* Bloomington: Indiana University Press, 1982.

Wallace, Antony F. C. St Clair. *A Nineteenth-century Coal Town's Experience with a Disaster-prone Industry.* New York: Knopf, 1987.

Weart, Spencer R. *Nuclear Fear: A History of Images.* Cambridge, MA: Harvard University Press, 1988.

Weindling, Paul (ed.). *The Social History of Occupational Health.* London: Croom Helm, 1985.

Whiteside, James. *Regulating Danger: The Struggle for Mine Safety in the Rocky Mountain Coal Industry.* Lincoln/London: University of Nebraska Press, 1990.

Wildavsky, Aaron. *Searching for Safety.* New Brunswick, N.J.: Transaction Books, 1988.

Williams, Rosalind. *Notes on the Underground: An Essay on Technology, Society, and the Imagination.* Cambridge, MA: MIT Press, 1990.

Wilson, Arnold and Hermann Levy. *Workmen's Compensation.* London: Oxford University Press, 1939. 2 volumes.

Wilson, Graham K. *The Politics of Safety and Health: Occupational Safety and Health in the United States and Britain.* Oxford: Clarendon Press, 1985.

Young, A.F. *Industrial Injuries Insurance: An Examination of British Policy.* London: Routledge & Kegan Paul, 1964. Chapter 3: 'Accident Prevention'.

Zelizer, Viviana A.R. 'Human Values and the Market: The Case of Life Insurance and Death in 19th-century America', *American Journal of Sociology*, 84 (1978), 591–610.

————. *Morals and Markets: The Development of Life Insurance in the United States.* New York: Columbia University Press, 1979.

————. *Pricing the Priceless Child: The Changing Social Value of Children.* New York: Basic Books, 1985.

Index